Practical Radiological Anatomy

Practical Radiological Anatomy

Sarah McWilliams

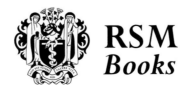

RSM *Books*

First published in Great Britain in 2011 by
Hodder Arnold, an imprint of Hodder Education, an Hachette UK Company
338 Euston Road, London NW1 3BH

http://www.hodderarnold.com

© 2011 Hodder & Stoughton Ltd

The logo of the Royal Society of Medicine is a registered trade mark, which it has licensed to Hodder Arnold.

Hachette UK's policy is to use papers that are natural, renewable and recyclable products and made from wood grown in sustainable forests. The logging and manufacturing processes are expected to conform to the environmental regulations of the country of origin.

Whilst the advice and information in this book are believed to be true and accurate at the date of going to press, neither the author[s] nor the publisher can accept any legal responsibility or liability for any errors or omissions that may be made. In particular (but without limiting the generality of the preceding disclaimer) every effort has been made to check drug dosages; however it is still possible that errors have been missed. Furthermore, dosage schedules are constantly being revised and new side-effects recognized. For these reasons the reader is strongly urged to consult the drug companies' printed instructions before administering any of the drugs recommended in this book.

British Library Cataloguing in Publication Data
A catalogue record for this book is available from the British Library

Library of Congress Cataloging-in-Publication Data
A catalog record for this book is available from the Library of Congress

ISBN: 978-1-85315-800-1

1 2 3 4 5 6 7 8 9 10

Commissioning Editor:	Hannah Applin
Project Editor:	Stephen Clausard
Production Controller:	Joanna Walker
Cover Designer:	Helen Townson
Index:	Indexing Specialists (UK) Ltd

Typeset in 10pt Palatino by Phoenix Photosetting, Chatham, Kent
Printed and bound in the UK by Antony Rowe

What do you think about this book? Or any other Hodder Arnold title?
Please visit our website: www.hodderarnold.com

Contents

Foreword

The most fundamental skill necessary for accurate interpretation of imaging investigations is a detailed knowledge of anatomy. The demonstration of anatomical structures made possible by modern cross-sectional imaging is superb. The features made visible by magnetic resonance imaging and computed tomography are shown much more clearly than is usually possible at post-mortem dissection. Imaging studies are performed on living patients and show the various tissues in their normal state, making it much easier to appreciate anatomical relationships.

Dr McWilliams' book is an excellent volume which sets new standards in radiological anatomy. It is comprehensive, covering all organ systems, using images from those imaging modalities most appropriate for the demonstration of the anatomy of each organ, often accompanied by high-quality diagrams. It combines exquisite radiological images with clear, concise, very readable accounts of the structures demonstrated. This outstanding text combines sufficient detail to be useful for even the most demanding expert diagnostic or interventional radiologist, physician or surgeon, whilst at the same time guiding the novice through the fundamentals of this most important of basic sciences.

This book will be used widely by radiology trainees and will also find its place in the libraries of all radiology departments and in many radiology reporting rooms.

Andy Adam
Professor of Interventional Radiology
Past President of the Royal College of Radiologists, UK

Preface

Having taught radiological anatomy for 17 years and – as a teacher, an FRCR examiner, a lecturer on the London FRCR Course and the organiser of the only established anatomy radiology course now in its 11th year – I strongly believe that a firm grounding in the normal appearances of the body on imaging, and of the normal anatomical variants, is critical in being a good radiologist. It enables a greater awareness of 'abnormality' and the ability to dismiss variants, which prevents the risk of over-investigation.

I wrote this book as a concise summary of my Radiology Anatomy Course and as a guide for 1st year Registrars in Radiology to parallel my anatomy tutorials. The application of radiological anatomy is also paramount in interpreting images in both a logical and organised fashion, and this book uniquely covers only the relevant anatomy that is required for reporting as a radiologist, with guides in each chapter as to the relevant application of this anatomy. The emphasis on providing images over text aims to make anatomical visualization easy; each chapter provides organised systems for interpreting and analysing both conventional and cross sectional anatomical images, including new multiplanar images relevant to the modern radiologist.

Practical Radiological Anatomy is divided into 10 chapters that cover each of the anatomical regions, covering the key radiological anatomy applicable to each imaging modality. The book also provides case histories for each modality with examples of how to assess key features using applied anatomy and how to write idealized reports. Also included is a chapter on the applied anatomy that is vital to the new trainee during their first few months on call.

Covering the essential anatomy required in all aspects of radiology, *Practical Radiological Anatomy* is the ideal framework for students preparing for the First FRCR Anatomy exam as well as Part 2A.

The book is aimed primarily at Radiology Specialist Registrars in their first two years, and F1 and F2 Radiologists. However, now that radiology has adopted a central role in patient management both at diagnosis and in subsequent care, this book will also be of use to Advanced Practitioners, Accident and Emergency doctors, surgeons, and anyone who is involved in reporting and interpreting imaging.

ACKNOWLEDGEMENTS

I wish to thank many of the Specialist Registrars at Guy's and St Thomas' who have helped me edit sections of this book, and particular thanks to Dr Sheila Rankin for helping me with editing.

1 Neuroimaging

RADIOLOGICAL ANATOMY

The skull (Figs 1.1–1.3)

- The skull is made up of the frontal bone, occipital bone, parietal bones, temporal bone and sphenoid bone.
- The lambdoid suture lies posteriorly between the occipital bone and the temporal and parietal bones.
- The sagittal suture lies in the midline.
- The coronal suture lies transversely between the frontal and parietal bones.
- The bregma is the most superior point at the junction of the coronal and sagittal sutures.
- The lambda is the junction of the lambdoid and sagittal sutures.
- The clivus forms the anterior wall of the foramen magnum and part of the skull base; it is formed by the occipit and the sphenoid. The superior aspect of the clivus forms the posterior clinoid processes or dorsum sellae.
- The anterior clinoid processes arise from either side of the anterior aspect of the pituitary fossa or sella turcica.

They are more widely spaced than the posterior clinoid processes.
- The crista galli is the perpendicular superior projection of the cribriform plate of the ethmoid bone seen on an anteroposterior (AP) view.
- The skull is divided into three cranial fossas: anterior, middle and posterior.

The skull at birth

There are several differences between the newborn skull and the adult skull:
- The maxillary sinus is not aerated until the age of 2–3 years. Imaging of the paranasal sinuses is indicated only once they have formed in young children.
- The face is only one-eighth of the entire skull volume in the newborn. In an adult the face volume equals the skull volume.
- The angle of the mandible is greater in the newborn as in edentulous adults, i.e. no teeth (Fig. 1.4).

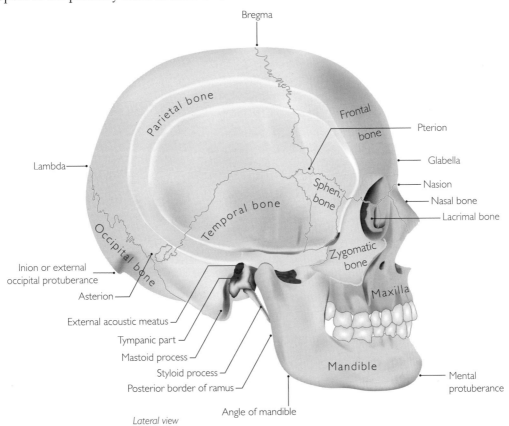

Lateral view

Fig. 1.1 Diagram of the skull: posteriorly the lambdoid suture joins the sagittal suture at the midline to form the lambda. Superiorly the coronal suture joins the temporal suture to form the bregma.

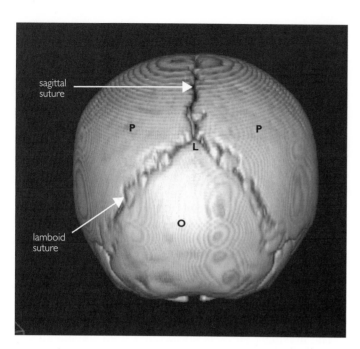

sagittal suture

P   P

L

lamboid suture

O

Fig. 1.2 Volume-rendered reconstruction of skull using bony window CT. Posterior view showing the lambdoid suture joining the sagittal suture at the midline, at the lambda (L), posteriorly the occipital bone (O) and on either side the parietal bone (P).

- Digital markings, i.e. convolutional markings, may be present in a newborn as a normal variant. They are round lucencies seen on the skull. They can be also be a sign of raised intracranial pressure in children, i.e. copper-beaten skull (Fig. 1.5).
- Fontanelles: the posterior fontanelle closes by 3 months and the anterior fontanelle by 18 months (Fig. 1.6). This is used for access to cranial ultrasound. The sutures and fontanelles are important to assess in a newborn to identify premature closing or widening that suggests raised intracranial pressure.
- The prevertebral soft tissues are wider at birth due to adenoidal tissue and can be very wide if an infant is crying.
- Sutures within the premature skull: various sutures are present that are fused by adult age, in addition to the standard sutures: sagittal, coronal and lambdoid. The extra sutures can, however, persist into adult life and are not to be confused with fractures:
  - mendosal suture – this runs posteriorly from the lambdoid suture
  - metopic suture lies within the frontal bone and usually disappears by age 2

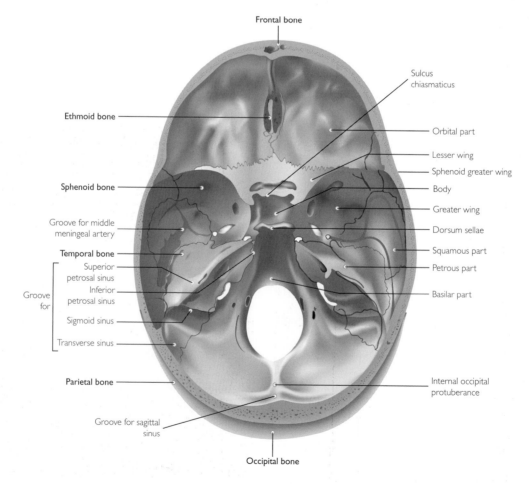

Frontal bone

Sulcus chiasmaticus

Ethmoid bone

Orbital part

Lesser wing

Sphenoid greater wing

Sphenoid bone

Body

Greater wing

Groove for middle meningeal artery

Dorsum sellae

Temporal bone

Squamous part

Superior petrosal sinus

Petrous part

Inferior petrosal sinus

Groove for

Basilar part

Sigmoid sinus

Transverse sinus

Parietal bone

Internal occipital protuberance

Groove for sagittal sinus

Occipital bone

Fig. 1.3 The skull base is divided into anterior cranial fossa, middle cranial fossa and posterior cranial fossa. The cranial nerves emerge through the skull base foramina.

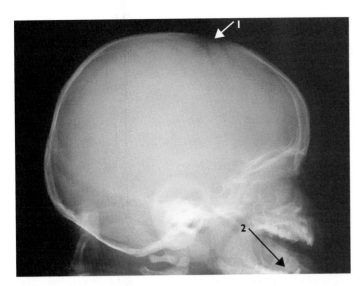

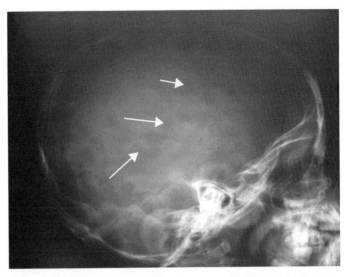

Fig. 1.4 Lateral skull radiograph of infant showing the anterior fontanelle (1) at the bregma, through which head ultrasound can be performed. This should close by age 2. (2) shows unerupted teeth in an infant

Fig. 1.5 Lateral skull radiograph: The circumscribed lucent lesions over the whole skull (arrows) are called digital markings or convolutional markings and can be a normal variant in a child. The teeth in the child are unerupted.

    – basispheno-basiocciput synchondrosis – a suture between the occipital bone inferiorly and the base of the sphenoid bone; it fuses by age 25 (Fig. 1.7)

    – interparietal suture: this can cause confusion with non-accidental injury (Fig. 1.8).

- Wormian bones are small sesamoid bones that lie within the lambdoid suture. Fewer than five wormian bones is a normal variant; more than five is associated with syndromes listed in Box 1.1 (Fig. 1.9).

Box 1.1 List of conditions associated with wormian bones ('pork chops')

Pyknodysostosis
Osteogenesis imperfecta
Rickets
Kinky hair – Menkes' syndrome
Cleidocranial dysostosis
Hypophosphatasia and hypothyroidism
Old age – progeria
Pachydermoperiostosis
Down's syndrome

Cranial nerves

In order to interpret computed tomography (CT) of the brain and know where to look for pathology, adequate knowledge of the cranial nerves is needed:

- The olfactory nerve emerges through the cribriform plate.
- The optic nerve passes through the optic canal to the optic chiasma, where the fibres from the nasal half of the retina cross the midline to join the optic tract of the

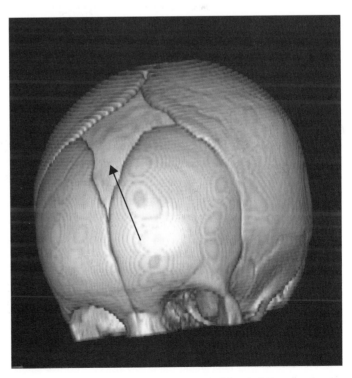

Fig. 1.6 Volume-rendered reconstruction of the skull showing the size and position of the normal anterior fontanelle in an infant (arrow).

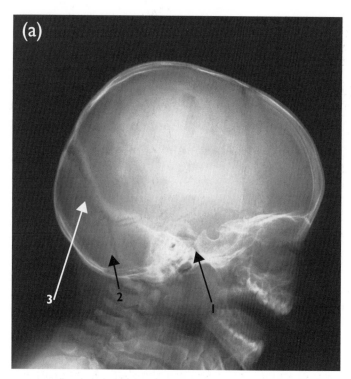

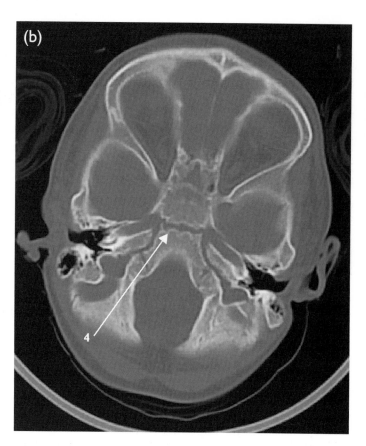

Fig. 1.7 (a) Lateral skull radiograph of infant. (1) marks the basispheno-basiocciput synchondrosis. The lambdoid suture and the mendosal suture are seen posteriorly. The coronal suture is seen anteriorly. Note that the sphenoid sinus has not aerated at this age and is dense bone underneath the sella. Mendosal (2) and lambdoid (1). (b) CT scan showing basipheno-basiocciput synchrondrosis marked by (4). This is an axial CT with bony windows.

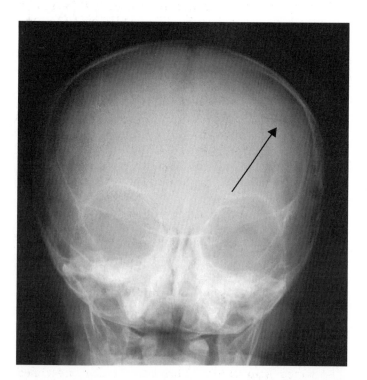

Fig. 1.8 Frontal skull radiograph: the arrow marks a normal suture called the interparietal suture. This can be confused with an interparietal fracture in non-accidental injury.

opposite side. The optic tracts pass back to the lateral geniculate body and then to the occipital visual cortex.

- The oculomotor nerve passes through the superior orbital fissure. It arises from the anterior midbrain and runs through the lateral wall of the cavernous sinus. The nerve supplies the five orbital muscles not supplied by abducens and trochlea.

- The trochlear nerve emerges from the posterior midbrain. The nerve passes through the lateral wall of the cavernous sinus and passes through the superior orbital fissure. It supplies the superior oblique muscle.

- The trigeminal nerve emerges from the anterior pons. The trigeminal ganglion lies in 'Meckel's cave' on either side of sella at the petrous apex (see Fig. 1.12). The nerve has three divisions: the ophthalmic passes through the lateral wall of the cavernous sinus and the superior orbital fissure; the maxillary passes through the lateral wall of the cavernous sinus and then into the foramen rotundum; and the mandibular passes through the foramen ovale.

- The abducens nerve emerges from the pons, and passes through the cavernous sinus and then the superior orbital fissure. It supplies the lateral rectus muscle: 'SO4 LR6'.

- The facial nerve emerges from the pons, and passes through the internal auditory canal, geniculate ganglion and stylomastoid foramen.

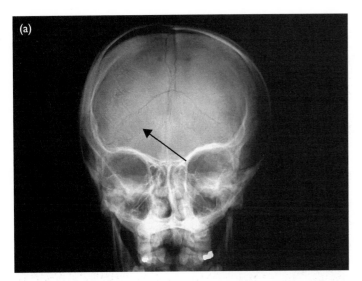 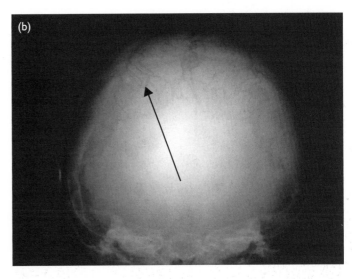

Fig. 1.9 Wormian bones: (a) posteroanterior (PA) 20 skull radiograph. (b) Towne's views: multiple small bones are seen within the lambdoid suture. Up to five bones is a normal variant. The arrows show multiple wormian bones.

- The vestibulocochlear nerve emerges from the pons and passes through the internal auditory canal.
- The glossopharyngeal nerve emerges from the medulla and passes through the jugular foramen.
- The vagus nerve emerges from the medulla and passes through the jugular foramen.
- The spinal accessory nerve arises from the spinal cord and the medulla. The spinal root runs up through the foramen magnum to join the cranial root. The two then join and pass through the jugular foramen.
- The hypoglossal nerve emerges from medulla and passes through the hypoglossal canal near the foramen magnum (Fig. 1.10).

The brain

- The brain is divided into the cerebellum, brain stem and cerebral hemispheres.
- The hemispheres themselves are divided into lobes:
  - The frontal lobe lies anterior to the central sulcus and above the lateral sulcus (Fig. 1.11).
  - The parietal lobes lie posterior to the central sulcus and above the lateral sulcus.
  - The temporal lobes lie in the middle cranial fossa, inferior to the lateral sulcus.
  - The occipital lobes are posterior to the temporoparietal lobes but there is no obvious surface landmark.
- The two halves of the brain are joined by the corpus callosum.
- The cerebellum lies in the posterior fossa with two hemispheres and a central vermis. If the vermis is absent a large cerebrospinal fluid (CSF) cyst occurs, called a Dandy–Walker cyst. The cerebellum has tonsils inferiorly

which should not project through the foramen magnum. Anterolaterally, the cerebellum has a flocculus (Fig. 1.12).
- The brain stem is made up of three parts: the midbrain, then inferiorly the pons and the medulla (Fig. 1.13).
- The midbrain has a characteristic shape. On the posterior or dorsal surface are the quadrigeminal bodies or superior and inferior colliculi, which are small elevations. Anterior are two broad convexities called the cerebral crus or cerebral peduncles. On axial T2-weighted magnetic resonance imaging (T2W MRI), the substantia nigra and red nuclei can be seen as low signal areas. The midbrain has the nuclei for cranial nerves III and IV (see Fig. 1.17).
- The pons has a characteristic shape, being almost round. It has the nuclei for cranial nerves V to VIII, which can be seen exiting on T2W MR axial images. The flocculus of the cerebellum lies lateral to the pons, behind the clivus
- The medulla is much smaller then the pons and has the nuclei for cranial nerves IX–XII. It has a characteristic shape of a cone with a median fissure on the anterior surface and pyramids on either side. The corticospinal tracts decussate in the pyramids. Posteriorly are the olives.
- The dura has a thick crescent-shaped fold called the tentorium cerebelli, or 'tent' for short, that separates the posterior fossa from the remaining brain (Fig. 1.14). This divides the brain into two compartments: the supratentorial compartment containing the cerebral hemispheres lies above the tentorium cerebelli; the cerebellum lies below the tentorium cerebelli or infratentorially.
- CSF spaces: the whole brain is bathed in CSF.
- Any surface of the brain that is surrounded by CSF is named as a cistern. Chambers of CSF are called ventricles.

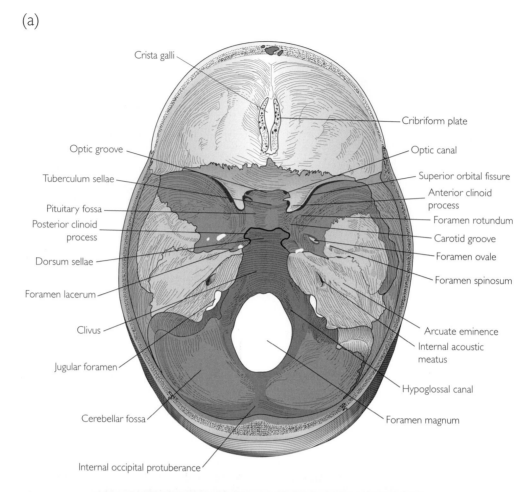

Crista galli

Cribriform plate

Optic groove

Optic canal

Tuberculum sellae

Superior orbital fissure

Pituitary fossa

Anterior clinoid process

Posterior clinoid process

Foramen rotundum

Dorsum sellae

Carotid groove

Foramen ovale

Foramen lacerum

Foramen spinosum

Clivus

Arcuate eminence

Jugular foramen

Internal acoustic meatus

Hypoglossal canal

Cerebellar fossa

Foramen magnum

Internal occipital protuberance

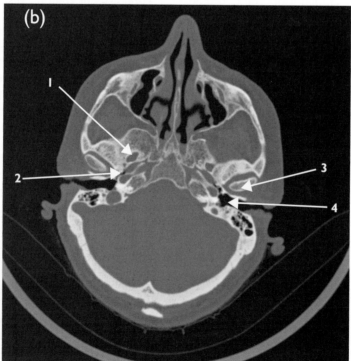

Fig. 1.10 Skull base: (a) diagram, showing the foramina of the skull base, with (b) a skull base CT. Foramen ovale (1), foramen spinosum (2), condylar process mandible (3), external auditory canal (4).

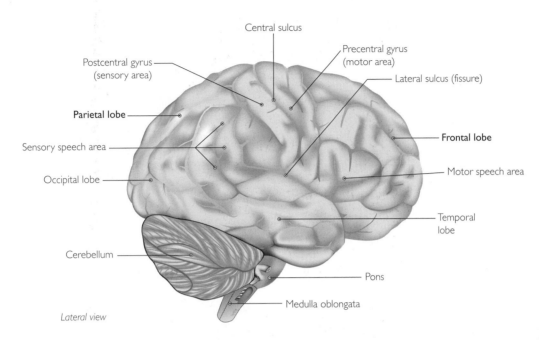

Fig. 1.11 Diagram of the lobes of the brain. The cerebrum is divided into frontal, parietal, occipital and temporal lobes. The brain stem and cerebellum lie posteriorly. Note the precentral gyrus dividing the temporal lobe from the parietal lobe and the central sulcus dividing the frontal lobe from the parietal lobe.

The ventricles

The fourth ventricle

This lies in the posterior fossa between the pons and the cerebellum. It connects inferiorly with the central canal in the spinal cord and superiorly with the aqueduct of Sylvius. The cerebellar vermis lies posterior to the fourth ventricle.

The openings in the roof of the fourth ventricle are called foramina of Magendie and Lushka (Fig. 1.15).

Aqueduct of Sylvius

This is a narrow canal connecting the third and fourth ventricles and is not normally visualized on CT.

The third ventricle

This is a slit-like structure lying in the midline supratentorially between the thalami. Posterior to the third ventricle lies the pineal gland. The third ventricle opens into the lateral ventricles through the foramen of Monro (Fig. 1.16).

The lateral ventricles

These are curved, 'C'-shaped structures with frontal, temporal and occipital horns joining at a body:

- The frontal horns contain no choroid and between them lies the septum pellucidum. This may be absent as a congenital abnormality.
- The temporal horns in the temporal lobe must be symmetrical – if one is unduly dilated this can be a sign of subuncal herniation. The hippocampus lies in the floor of the temporal horn and hippocampal atrophy in dementia can be detected by looking at the temporal horn (Fig. 1.16).
- The occipital horns arise from the posterior body called the trigone. The calcified choroid plexus lies within the trigone of the lateral ventricles. There is no choroid in the occipital horns themselves which are often asymmetrical (Fig. 1.16d).

The cisterns

- Ambient cistern and quadrigeminal cisterns surround the midbrain. The quadrigeminal cistern is the CSF space surrounding the quadrigeminal bodies, which are also called the superior and inferior colliculi. The vein of Galen lies in the quadrigeminal cistern. The ambient cistern is the CSF continuation around the side of the midbrain (Fig. 1.17).
- Prepontine cistern and basal cisterns are the CSF space anterior to the pons and around the brain stem. The basilar artery runs through the prepontine cistern.
- The cisterna magna lies behind the medulla and cerebellum (Fig. 1.17c).
- Suprasellar cistern: lies above the sella, i.e. the pituitary gland. Pathology in this site has a narrow differential, which is why it is important to assess this area (Fig. 1.18).

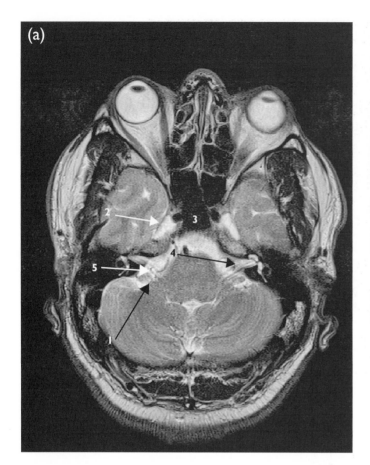

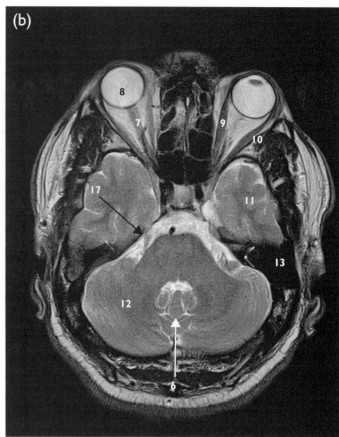

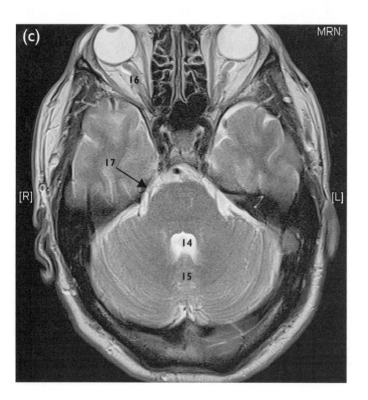

Fig. 1.12 (a) Axial T2-weighted images through the brain showing the flocculus of the cerebellum (1). Meckel's cave is seen on either side of the petrous bone as a high-signal CSF-containing space. The trigeminal ganglion lies within this (2). Signal voids from the basilar artery and the carotid arteries are seen (3). (4) Nerves VII and VIII are seen entering the internal auditory canal. (5) The anterior inferior cerebellar artery is seen winding around the cerebellopontine angle. (b) A slightly higher section of the brain stem, again showing the pons. The basilar artery is seen as a signal void within the prepontine cistern. Nerves V are seen (17) originating from the pons, running anteriorly. The cerebella vermis (6) is marked posteriorly: globe (7), optic nerves (8), medial rectus (9), lateral rectus (10), temporal lobe (11), cerebellum (12) and petrous bone (13). (c) An axial T2-weighted image showing the nerves V (17) bilaterally as they originate from the anterior aspect of the pons: fourth ventricle (14), cerebella vermis (15) and serpiginous superior ophthalmic vein (16).

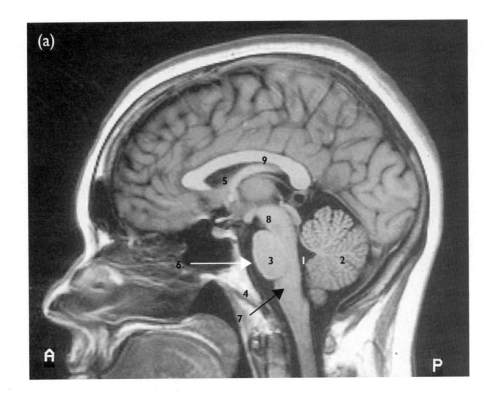

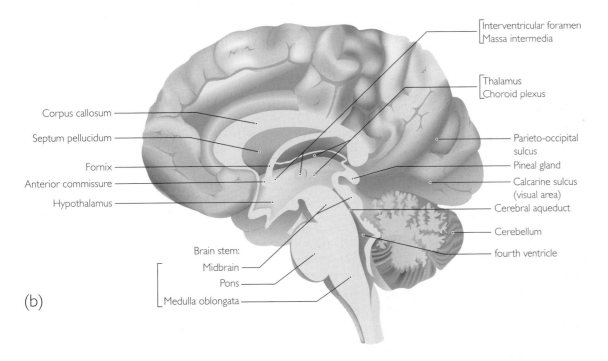

Fig. 1.13 (a) Sagittal T1-weighted image of the brain with (b) sagittal diagram of the brain. The corpus callosum can be seen uniting the two halves of the brain. The pons is marked (3). The medulla lies inferior to this. The corpus callosum is seen as a C-shaped structure which connects the two halves of the brain. The three parts of the brain stem, the midbrain, the pons and the medulla, are well seen. The cerebellum is seen posteriorly. Fourth ventricle (1), cerebellum (2), pons (3), clivus (4), third ventrical (5), prepontine cistern (6), medulla (7), mid brain (8), corpus collosum (9).

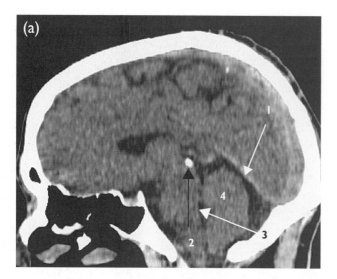

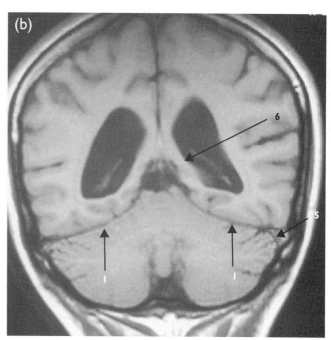

Fig. 1.14 (a) Sagittal reconstructed CT, (b) coronal T1-weighted image, unenhanced. The tentorium cerebelli (1) can be seen on CT as a very high-density line in relation to the fourth ventricle. The calcified pineal gland is seen posterior to the third ventricle (2). Fourth ventricle triangular diamond shape (3), cerebellum (4), tentorium cerebelli. Coronal T1-weighted image shows the tentorium cerebelli (1). The transverse sinuses can be seen (5) and the trigone of the lateral ventricles containing choroid plexus (6).

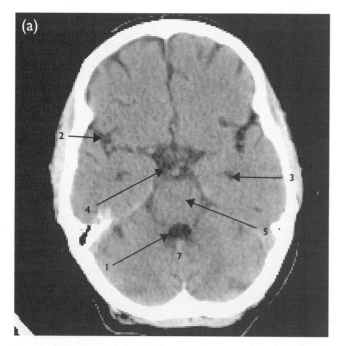

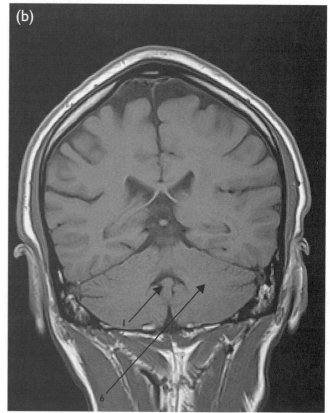

Fig. 1.15 (a) Axial CT, (b) Coronal T1-weighted MRI. The fourth ventricle (1) is seen within the posterior fossa between the pons (5) and the cerebellar vermis (7). It communicates with the remaining ventricles via the aqueduct: sylvian fissure (2), temporal horn (3), suprasellar cistern (4), pons (5) and left cerebellar hemisphere (6).

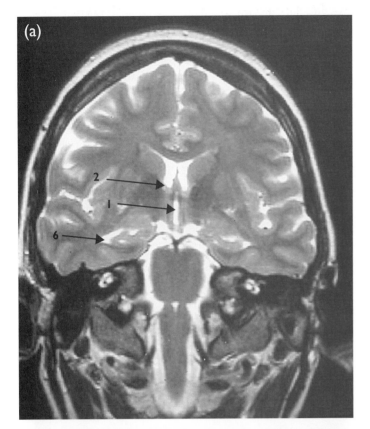

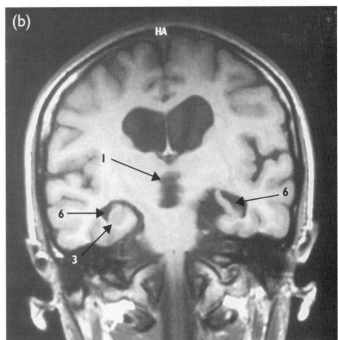

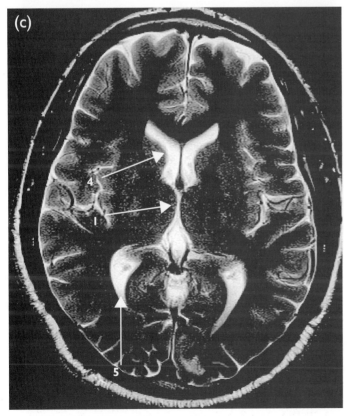

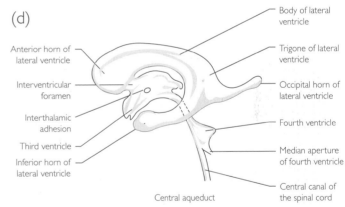

Fig. 1.16 Third ventricle: (a) coronal T2-weighted MRI; (b) T1-weighted MRI. The third ventricle is marked (1) as a slit-like structure in the midline. The third ventricle communicates, via the foramen of Monro (2), with the lateral ventricles. The hippocampus (3) is seen in the floor of the temporal horn of the lateral ventricles (6). (c) Axial T2-weighted MRI. (d) Diagram of ventricles. The lateral ventricle is a curved C-shaped structure. The frontal horns are seen anteriorly (4); the lateral ventricle communicates with the third ventricle (2) via the foramen of Monro. The occipital horn is seen posteriorly (5).

Parts of the brain

The pineal gland

- Under the age of 10 years the pineal gland should not be calcified.
- The pineal gland may be calcified by up to 1 cm in diameter in a normal individual over the age of 20.
- The age range 10–20 years is indeterminate. If a child in this age range has a calcified pineal gland it may be due to a pinealoma (Fig. 1.19 and see Fig. 1.14).

The internal capsule

This is a V-shaped structure made up of white matter. The anterior limb is smaller than the posterior limb. The right-sided fibres supply the left side of the body. A right internal capsule infarct leads to a corresponding left hemiplegia. Superiorly the fibres of the internal capsule fan out into the corona radiata or centrum semiovale (Fig. 1.20).

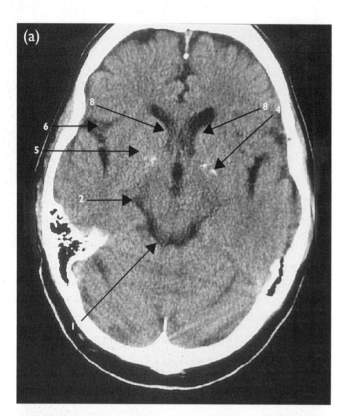

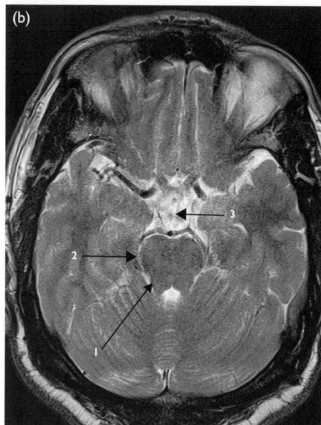

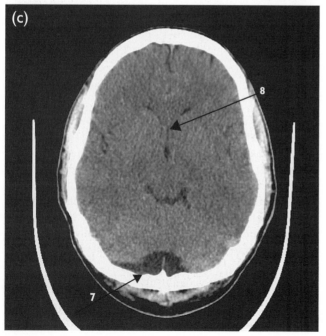

Fig. 1.17 (a) Axial CT unenhanced. (b) Axial T2-weighted MRI. The quadrigeminal system lies around the quadrigeminal bodies (1). The continuation around the edge of the midbrain is called the ambient cistern (2). The suprasellar cistern (3) can be seen on the MRI with the circle of Willis around it. On the CT, the third ventricle is seen with some incidental calcification in the basal ganglia (4). The head of caudate nucleus (8); lentiform nucleus (5) and sylvian fissure (6). (c) Axial CT of the brain shows a large cisterna magna posteriorly (7).

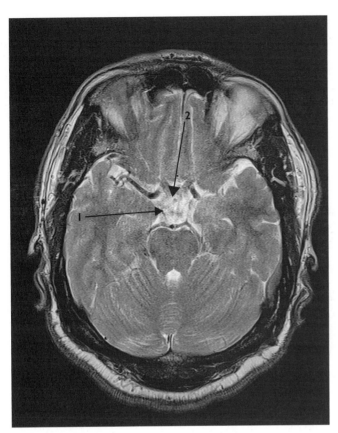

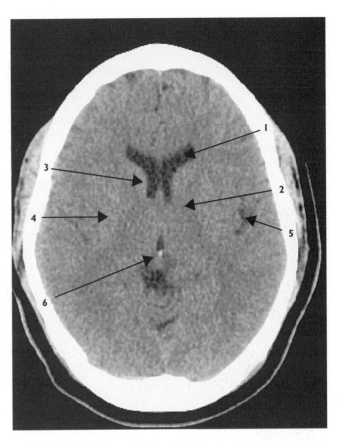

Fig. 1.18 Axial T2-weighted MRI of the brain shows the suprasellar cistern (1), which is the cerebrospinal fluid space above the pituitary gland. The circle of Willis is closed opposed to this, as is the optic chiasma (2).

Fig. 1.19 Axial CT scan showing the normal calcified pineal gland at the posterior aspect of the third ventricle (6): (1) anterior horns of lateral ventricles, (2) internal capsule, (3) head of caudate nucleus, (4) lentiform nucleus and (5) sylvian fissure.

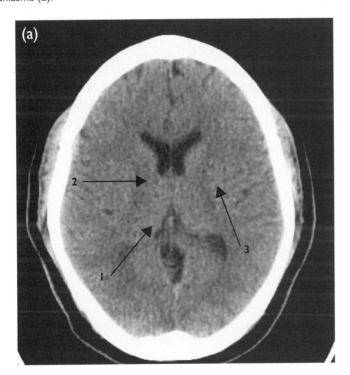

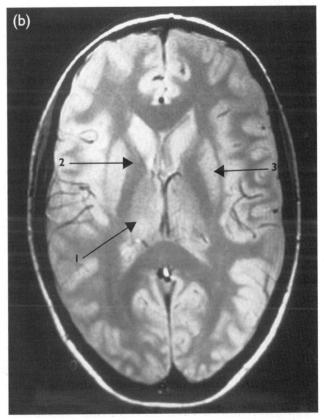

Fig. 1.20 (a) Axial CT and (b) proton density MRI of the brain showing the same anatomy: thalamus (1), anterior internal capsule (2) and lentiform nucleus (3).

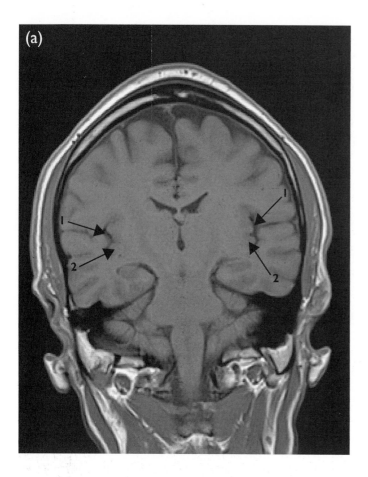

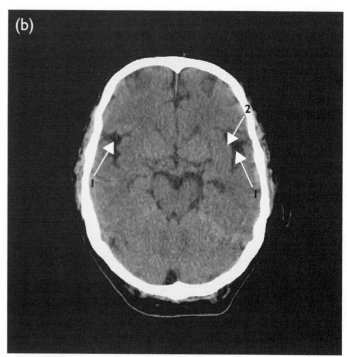

Fig. 1.21 (a) Coronal T1-weighted MRI and (b) axial CT scan of the brain. (a) Coronal MRI shows the sylvian fissure (1), deep to the sylvian is a rim of cortex called the claustrum (2). This is also marked on the CT (b). Note on CT there is reversal of grey–white matter differentiation, which is also seen on T1-weighted MRI.

The basal ganglia

- The basal ganglia consist of the caudate nucleus which abuts the internal capsule medially and the lentiform nucleus which is lateral to the genu of the internal capsule. These are supplied by the lenticulostriate vessels, which are small end-arteries coming off the middle cerebral artery. Small-vessel ischaemia affects these and leads to small lacunar infarcts within the basal ganglia.
- The caudate is a C shape with a head that sits in the convexity of the anterior horn of the lateral ventricle. The tail lies in the temporal lobe (see Fig. 1.20).
- The lentiform nucleus contains the putamen and globus pallidus and is shaped like a slice of cake with a V-shaped inner surface and a convex outer surface.
- Over age 45 years the basal ganglia can calcify as a normal variant.

The thalamus

This is an oval paired structure that abuts the third ventricle. The most medial part is called the pulvinar (see Fig. 1.20).

The claustrum and insula

These areas represent the area inside the sylvian fissure. The claustrum is also called the external capsule, and its territory is supplied by the middle cerebral artery. The sylvian fissures are usually symmetrical and asymmetry or loss of visualization of the fissure may be the only clue to a subarachnoid haemorrhage or pathology (Fig. 1.21).

The corpus callosum

The corpus callosum is made up of the following four parts: anteriorly rostrum, genu, body and splenium. Congenital anomalies of the corpus callosum may be associated with its partial or complete absence. Demyelination has a predilection for the corpus callosum. In utero the anterior part of the rostrum develops first, followed by the body and splenium (see Fig. 1.13).

Centrum semiovale or corona radiata

This is the spanning out of the deep white matter. The internal capsule fibres continue into the centrum semiovale where small vessel ischaemia is commonly seen.

Limbic system

This comprises the hippocampus, the parahippocampus and the fornix. Its function is emotion and short-term memory. The hippocampus lies in the floor of the temporal horn of the lateral ventricle (Fig. 1.22).

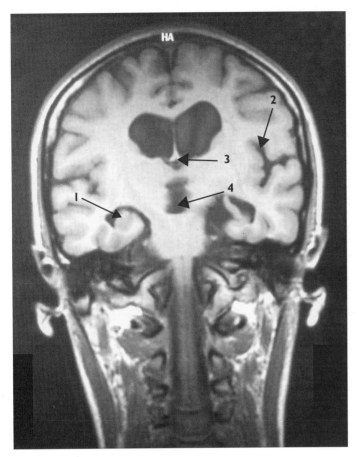

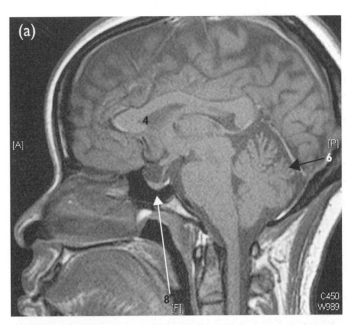

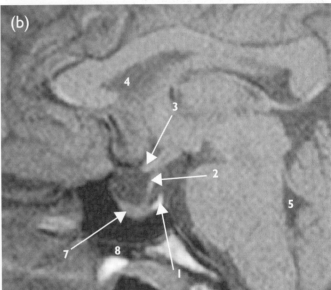

Fig. 1.22 Coronal T1-weighted MRI of the temporal lobe showing the hippocampus (1) in the floor of the temporal horn of the lateral ventricle: sylvian fissure (2), foramen of Monro (3) and third ventricle (4).

The pituitary gland
- It has an large anterior and a small posterior lobe.
- The gland lies in the sella. The sphenoid sinus lies underneath the sella and the cavernous sinuses on either side.
- The pituitary stalk or infundibulum connects the hypothalamus to the posterior lobe.
- The optic chiasma lies above the pituitary gland and pituitary tumours or adenomas can compress the chiasma, causing bitemporal hemianopia (Fig 1.23).
- The pituitary measures 12 mm in transverse, 9 mm in height and 8 mm in AP diameter.

The hypothalamus
- This comprises the infundibulum or pituitary stalk, the mammillary bodies and the optic chiasma.
- It lies in the floor of the third ventricle.

Fig 1.23 MRI of the pituitary: (a) sagittal image of the brain. (b) is a zoomed image, sagittally unenhanced, of the pituitary gland. The pituitary gland is seen in the floor of the sella. The posterior pituitary (1) is of high signal intensity in T1. The infundibulum (2) is seen running to the base of the pituitary gland. The optic chiasma is seen superiorly to this (3); third ventricle (4), fourth ventricle (5) and tentorium cerebelli (6), anterior pituitary (7), sphenoid sinus (8).

Facial bones

The mandible, the zygoma, the nasal bones, the maxilla and the bony orbit form the face:
- The mandible is the union of two bones at the symphysis menti. Each side had a vertical ramus, a horizontal body, a coronoid process anteriorly and a condylar process posteriorly that articulates with the temporomandibular joint.
- The zygoma has several processes that articulate with the frontal bone, the maxilla and the temporal bone (Fig. 1.24).

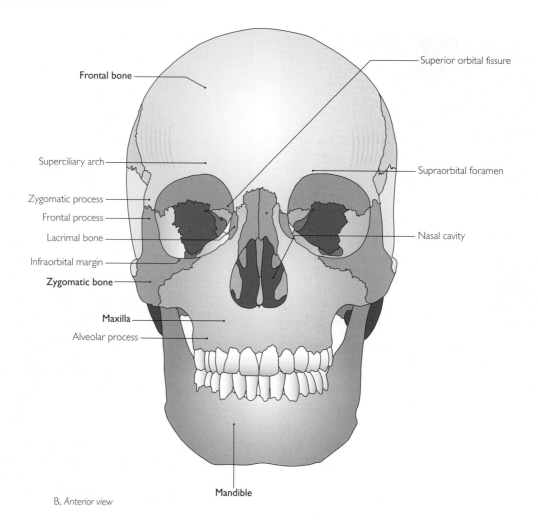

Frontal bone

Superior orbital fissure

Superciliary arch

Supraorbital foramen

Zygomatic process

Frontal process

Lacrimal bone

Nasal cavity

Infraorbital margin

Zygomatic bone

Maxilla

Alveolar process

Mandible

B, *Anterior view*

Fig. 1.24 Diagram of the facial bones. The frontal view of the facial bones is noted. The very thin lacrimal bone is noted medially, which is very prone to fracture. The infraorbital foramen is seen, which again can be affected by a blow-out fracture of the orbit.

Vascular supply to the brain

- The brain is supplied by branches of the internal carotid arteries and the basilar artery.
- The common carotid arteries arise on the left side from the aortic arch and on the right side from the brachiocephalic trunk in most individuals (Fig. 1.25).
- The common carotid arteries run up in the carotid sheath with the jugular vein and vagus nerves.
- At C4 the common carotid bifurcates into the internal and external carotid arteries. The internal carotid artery usually runs deeper or more posteriorly and in its cervical portion has no branches. It also has a different Doppler waveform from the external carotid artery.
- The external carotid artery has branches in the neck: ascending pharyngeal, superior thyroid, lingual, facial and occipital, posterior auricular, superficial temporal and maxillary (Fig. 1.26). This mnemonic may help memory:

  As Sally Lay Faint Oscar Pinched Some Money

- The external carotid has its terminal divisions into the superficial temporal and maxillary artery in the parotid gland.
- The internal carotid artery has a bulb or sinus, which is a slight dilatation of its origin. It has no branches in the neck.
- The internal carotid enters the skull through the carotid canal of the petrous bone. The artery has four portions: cervical before entering the skull, petrous in the temporal bone passing into the foramen lacerum, cavernous within the venous sinus and intracerebral within the subarachnoid space (Fig. 1.27).
- The internal carotid artery gives off the ophthalmic artery anteriorly as its first large visible branch and the posterior communicating artery posteriorly before dividing into the middle and anterior cerebral arteries.
- The middle cerebral artery is divided into two main portions: M1, the transverse section, and M2 in the insula. The middle cerebral artery gives rise to the lenticulostriate arteries from its M1 portion and then the angular and temporal from the M2 portion.

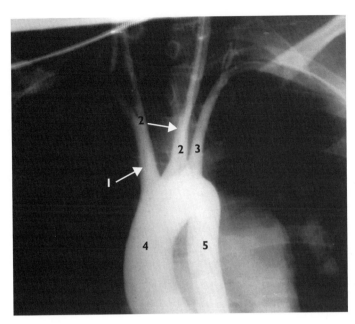

Fig. 1.25 Conventional aortic arteriogram: shows the normal conventional origin of the three great vessels to the head and neck: brachiocephalic artery (1), left common carotid (2), left subclavian artery (3), ascending aorta (4), descending aorta (5). This is the standard arrangement and is the most common.

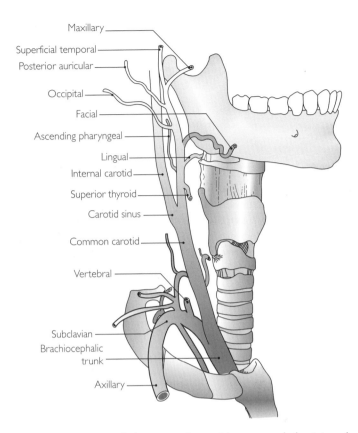

Fig. 1.26 Diagram of the external carotid artery and the internal carotid artery. Note that the internal carotid artery has no branches in the cervical region. The external carotid artery has multiple vessels arising from it, starting with the superior thyroid artery, then the lingual and facial arteries.

- The anterior cerebral artery is divided into two main portions: A1, the transverse section, and A2, the vertical section. The anterior cerebral artery gives rise to the pericallosal, the callosomarginal and the frontopolar arteries (Fig. 1.28).
- The circle of Willis is formed by the three arteries through links via the anterior communicating arteries between the two anterior cerebral and the two posterior communicating arteries (Fig. 1.29).
- The basilar artery is formed from two vertebral arteries: the vertebral arteries are usually the first branch of the subclavian artery and run up through the foramen transversarium, looping around C1 and passing up into the foramen magnum. They give rise to the posterior inferior cerebellar artery (PICA) before joining to form the basilar artery.
- The basilar artery runs up anterior to the pons in the prepontine cistern; it gives rise to the anterior inferior cerebellar artery or AICA near the IAM (internal auditary meatus), the superior cerebellar arteries, and then terminates in the posterior cerebral arteries which run back posteriorly to supply the occipital lobes and ocular cortex (Fig. 1.30).

Veins/cerebral venous system

- In the neck the jugular veins run from the jugular foramen to the thoracic inlet.
- The jugular veins run in the carotid sheath with the carotid arteries.

- There may be marked asymmetry in the normal size of the jugular.
- The internal jugular veins drain into the brachiocephalic veins with the subclavian veins.
- In the head there are deep veins and venous sinuses. The main venous sinuses are superior and inferior sagittal, transverse, petrosal and sigmoid sinuses. The sigmoid sinuses drain into the jugular veins at the jugular foramen (Fig. 1.31).
- The cerebral venous sinuses lie within the dura.
- The superior sagittal sinus is a large midline structure that runs posteriorly in the falx cerebri and then drains, usually to the right into the transverse sinuses at the torcula herophili or is more commonly called confluence of sinuses. It usually becomes the right transverse sinus, and right sigmoid and right jugular veins.
- The inferior sagittal sinus is small and lies in the lower falx in its free edge in the midline.
- The straight sinus runs in the tentorium and usually becomes the left transverse sinus at the torcula, and left sigmoid and left jugular veins.

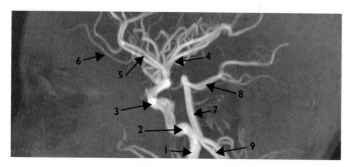

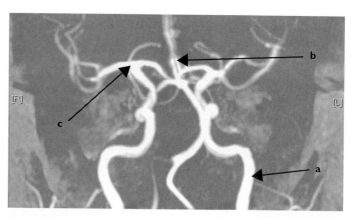

Fig. 1.27 Time of Flight 3D circle of Willis MIP sagittal image to demonstrate anatomy. The four portions of the internal carotids are marked: cervical (1), petrous (2), cavernous (3) and intracerebral. The internal carotid artery divides into the middle cerebral artery (4) and the anterior cerebral artery (5), callosomarginal (6), pericallosal (7), frontopolar artery.

Fig. 1.28 Frontal view of a middle and cerebral artery angiogram: (a) internal carotid artery; (b) anterior cerebral artery; (c) middle cerebral artery.

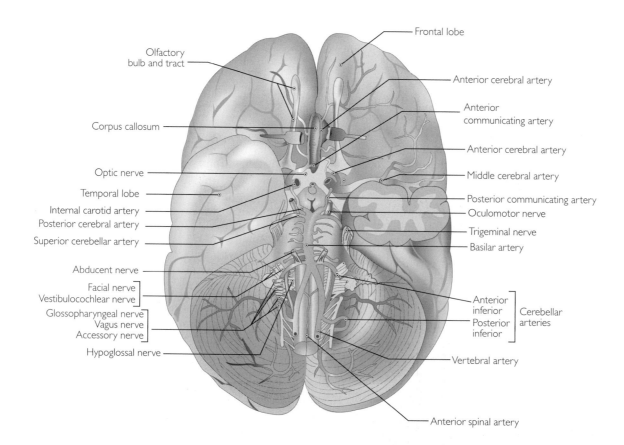

Fig. 1.29 Diagram of the base of the skull showing the vertebral arteries joining to form the basilar artery and the circle of Willis: optic chiasma (1); internal carotid artery (2); anterior cerebral artery (3); and posterior communicating artery (4).

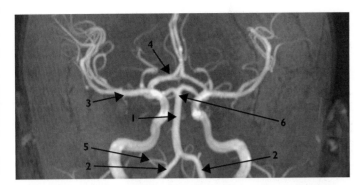

Fig. 1.30 Time of Flight 3D circle of Willis MIP coronal image showing the normal basilar artery (1), vertebral arteries (2), middle cerebral artery (3), anterior cerebral arteries (4), PICA (5) and superior cerebella (6).

- The transverse sinuses become the sigmoid sinus and drain into the jugular vein at the jugular foramen (Fig. 1.32).
- The superior and inferior petrosal sinuses also drain into the jugular veins at the jugular foramen.
- The deep cerebral veins: the internal cerebral veins that run in the roof of the third ventricle and join to form the vein of Galen. This short vein lies in the quadrigeminal cistern. The vein of Galen joins the inferior sagittal sinus to become the straight sinus.
- The cavernous sinus communicates with the facial veins via the ophthalmic veins and empties into the petrosal sinuses.

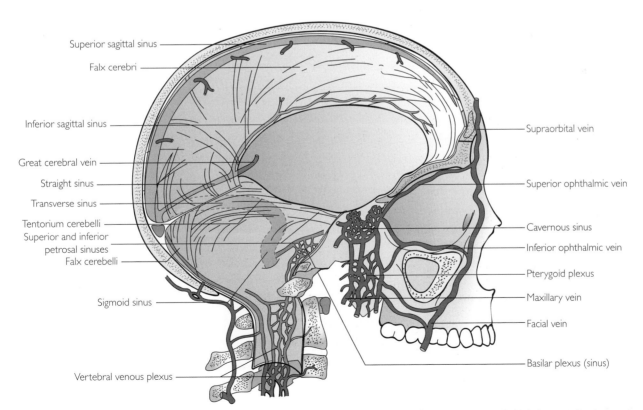

Fig. 1.31 Diagram of venous sinuses. The superior sagittal sinus is seen joining the transverse sinuses posteriorly and the straight sinus posteriorly at the confluence of venous sinuses.

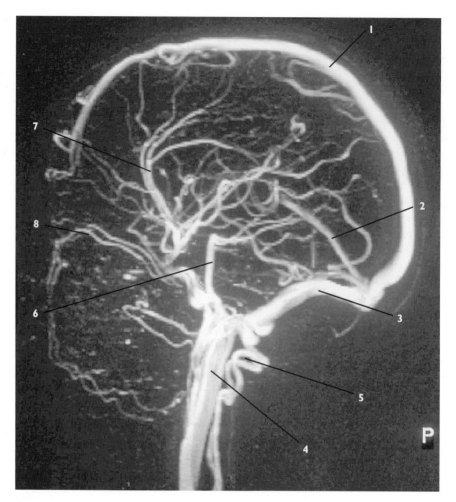

Fig. 1.32 MIP (maximum intensity projection) image of the venous sinuses on MRI: superior sagittal sinus (1); straight sinus (2); transverse sinus (3); jugular vein (4). The arteries are also shown on: vertebral arteries (5), basilar (6), anterior cerebral (7) and ophthalmic (8).

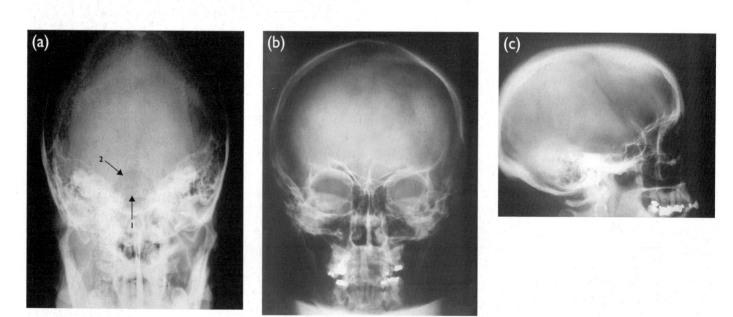

Fig. 1.33 Standard skull radiograph series: (a) Towne's views. The dorsum sellae (1) should be visible through the foramen magnum (2), as marked. (b) This shows the posteroanterior (PA) 20 skull radiograph; the petrous bone should be projected to the lower edge of the orbits. (c) Lateral skull radiograph.

IMAGING

Imaging of the skull

Standard skull radiograph series

Indication
Metastatic skull involvement, myeloma screen, non-accidental injury, skeletal syndromes.

Technique
This includes three views (Fig. 1.33):
1. Towne's view: the dorsum sellae should be visualized though the foramen magnum.
2. PA20 view: this is a frontal view when the petrous bone should lie at the lower limit of the orbit. Good views of the orbit are obtained.
3. Lateral skull radiograph: the pituitary fossa is seen and the sphenoid sinus, foramen magnum and orbital roofs.

Findings
Various other normal skull markings are present on the skull, of which the radiologist should be aware so not to be confused with fractures and pathology.

Skull radiographs are uncommonly performed but are used in paediatrics and for skeletal surveys.
- The parietal star is seen in the parietal bone on a lateral view due to a complex of veins (Fig. 1.34).
- Hair braids: structures outside the skull such as hair braids can mimic pathology, in this case sclerotic bony metastasis (Fig. 1.35).

- Chamberlain's line and McGregor's line: the lines are taken from the hard palate to the inner and outer tables of the skull at the foramen magnum, respectively. These lines are important to assess for softening of the bone when basilar invagination can occur. In Chamberlain's line <2 mm of the odontoid peg should be above the line and <5 mm with Macgregor's line (Fig. 1.36).
- Skull calcifications have decreased in importance due to the ubiquitous nature of CT. Multiple structures can normally calcify within the brain and this could show up on the skull radiograph: pineal gland, dura, habenular commissure, falx cerebri, basal ganglia and choroid plexus (Fig. 1.37).
- The middle meningeal vessels form a groove over the temporal bone on a lateral view (Fig. 1.38).
- The superior orbital fissures (SOFs) can be seen on a PA20 view. They lie between the greater and lesser wings of sphenoid (Fig. 1.39). The following mnemonic lists the cranial nerves and structures that pass through the SOFs – Loud French Toads Sit Noisily In Alaska:

Lacrimal V	**L**oud
Frontal V	**F**rench
Trochlea IV	**T**oads
Superior division of III	**S**it
Nasociliary V	**N**oisily
Inferior division of III	**I**n
Abducens VI	**A**laska

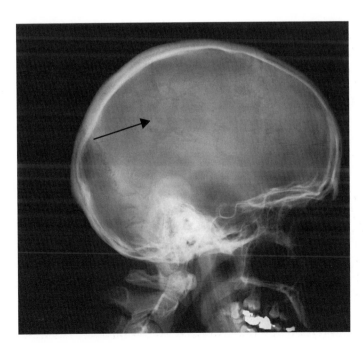

Fig. 1.34 A venous plexus on the lateral skull, which can mimic pathology called a parietal star (arrow).

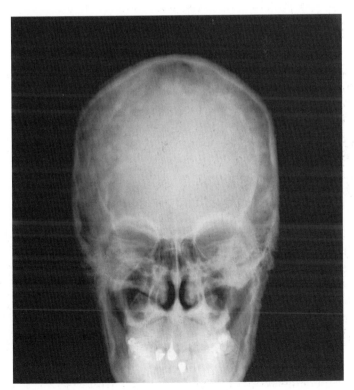

Fig. 1.35 PA20 radiograph showing hair braids, which can mimic sclerotic metastasis.

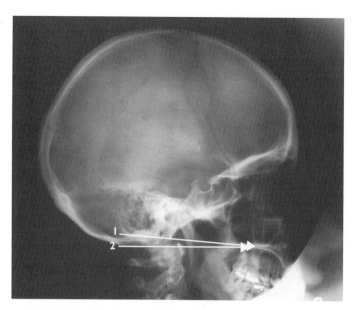

Fig. 1.36 Lateral skull radiograph showing Chamberlain's (1) and McGregor's (2) lines. The tip of the odontoid peg in Chamberlain's line (<2 mm) should be above the line and in McGregor's line (<5 mm) should be above the line.

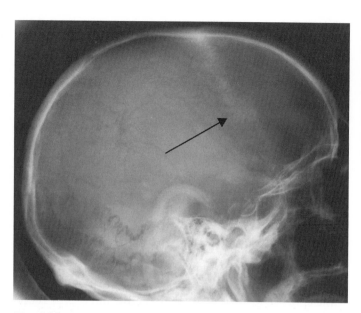

Fig. 1.38 Vascular markings of the skull on a lateral skull radiograph can mimic fractures. Awareness of the normal arterial pathways on the skull can help differentiate from fractures. The arrow marks the groove for the middle meningeal artery.

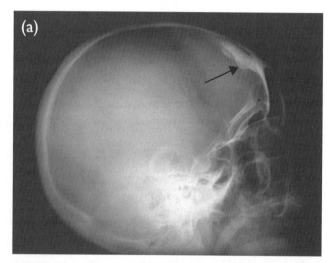

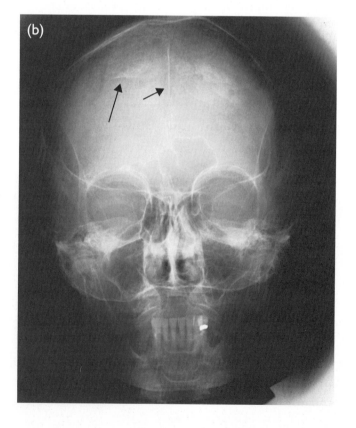

Fig. 1.37 (a) Lateral skull radiograph. (b) PA20 skull radiograph shows dural calcification-caused hyperostosis frontalis interna and calcification of the falx, which is a normal finding (arrows mark dural calcification).

Facial views

Indication
Facial trauma, sinusitis.

Technique
Facial views include the following:

- OM (occipitomental): on the frontal views the petrous bone is thrown below the maxillary antrum which can therefore be adequately visualized.
- OM30 (Fig. 1.40).
- Lateral.

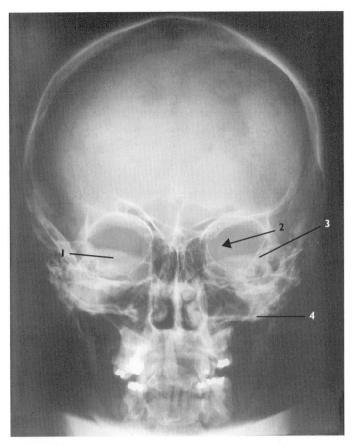

Fig. 1.39 The superior orbital fissure (1), which can be seen on PA20 skull radiograph. The ophthalmic division of the trigeminal nerve, the superior and inferior divisions of the oculomotor nerve, the abducens and the trochlear nerves all pass through the superior orbital fissure: petrous bone (2), internal auditory canal (3) and basiocciput (4).

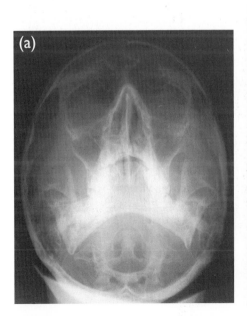

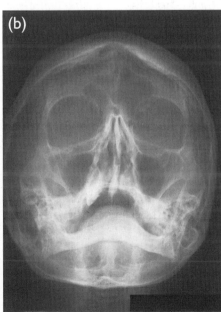

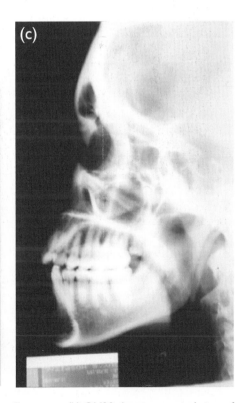

Fig. 1.40 Standard facial series: (a) OM showing the petrous bone at the lower margin of the maxillary antra. (b) OM30 showing a typical view of the mandible with prolonged coronoid processes. The odontoid peg is seen on this view. (c) Lateral facial series: a coned lateral view of the skull showing the facial views only.

Findings

Interpreting facial views:

- Look for soft-tissue swelling around orbit and cheek.
- Look for fluid levels/soft tissue in the sinuses, antra that are seen when facial fractures, blow-out fractures, present.
- The innominate line is a straight line seen within the orbit.

Imaging of the Brain

CT of the brain

Indications

CT of the brain has become the workhorse of the accident and emergency department (A&E):

- In trauma CT is the best for fresh haemorrhage and is a quick safe investigation if the patient is sick and unable to keep still.
- CT is indicated if the patient has pacemaker clips or when MRI is contraindicated.
- Calcification is better seen on CT. MRI is, however, superior for cerebral metastases, HIV-related disease, epilepsy and ischaemia.

Technique

Scans are now taken supine with the multislice CT and reconstructed into coronal and sagittal planes (Fig. 1.41).

Findings

- A good knowledge of the anatomy is required in order to assess pathology.

- CSF has the same CT number as water, i.e. 0. The cisterns and ventricles must be identified on every scan to assess for compression of the chambers or shift of their normal anatomical position.

Hounsfield units

- All CT images are based on a grey scale centred around water where tissues in the body are ascribed a Hounsfield unit (HU) depending on their ability to stop X-rays, i.e. their density (Fig. 1.42). The scale ranges from −1000, which is air density, does not stop X-rays and therefore gives a very black image, to ≥+1000 with bone, which completely stops X-rays and so appears white.
- Fat is lighter than water and so has a negative CT number of approximately −40 HU to −100 HU.
- Fresh blood which is denser than soft tissues has a CT number of +100 HU. In brain CT this means that fresh blood is denser than normal brain and so appears white on a standard brain window setting (Fig. 1.43).
- The image obtained from a CT is displayed on a grey scale; the values can be manipulated after the scan to display different tissues to advantage. A standard brain setting has a centre point on grey matter and a narrow window width to maximize the contrast between grey and white matter, which is very subtle, being a difference of only 10 HU. The settings can be altered using standard presets to show, for example, the bones if looking for fractures. Different window settings are used for different parts of the body.
- On CT there is reversal of the grey–white matter. This is due to the higher fatty content of white matter as a

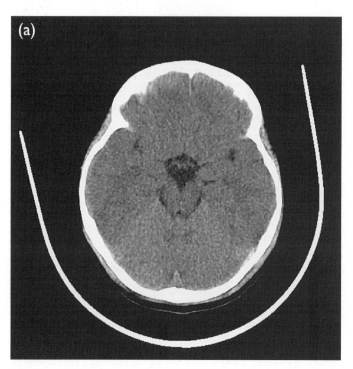

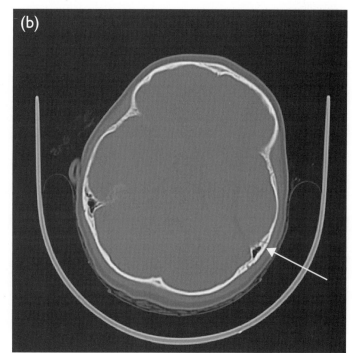

Fig. 1.41 Axial CT of the brain, with bony and standard windows. (a) Standard window setting. On the standard CT, no definite fracture is visible. On the correct bony windows (b), using a sharp filter, a fracture can be identified (arrow).

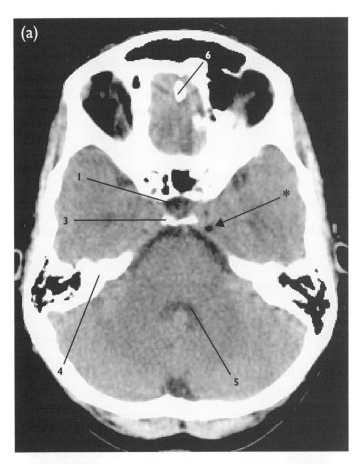

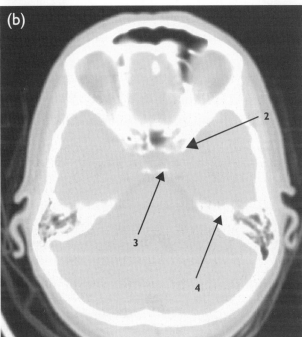

result of the presence of sphingomyelin. Sphingomyelin is fatty and therefore reduces the CT number of white matter, so that it appears greyer than grey matter. The CT number of white matter is 25 HU and of grey matter 35 HU (Fig. 1.44):

- Therefore on brain settings of 40/80, fat will appear black similar to air and fresh blood will appear white.
- Things on brain settings that appear white, i.e. hyperdense:
  - fresh blood <2 weeks' old
  - intravenous contrast
  - calcification: the pineal gland and choroid plexus are calcified and hence appear white, i.e. hyperdense on this setting.

Box 1.2 CT numbers

White matter = 25 HU
Grey matter = 35 HU
Fat = −40 HU
Fresh blood = +100 HU

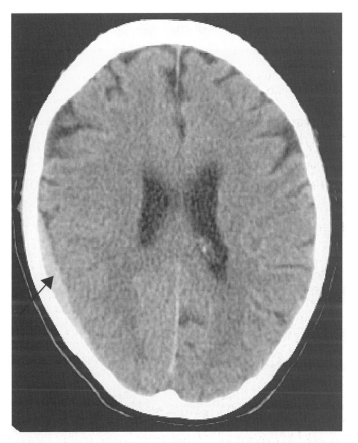

Fig. 1.42 (a) Axial CT of the brain and (b) lung windows of CT of the brain. The axial brain on normal windows shows a small focal low-density lesion which gives the impression of intracerebral air*. However, when put on lung windows, this should appear low density whereas it merges with the remaining brain structures. This is a small focus of fat that can mimic air on brain windows: sella (1), anterior clinoid (2), clivus (3), petrous bone (4), fourth ventricle (5) and crista galli (6).

Fig. 1.43 CT scan, axial standard brain settings (no contrast), shows a high-density extra-axial collection (arrow). Blood appears hyperdense on brain windows as the Hounsfield unit number of blood is =100. The window range is from −45 to +35 HU.

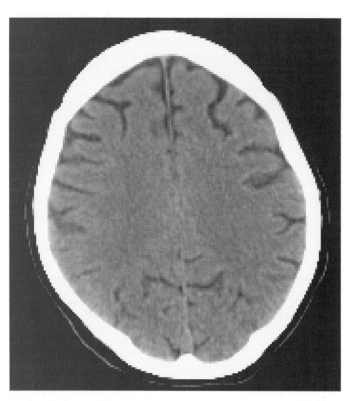

Normal variants

- Cavum septum pellucidum lies between the frontal horns of the lateral ventricles, a CSF chamber that persists into adult life (Fig. 1.45).
- Cavum septum vergae (Fig. 1.45).
- Idiopathic basal ganglia calcification (Fig. 1.46).

> **Box 1.3 Differences in what can be imaged on CT and MRI**
>
> | CT | MRI |
> |---|---|
> | Trauma | White matter disease |
> | Fresh haemorrhage | Posterior fossa |
> | Calcification | Cranial nerves |
> | Metastatic disease | |

Fig. 1.44 CT scan of the brain showing grey–white matter differentiation. On CT the cortex is high density and the white matter is low density due to the presence of fat from sphingomyelin in the white matter.

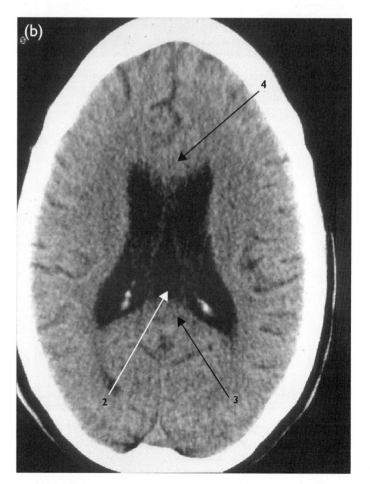

Fig. 1.45 Axial CT: (a) a cavum septum pellucidum (1), which lies in between the frontal horns of the lateral ventricles. (b) Cavum velum interpositum, with extension of the chamber posteriorly between the lateral ventricles (2), Splenium of corpus callosum (3), genu corpus callosum (4), internal capsule (5), pineal gland (6) and thalamus (7).

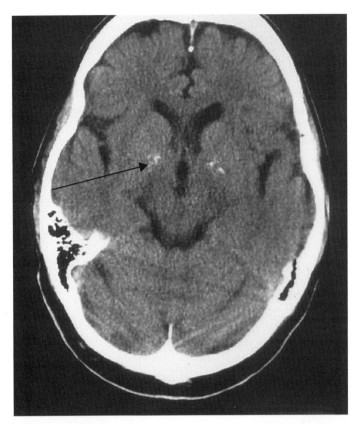

Fig. 1.46 Axial unenhanced CT shows symmetrical high density in the lentiform nucleus. This is basal ganglia calcification which is normal over age 45 (black arrow).

Table 1.1 Advantages and disadvantages of CT/MRI

	CT	MRI
Advantages	• Widely available. • Virtually no claustrophobia.	• No ionizing radiation involved. • Vessels are shown without intravenous contrast enhancement.
Disadvantages	• Large radiation dose. • Moderately expensive. • In order to see vessels intravenous contrast enhancement is necessary.	• Access and availability still problematic. • Claustrophobia. • Restrictions such as pacemakers, and magnetic clips contraindicate MRI.

MR of the brain

Indications

MR of the brain is superior in evaluating the posterior fossa, white matter disease, metastatic disease and meningeal disease. The cranial nerves are visualized with MRI, particularly nerves VII and VIII. With modern-day CT multislice scanning, both MRI and CT have a multiplanar capability.

Technique

A standard MR scan of the brain includes an axial T2-weighted image and coronal T1-weighted image. Flair and enhanced T1-weighted images may be used. For subtle haemorrhage T2-weighted gradient echo images are indicated.

Findings

The anatomy is the same in CT and MRI. MRI is more difficult initially to grasp and interpret because the bony landmarks are harder to see (Fig. 1.47):

- The midbrain is well visualized and MRI identifies the substantia nigra and red nuclei, unlike CT (Fig. 1.48).
- The internal capsule is well seen on MRI (Fig. 1.49).
- Nerves VII, VIII and V are well visualized on MRI as seen on the T2-weighted image in Fig. 1.50. If an acoustic neuroma is being searched for then T1-weighted images with gadolinium are complementary.
- The corpus callosum is seen on sagittal MRI (see Fig. 1.13). The third ventricle is well seen underneath the corpus callosum.
- The posterior fossa and temporal horns are better seen than on CT (Fig. 1.52).
- The meninges are identified on MRI. A coronal image shows the meninges clearly and thickening can be detected clearly, but may need gadolinium (Fig. 1.53).
- The pituitary gland is superiorly investigated with MRI with T1-weighted images before and after intravenous gadolinium in the coronal and sagittal planes.
- The superior aspect of the pituitary is normally flat or concave but can normally be convex in the menstruating female (Fig. 1.54). Note the concave surface of the pituitary bordered by the cavernous sinus. The signal voids within it are the carotid vessels.
- The posterior pituitary is of higher signal intensity than the anterior pituitary on T1-weighted and T2-weighted imaging.
- The pituitary stalk normally enhances after contrast.
- The pituitary gland enhances homogeneously after contrast. Adenomas show up areas of relative lack of enhancement compared with the normal gland.
- The cavernous sinus lies adjacent to the pituitary, with the internal carotid traversing it; flow within the carotid should be assessed by looking for flow voids.
- The optic chiasma lies above the pituitary gland and is best seen on coronal imaging. The optic nerves and chiasma can be clearly evaluated with MRI (Fig. 1.55).

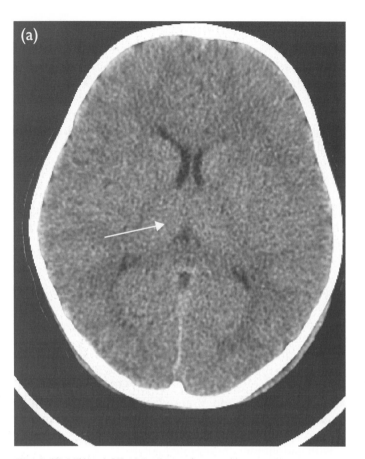

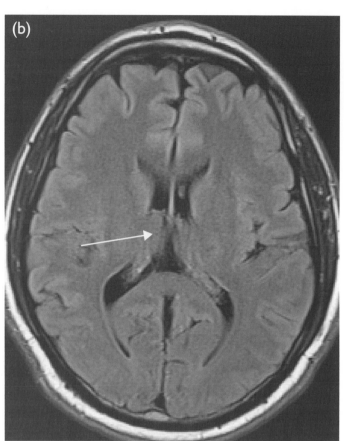

Fig. 1.47 MRI and CT of the brain. Comparison is made between the MRI and the CT: (a) CT and (b) MRI. The anatomy is the same. The thalami can be identified on both images (arrow). No abnormality seen.

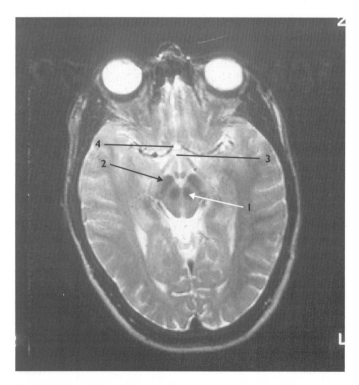

Fig. 1.48 Axial T2-weighted MRI shows the anatomy of the midbrain. The red nuclei (1) and the substantia nigra (2) can be well visualized in the midbrain on CT. Optic chiasma (3) and circle of Willis (4).

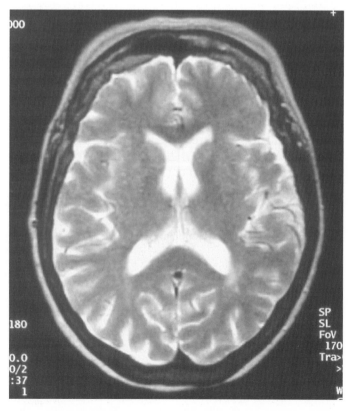

Fig. 1.49 Axial T2-weighted image showing the lateral ventricles. There is normal grey–white matter reversal on T2-weighted imaging.

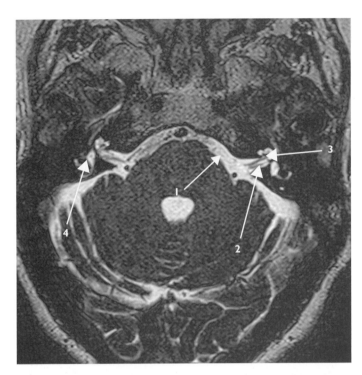

Fig. 1.50 Axial T2-weighted image shows nerves VII and VIII clearly as they leave the pons and travel into the internal auditory meatus. The anterior inferior cerebellar artery (1) can loop around the nerves in the cerebellar pontine angle and mimic a neuroma. Internal auditory canal (2), cochlea (3) and vestibule (4).

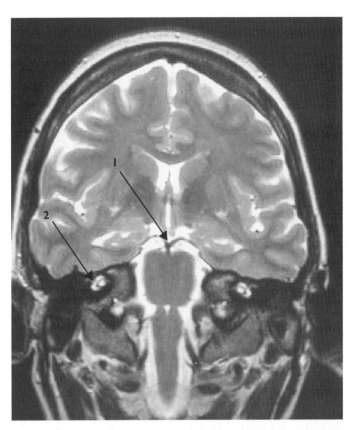

Fig. 1.52 Coronal T2-weighted image through the brain shows the normal pons and pyramids of the medulla. The terminal division of the basilar artery can be seen (1). The cochlea is well seen bilaterally in the petrous bone as a small snail shape (2).

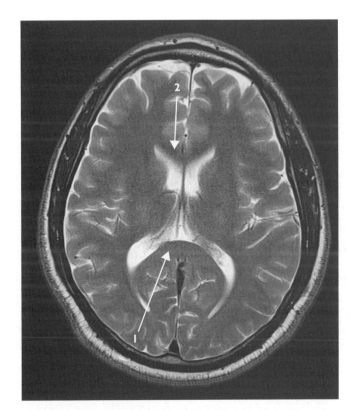

Fig. 1.51 Axial T2-weighted MRI: the anatomy of the corpus callosum can be well seen with the splenium posteriorly (1) and the genu (2) anteriorly.

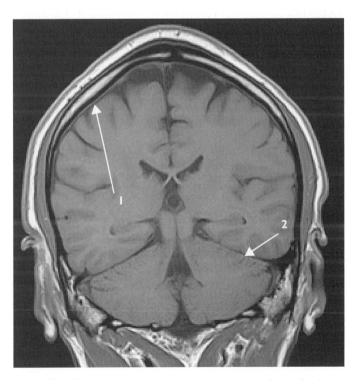

Fig. 1.53 MRI of the meninges: the meninges are well visualized normally on MRI (1). The tentorium cerebelli (2) is a good site to search for metastases.

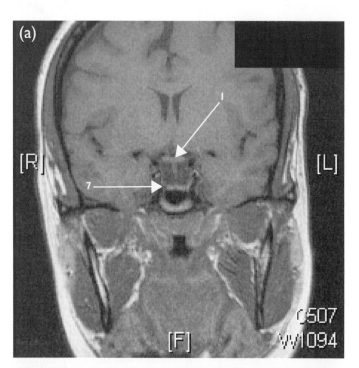

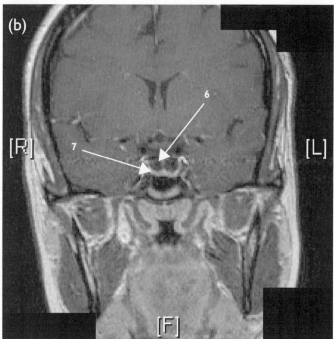

- The cavernous sinus is clearly evaluated with MRI. Cranial nerves III, IV, VI and V2 lie in the side wall. Nerve VI runs through the cavernous sinus, as does the internal carotid artery. Coronal images are used (Fig. 1.56).

Cerebral angiography, both MR and CT, and interventional

Indications
Subarachnoid haemorrhage, venous sinus thrombosis.

Technique
Now non-invasive techniques are used as much as possible because of the complications that can occur with direct neuro angiography.

Findings
- The internal carotid artery starts at C4 following division of the common carotid artery. There are four portions of the internal carotid artery:
  (1) cervical – no branches
  (2) petrous – no branches
  (3) cavernous
  (4) intracranial – first branch ophthalmic = intradural.
- Then the internal carotid artery divides into the anterior cerebral and middle cerebral arteries.

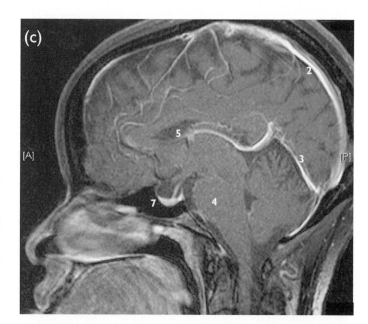

Fig. 1.54 MRI of the pituitary: (a) coronal T1-weighted images before contrast, (b) coronal T1-weighted post-contrast images and (c) sagittal post-contrast T1-weighted images demonstrate the pituitary gland. This normally enhances after contrast and the infundibulum normally enhances after contrast. The optic chiasm (1) can be seen above the sella. The superior sagittal sinus (2) and straight sinus (3) are well seen on the sagittal image. Pons (4), third ventricle (5), infundibulum (6), pituitary (7).

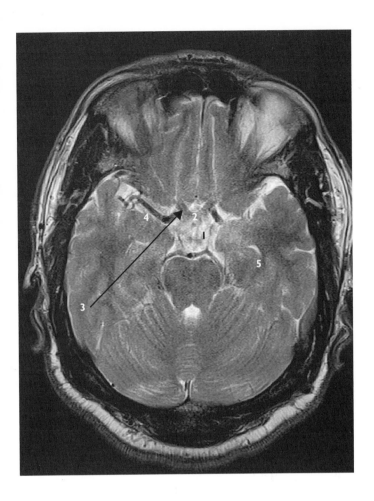

Fig. 1.55 Optic nerves in the suprasellar cistern (1). The optic tracts run posteriorly from the optic chiasm (2) and the optic nerves (3) themselves are well seen in the suprasellar cistern on MRI on T2-weighted imaging. Middle cerebral artery (4), temporal horn of lateral ventricle (5).

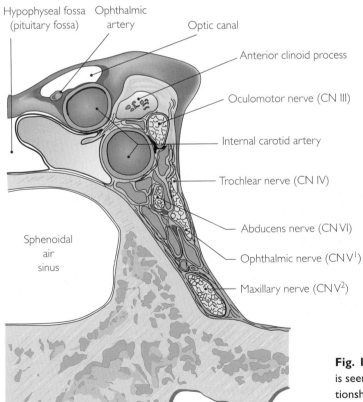

Hypophyseal fossa (pituitary fossa)

Ophthalmic artery

Optic canal

Anterior clinoid process

Oculomotor nerve (CN III)

Internal carotid artery

Trochlear nerve (CN IV)

Sphenoidal air sinus

Abducens nerve (CN VI)

Ophthalmic nerve (CN V^1)

Maxillary nerve (CN V^2)

Fig. 1.56 Diagram of the cavernous sinus. The internal carotid artery is seen within the cavernous sinus and the cranial nerves and their relationships are noted.

- The anterior cerebral is divided into A1 and A2 segments and gives off these branches. At this stage learn these three: pericallosal, callosomarginal, frontopolar (Fig. 1.57).
- The basilar artery is intradural, i.e. subarachnoid throughout its length.
- It is formed by convergence of the two vertebral arteries.
- The branches that it gives off are the anterior inferior cerebellar artery (AICA) and the superior cerebellar arteries.

- It becomes the posterior cerebral arteries, which supply the occipital lobes and most importantly the visual cortex. An embolism or infarct in this territory will lead to occipital blindness.
- It does not supply the PICA; this is supplied by the vertebral artery (Fig. 1.58).
- The left vertebral artery is usually dominant. When doing angiography contrast usually refluxes down the right artery and therefore only the left has to be assessed (Fig. 1.59).

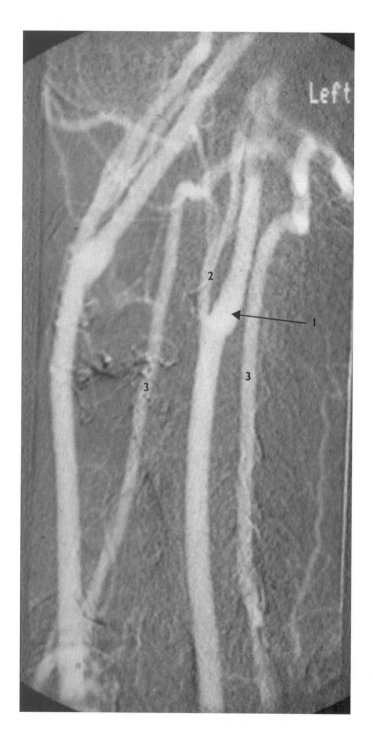

Fig. 1.57 Carotid angiogram: digital subtraction on two different patients. The internal carotid artery is seen with its sinus at its origin, which is a slight dilatation (1). Only the external carotid artery has branches (2). The smaller vertebral arteries (3) running through the foramen transversarium can be seen.

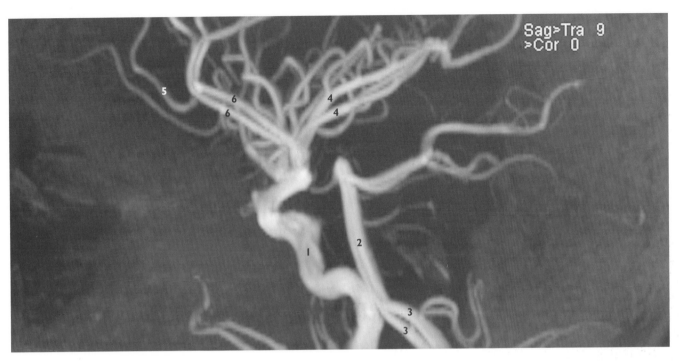

Fig. 1.58 MRI Time of flight (ToF). 3D circle of Willis MIP sagittal image showing the carotid and basilar arteries. (1) Carotid internal, (2) basilar, (3) vertebrals, (4) middle cerebral, (5) frontopolar, (6) anterior cerebra.

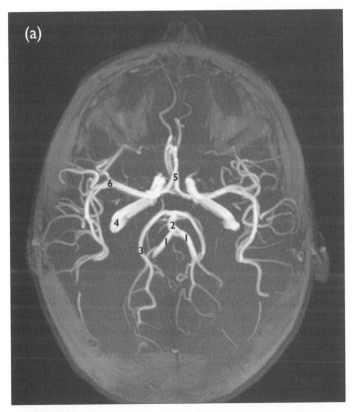 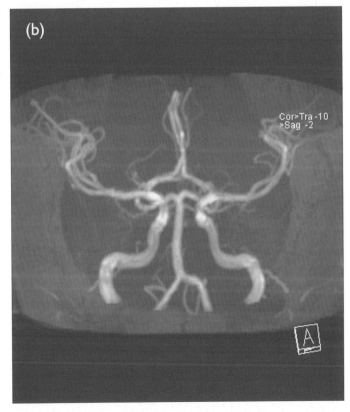

Fig. 1.59 (a) Time of flight (TDF) 3D circle of Willis MIP Transverse image showing the normal vertebral arteries (1) joining to form the basilar artery (2). The posterior cerebrals (3) arise from the basilar artery, (4) internal carotid artery, (5) anterior cerebral artery and (6) middle cerebral artery. (b) TDF 3D circle of Willis MIP coronal image.

- The cerebral venous sinuses are well seen by MR vascular imaging. MR vascular studies can also assess the arteries within the brain when arteries and veins, i.e. sinuses, are superimposed (Fig. 1.60).

Cerebral ultrasound

Indications
Neonatal suspected haemorrhage, neonatal irritability, premature neonates.

Technique
- Use the anterior fontanelle, which closes at 18 months, or the posterior fontanelle, which closes at 3 months. The probe must have a small foot to fit the small size of the anterior fontanelle and a wide curvilinear array to cover the brain inside (Fig. 1.61).

- Ultrasound is a portable technique avoiding ionizing radiation.
- Scans are taken in the coronal (Fig. 1.62), sagittal and parasagittal planes. In the parasagittal plane the caudate, the thalamus and the caudothalamic groove are seen.

Findings
- The caudothalamic grove is seen parasagittally where the germinal matrix occurs and it is an important site to assess for haemorrhage. The size of the ventricles can be seen.
- The presence of echogenic haemorrhage in the ventricles or brain.
- The presence of collections in the falx.
- Doppler ultrasound of the vessels can be performed.

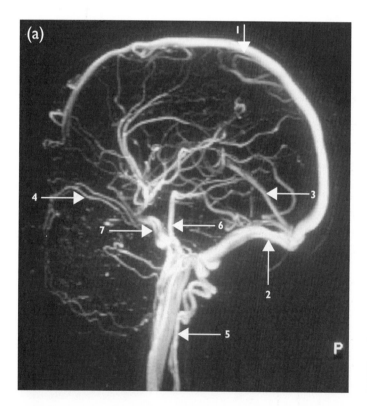
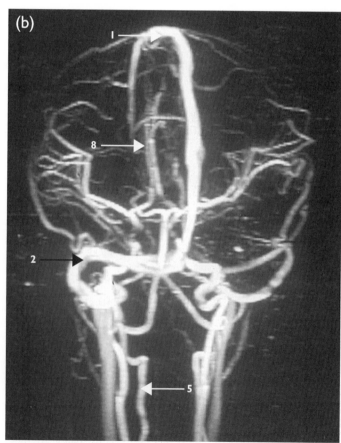

Fig. 1.60 The MIP (maximum intensity projection) image shows the venous sinuses with the cerebral arterial supply superimposed. (a) Sagittal image; (b) coronal image: superior sagittal sinus (1), transverse sinus (2), straight sinus (3), ophthalmic artery (4), vertebral artery (5), basilar artery (6), internal carotid artery (7) and anterior cerebral artery (8).

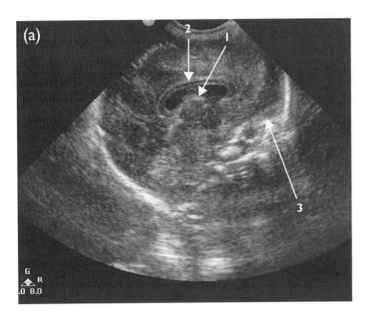

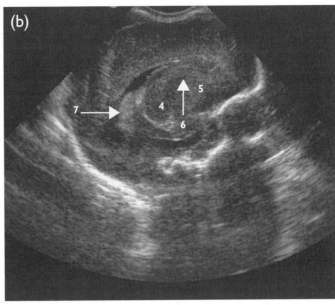

Fig. 1.61 Neonatal head ultrasound: (a) midline sagittal section shows the third ventricle (1) in the midline which appears large on a sagittal image. Corpus callosum (2). The floor of the orbits can be seen anteriorly (3). (b) A parasagittal image showing the thalamus (4) and the caudate (5). The caudothalamic groove (6) lies between the two. Choroid plexus can be seen (7) in the trigone of the lateral ventricle.

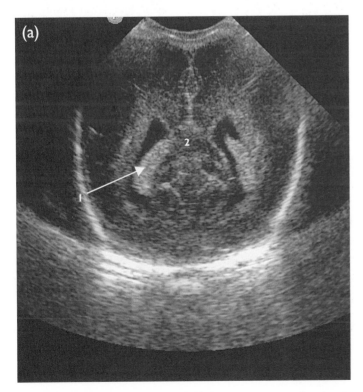

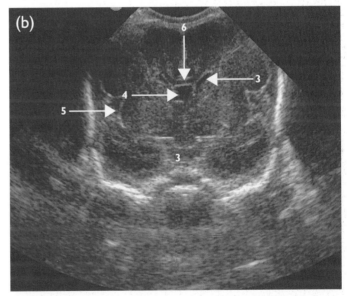

Fig. 1.62 Coronal head ultrasound: (a) A posterior image showing the trigone of the lateral ventricles containing normal choroid plexus (1); splenium of the corpus callosum (2). (b) Anterior horns of lateral ventricles (3). A coronal image anteriorly showing the cavum septum pellucidum (4). sylvian fissure (5) and corpus callosum (6).

Imaging the carotid arteries

Carotid Doppler ultrasonography

Indications
Atheroma, previous cerebrovascular accident (CVA), transient ischaemic attacks (TIAs), bruits.

Technique
A high-frequency linear-array probe, either 7 MHz or 10 MHz (Fig. 1.63).

Findings
- The intima can be seen in the vessels.
- The external carotid has branches.
- The internal carotid artery has the sinus at its origin.

CT and MR angiography

Non-invasive techniques. CT uses iodine-based contrast. CT angiography is being used increasingly with multislice CT.

Head angiography

Mainly performed for intervention and problem-solving.

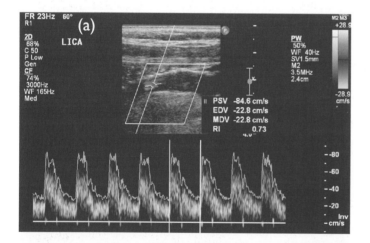

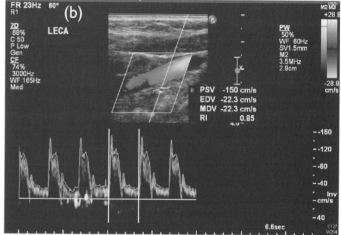

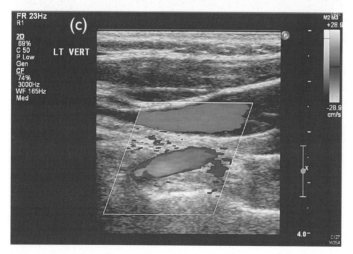

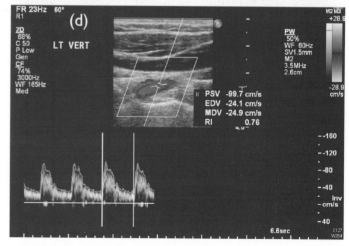

Fig. 1.63 Carotid ultrasound. (a) The normal Doppler wave from the internal carotid artery with high flow throughout the cardiac cycle to the brain in systole and diastole. (b) Doppler waveform of the external carotid artery with a notch and less flow in diastole. (c) The left vertebral artery also gives a Doppler signal when imaged in between the foramen transversarium. (d) The Doppler waveform of the vertebral arteries.

CASES

Case 1.1

A patient presents with a first fit. An MRI of the brain is performed because it is superior for the investigation of first fits. However, in the emergency setting, if MRI is not available and there is any evidence of focal fitting, or history of headache or focal neurology, a CT of the brain may be performed.

Anatomy review: name 1–5 (see Fig. 1.64 for answers)

- Review the brain scan with a system.
- Start with T2W axial series. Are there any high signal abnormalities on T2? An abnormality could be due to oedema or pathology.

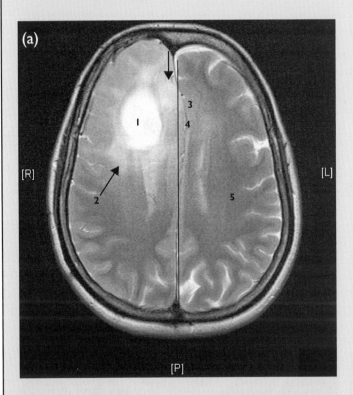

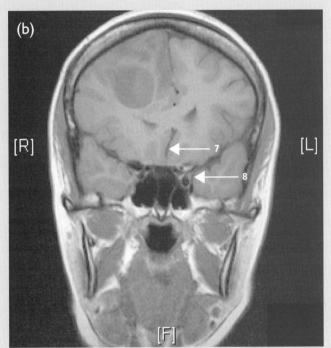

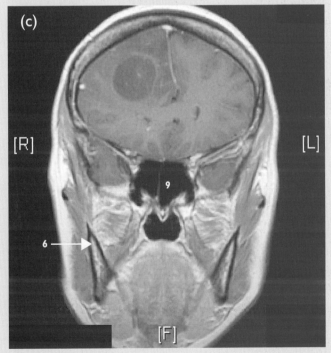

Fig. 1.64 (a) Axial T2W MRI; (b) coronal T1W MRI; (c) coronal post-contrast T1W MRI. The MRI shows a mass (1) with minimal enhancement in the right frontal lobe, with marked surrounding oedema (2). There is a small amount of midline shift (3). the amount of midline shift (4), which was 4 mm. This is usually measured at the level of the foramen of Monro. The differential would include a glioma, primary brain tumour, malignancy or infection. Centrum semiovale (5), ramus mandible (6), third ventricle (7), cavernous sinus (8) and sphenoid sinus (9).

- Look at the ventricles and sulci as if looking at a CT scan. Look for loss of sulci.
- Look at the T1W images for any high signal, usually suggesting methaemoglobin from blood, and at the T1W post-contrast for any abnormal enhancement.
- Check the review area: the orbits, the petrous bones, the chiasma, the cavernous sinus and Meckel's cave, for loss of sulci, the circle of Willis for an abnormality.

Findings

- There is a well-circumscribed high-signal lesion in the right frontal lobe on T2W image. It has some surrounding intermediate signal on T2W which is oedema. It is a solitary lesion.
- On the T1W images the mass is seen in the frontal lobe and shows only minimal enhancement after contrast.
- The mass is displacing the midline to the left and effacing and depressing the right frontal horn of the lateral ventricle.
- The appearance is that of a solid mass in the brain. The differential includes a primary or secondary tumour.

Diagnosis

Primary glioblastoma. Most first fits show no abnormality on a standard MRI, but occasionally a cerebral abnormality is present and the history may reveal recent headache or personality change.

The idealized report reads: There is a minimally enhancing mass in the right frontal lobe with surrounding oedema and some mass effect. There is 4 mm of midline shift. This is a solitary lesion and the most likely diagnosis is a primary glioma or a secondary deposit.

Case 1.2

A patient presents after a fall with vomiting and slight confusion. The patient is taking warfarin. A CT scan of the brain is performed. Using a system approach the brain is reviewed:

- The soft tissues show no scalp swelling.
- The skull on bony windows with a sharp filter applied shows no skull fracture.
- The ventricles appear normal but there is effacement of the posterior sulci in the left frontoparietal region. The sulci do not extend to the skull on the left side.
- Is the abnormality in the brain or outside the brain, i.e. intra-axial or extra-axial?

Findings

- There is a slightly dense extra-axial collection on the left. It is less than 2 weeks' old due to its density.
- Fresh blood is denser than brain on brain windows if less than 2 weeks' old. At 2 weeks the blood becomes isodense and at 4 weeks it becomes hypodense.
- There is some effacement of the sulci on the left, but no midline shift.
- Go through the review areas.
- Fresh blood is high density on CT due to the window used. The Hounsfield unit number of fresh blood is 100 and therefore, because of the narrow window width of 80 HU centred on 35 HU, fresh blood appears hyperdense.

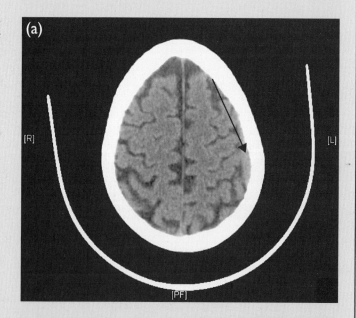

Fig. 1.65 Subdural haemorrhage in patient on warfarin. The three images are more or less taken at the same level towards the vertex of the skull. A checklist is to check that the sulci all run to the calvarium. If the sulci stop then this may indicate an isodense subdural or in this case a subacute haemorrhage (arrow).

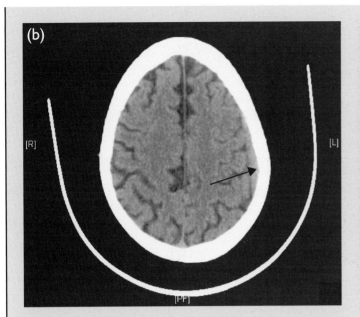

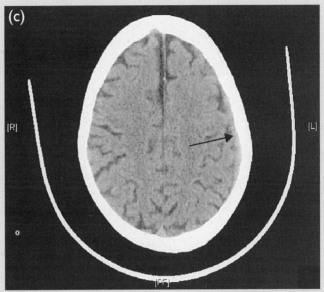

- When looking for extra-axial collections remember that blood becomes isodense to the normal brain at 2 weeks. In order to detect it, the sulci must be assessed. If the sulci are not apparent and if they do not go to the edge of the skull, suspect an isodense subdural.

Diagnosis

Subacute left subdural haemorrhage.

Case 1.3

A patient presents with acute onset of right-sided weakness. The new guidelines for acute stroke indicate that an urgent CT of the brain is required. This should be performed immediately or within an hour, whichever is sooner. A CT scan was performed at 01:00.

Review (Fig. 1.66)

- The scalp and bones are normal.
- The ventricles and sulci are normal.
- Assess for haemorrhage – intra- or extra-axial.
- Assess every sulcus carefully – can all the sulci be traced to the skull? Are any sulci effaced?
- Are there any focal lesions?

Review the images within CVA windows which are centre 40 HU, window width 40 HU for subtle grey/white matter loss of differentiation or low density.
- The history is one of a CVA so look at review areas for a hyperdense vessel around the circle of Willis. The

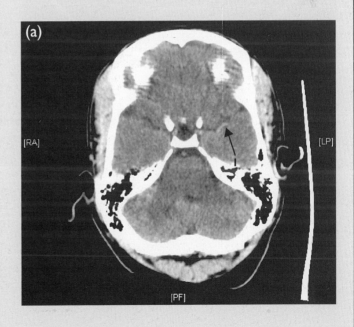

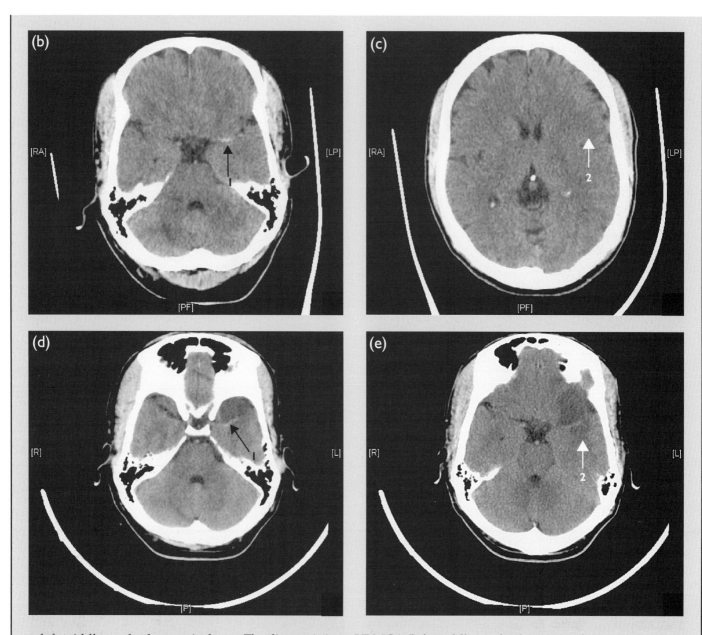

left middle cerebral artery is dense. The diagnosis is an LT MCA (left middle cerebral artery) infarct.

- Thrombolysis is given and the scan is repeated at 16:00 to look for a complication of thrombolysis.
- The repeat CT of the brain shows an evolving infarct with a hyperdense vessel, left MCA and an infarct seen as a wedge-shaped low-density lesion in the left frontotemporal region. The lesion is well demarcated, extends to the cortex and has a wedge shape.

Diagnosis

Left middle cerebral artery infarct.

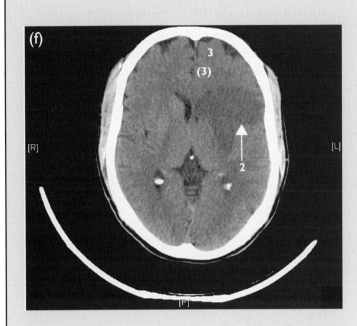

Fig. 1.66 (a–c) Taken at 01:35; (d–f) taken at 16:07. There was 14 hours between the two scans. (a) Image through posterior fossa; (b) suprasellar level; (c) anterior horn level. This show a hyperdense left middle cerebral artery (1). The (2) shows a subtle low-density area. Scan at 16:07, 14 hours later: (d) level of sella; (e) suprasellar fossa; (f) level of anterior horns. (d–f) These images show extensive low density in the left middle cranial fossa, consistent with an infarct (2). (a) This image shows a hyperdense left middle cerebral artery (1). The infarct has surrounding oedema and is effacing the frontal horn on the left (3).

Case 1.4

A patient presents to A&E after collapsing. There is no other history and there are no clinical signs. A CT of the brain is performed. Two images are shown from the skull base region (Fig. 1.67).

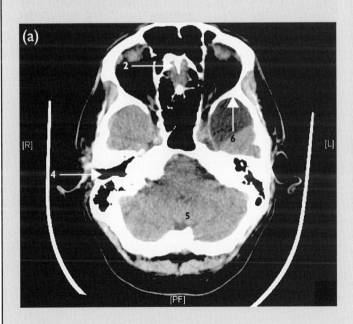

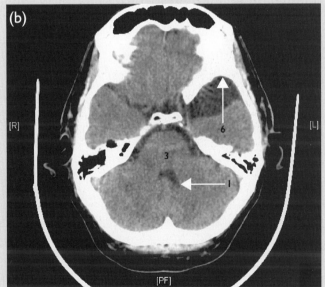

Fig. 1.67 In the left middle cranial fossa, there is a CSF density structure with the appearance of fluid (6). This is a typical site for an arachnoid cyst. There may be associated scalloping of the immediate adjacent bone. Fourth ventricle (1), crista galli (2), pons (3), external auditory canal (4) and cerebellar vermis (5).

Anatomy review: name 1–5 (see Fig. 1.67 for answers)

- Using the systematic review:
  - the scalp and skull are normal.
  - the ventricles are normal
  - sulci: there is abnormality in the left temporal lobe where a well-demarcated fluid density lesion is seen with no mass effect; looking carefully the bone is slightly thinner at this site
  - no high density or haemorrhage is seen.

Diagnosis

The diagnosis is of a left arachnoid cyst. This is an incidental finding and usually of no clinical significance. The lesion is made up of water-density fluid. It is worth putting a cursor on if unsure to check the density of structures and familiarize yourself with the appearance of cysts and water-based abnormalities.

The idealized report reads: The ventricles and sulci appear normal. There is an incidental arachnoid cyst in the left temporal lobe. No haemorrhage or extra-axial collection. No skull fracture. No significant abnormality.

Case 1.5

A female presents after an assault. There is a bruise over her cheek. This is the facial series.

Facial series

There is no fluid in the sinuses and no evidence of a facial fracture. There is an abnormal appearance to the bones. This is due to superimposed density from hair braids mimicking sclerotic metastases.

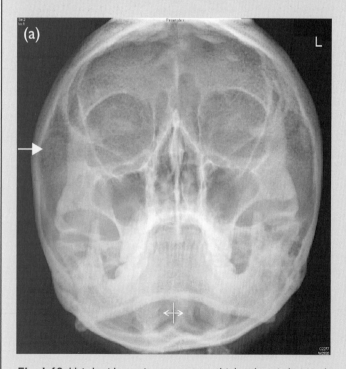
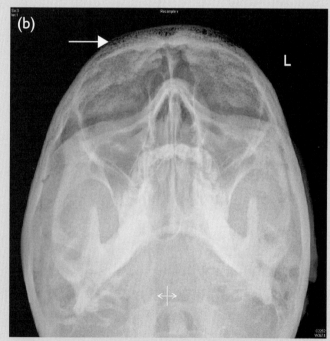

Fig. 1.68 Hair braids causing apparent multiple sclerotic lesions (arrow) over the bones contiguous with hair braids on this facial series.

Case 1.6

An infant presents with fits and delayed milestones. An MRI is requested. MRI is superior in the investigation of congenital and paediatric abnormalities and avoids radiation. Infants may not need a general anaesthetic if recently fed.

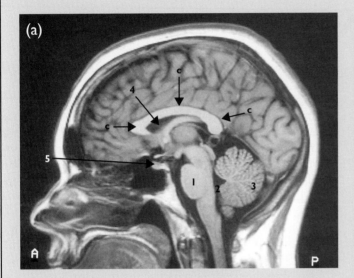

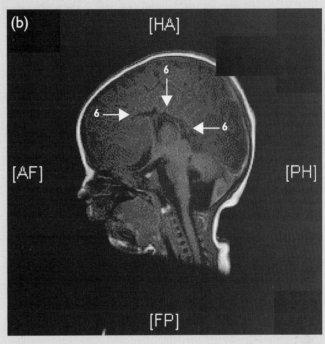

Do anatomy review on Fig. 1.69a first. The corpus callosum normally runs over the roof of the third ventricle. In paediatrics the presence of a normal corpus callosum should be a review area. It may be partially absent. On a coronal image the lateral ventricles are characteristically widely spaced. By comparing with the normal image the abnormality (Fig. 1.69b) becomes more apparent. The third ventricle, which normally lies under the corpus callosum, appears irregular.

Fig. 1.69 (a) Sagittal TIW MRI of the brain showing the normal corpus callosum (c). Pons (1), fourth ventricle (2), cerebellum (3), third ventricle (4) and pituitary gland (5). (b) Sagittal TIW MRI of a child showing absence of the whole corpus callosum (6).

Diagnosis

Absence of corpus callosum.

2 Imaging of the nasopharynx, face and neck

RADIOLOGICAL ANATOMY

Pharynx

The pharynx is divided into the nasopharynx, oropharynx and hypopharynx.

Nasopharynx

- The nasopharynx lies behind the nasal cavity and above the soft palate. Lateral to the nasopharynx is the lateral parapharyngeal fat space, which communicates with the infratemporal fossa. It is important to identify the fat within this slit-like space on CT, as loss of this fat plane may indicate a subtle tumour.
- Posterior to the nasopharynx lie the upper cervical vertebrae and muscles (Fig. 2.1).

- The eustachian tube opens on to the lateral wall of the nasopharynx. A slight bulge can be seen on CT where the tube opens and terminates as a result of the cartilaginous end of the tube; this is called the torus tubarius. Behind this bulge is a pair of recesses called the fossa of Rosenmüller or pharyngeal recess. Asymmetry of the fossa of Rosenmüller may indicate a subtle nasopharyngeal mass. Within the nasopharynx lies lymphoid tissue called the adenoids, which may be hypertrophied in young children (Fig. 2.2).
- Lateral to the nasopharynx lies the infratemporal space, anteriorly lies the pterygoid plate.
- A small space is seen between the pterygoid plate and the posterior wall of the maxillary antrum called the pterygomaxillary fissure. The fissure communicates through the inferior orbital fissure with the orbit and through the foramen rotundum with the middle cranial fossa, and

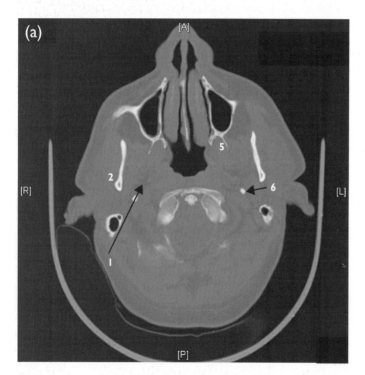
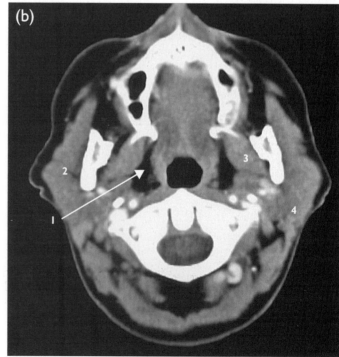

Fig. 2.1 (a) Axial CT of the nasopharynx, bony windows. (b) Axial CT of the nasopharynx, soft-tissue windows. The lateral pharyngeal fat space lies on either side of the nasopharynx (1). Masseter muscle (2), lateral pterygoid muscle (3), parotid gland related to the mandible (4), pterygoid plates (5) and styloid process (6).

laterally with the infratemporal fossa. It is therefore easy for cancer to spread into this space and then into the orbit and the brain (Fig. 2.3).

- Lateral to the parapharyngeal fat space are the parotid glands. The parotid glands are closely related to the angle of the mandible and are low density on CT due to their serous nature.

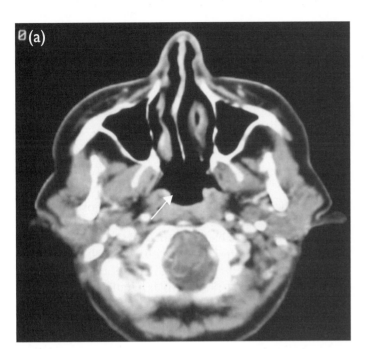

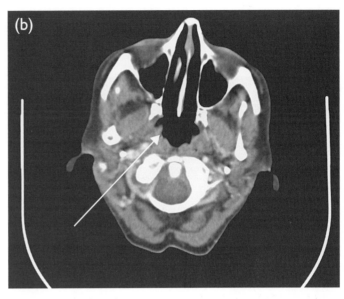

Fig. 2.2 Axial CT of the nasopharynx in two different patients: fossa of Rosenmüller, which is the recess behind the opening of the eustachian tube (arrow). Asymmetry of the fossa of Rosenmüller may indicate subtle malignancy.

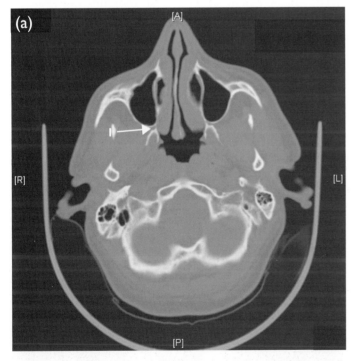

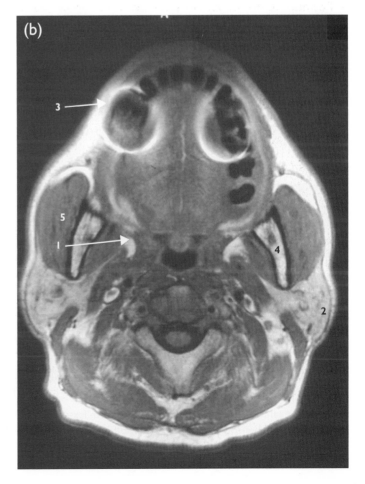

Fig. 2.3 (a) Axial CT of the nasopharynx: the pterygomaxillary fissure is an important communication with the brain through the foramen rotundum and orbit through the inferior orbital fissure (1). This is seen on the CT scan and (b) the T1-weighted MR image. The parotid gland (2), metallic artefact from dental amalgam (3), mandible (4) and masseter muscle (5).

Oropharynx

The nasopharynx becomes the oropharynx at the lower part of the soft palete down to the epiglottis. The palatine tonsils lie in the oropharnyx. Between the posterior third of the tongue and the epiglottis is the medial epiglottic fold and two recesses, one on each side of the fold, called the valleculae (Fig. 2.4).

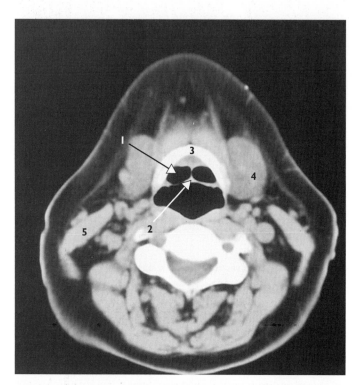

Fig. 2.4 Axial CT at level C3 with contrast: the valleculae (1) are seen anterior to the epiglottis (2). Hyoid bone is a U shape (3); the submandibular glands seen either side of the hyoid bone (4) and sternocleiodomastoid muscle (5).

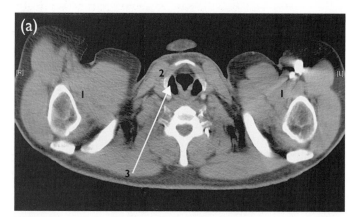

Fig. 2.5 (a) CT at axial level of hyoid bone C3 with arms up. (b) different patient same level with arms down. The piriform fossae are seen deep to the hyoid bone formed by the aryepiglottic fold (3). The arms are seen elevated (1) and sternomastoid muscle (2).

Hypopharynx

- Below the oropharnyx lies the hypopharynx, which lies behind the larynx itself.
- This extends from the level of the epiglottis to the level of C6, from where it continues inferiorly as the oesophagus.
- Two deep recesses are seen on either side of the laryngeal inlet called the piriform fossae. Food and drink pass from the back of the tongue through the piriform fossae into the oesophagus, avoiding the larynx.
- Normally there can be marked asymmetry between the piriform fossae (Fig. 2.5).

The larynx

- Behind the tongue lies the epiglottis and just in front of this are the valleculae.
- Attached between the epiglottis and the arytenoid cartilages is a membrane called the quadrangular membrane or aryepiglottic fold. This has a free inferior margin called the false vocal folds or vestibular ligaments (Fig. 2.6).
- The aryepiglottic folds form the boundary of the piriform fossae.
- The false vocal folds lie above the true vocal folds. The chamber in between the true and the false folds is called the vestibule of the larynx.
- The true folds attach to the arytenoid cartilages.
- The management of laryngeal tumours depends on whether the tumour involves the true vocal folds, the ventricle, or the subglottic or supraglottic region.
- The corniculate and cuneiform cartilages lie on top of the arytenoid cartilages and are attached to the aryepiglottic folds.

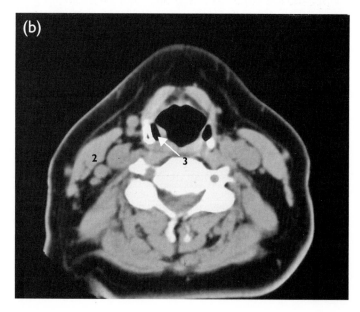

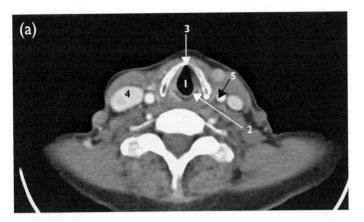 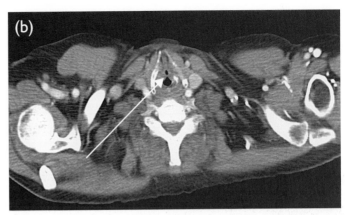

Fig. 2.6 Axial CT of the larynx at the level of the thyroid cartilage: (1) the true larynx is seen. The CT images show (a) the vocal folds abducted and (b) the vocal folds adducted. The cricoid cartilage lies posterior to the vocal folds (2), the anterior commissure is the small anterior soft tissue adjoining the folds (3), which should measure less than 2 mm, internal jugular vein (4) and common carotid artery (5).

Anatomy of the parotid gland

- The parotid gland has a deep lobe and a superficial lobe. which are closely related to the angle of the mandible.
- Three structures run through the parotid glands which are, from superficial to deep: the facial nerve, the retromandibular vein, and the terminal division of the external carotid artery into the superficial temporal artery and the maxillary artery.
- The parotids are the largest salivary glands and predominantly serous.
- The parotid gland drains via Stensen's duct, opening opposite the upper second molar tooth (Fig. 2.7).
- The parotid gland has an accessory duct that lies above the main duct. The duct runs along the masseter muscle and pierces the buccinator muscle before opening.
- Deep to the parotid gland is the lateral parapharyngeal fat space.
- The stylomandibular ligament separates the parotid and submandibular glands.

Submandibular gland

- The submandibular gland is paired and closely related to the mylohyoid muscle and hyoid bone.
- The gland has a large superficial and a small deep part, which communicate around the posterior border of the mylohyoid muscle.
- The submandibular gland drains via Wharton's duct, which opens lateral to the frenulum at the base of the tongue (Fig. 2.8).

- The submandibular gland is related to the facial artery and the lingual and hypoglossal nerves.
- The parotid gland is more serous than the submandibular gland which is mixed serous and mucous acini and hence denser on CT.
- The sublingual gland is the smallest of the three salivary glands lying under the floor of the mouth.

The infratemporal fossa

- Lies between the skull base, pharynx and ramus of the mandible.
- The space communicates with the temporal region deep to the zygomatic arch.
- The medial and lateral pterygoids, mandibular nerve, otic ganglion, chorda tympani, maxillary artery and pterygoid venous plexus lie in the space.

The temporomandibular joint (TMJ)

- The TMJ is the joint between the condylar process of the mandible and the articular tubercle and mandibular fossa of the temporal bone.
- There is a fibrocartilaginous disc in the joint dividing it into upper and lower cavities. The disc moves forwards and backwards with protraction and retraction of the mandible.
- The cavities have a synovial lining (Fig. 2.9).

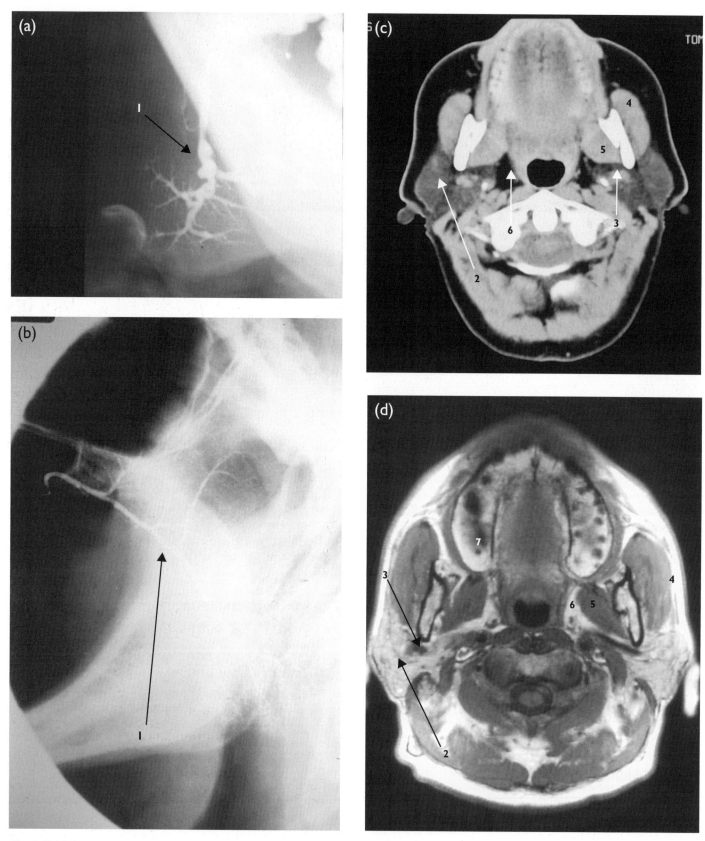

Fig. 2.7 (a) Parotid sialogram, frontal or AP view, with Stensen's duct (1); (b) lateral view with Stensen's duct marked (1). (c) Axial CT of the parotids shows the serous low-density parotid gland related to the ramus of the mandible (2). The terminal division of the external common carotid artery into superficial temple and maxillary vessels is seen within the deep part of the parotid gland (3). Masseter (4), lateral pterygoid muscle (5) and lateral pharyngeal fat space (6). (d) MRI of the parotid glands, alveolar ridge of the maxilla (7).

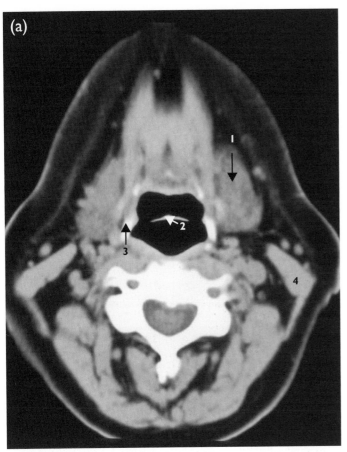

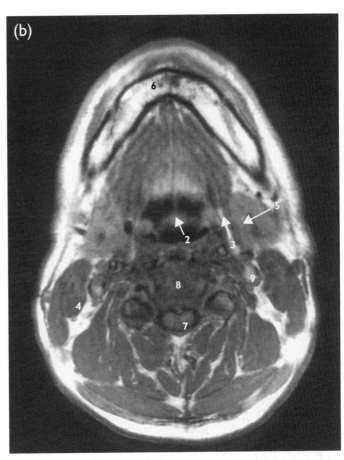

Fig. 2.8 (a) Axial CT – submandibular glands are seen on either side of the hyoid bone (1): epiglottis (2); hyoid bone (3); sternocleidomastoid (4). (b) Axial MRI of the submandibular glands. The submandibular glands are shown (5): epiglottis (2), hyoid bone (3), sternocleidomastoid (4), mandible (6), theca (7), cervical vertebral body (8) and jugular vein (9).

The thyroid gland

- The thyroid gland consists of two lateral lobes joined by a midline isthmus. It lies anterior and lateral to the trachea. The lobes may be asymmetrical with the right being larger than the left (Fig. 2.10).
- In 10–40% of individuals a third lobe or pyramidal lobe extends upward close to the midline.
- The isthmus lies anterior to the second to fourth tracheal rings at the level of C6.
- Posterolaterally lies the carotid sheath containing the carotid artery and the internal jugular vein.
- The strap muscles of the neck lie anterior to the thyroid gland.
- The parathyroid glands are closely related to the deep surface and may lie within the capsule itself.
- The thyroid gland is supplied by the superior thyroid artery, the first branch of the external carotid artery and the inferior thyroid artery from the thyrocervical trunk, a branch of the subclavian artery. Three per cent of individuals may have a third artery, the thyroidia ima, arising from the brachial cephalic artery.

The muscles of mastication

- Temporalis muscle.
- Masseter muscle.
- The medial and lateral pterygoid muscles (Fig. 2.11)
- Supplied by the mandibular division of the trigeminal nerve.
- Not the buccinator muscle, which is supplied by VIII as a muscle of facial expression.

The lacrimal apparatus

- This consists of the large lacrimal glands, which lie in the superolateral part of the orbit and produce tears, lacrimal canaliculi, lacrimal sac and nasolacrimal duct. The tears run over the conjunctiva and drain into the puncta and then into the lacrimal sac. The sac then drains into the nasolacrimal duct (Fig. 2. 12).
- The nasolacrimal duct extends from the lacrimal sac through a bony canal to the inferior meatus. The narrowings are:
  - orbicularis oculi
  - the valves of Hasner, Krause and Taillefer.
- The duct opens into the inferior meatus.

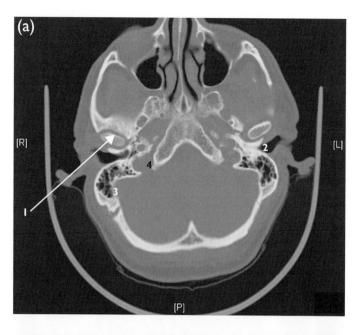

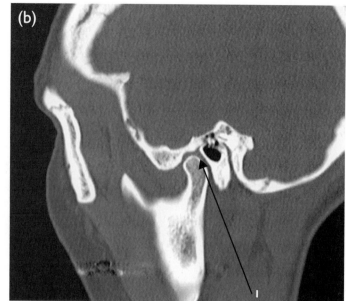

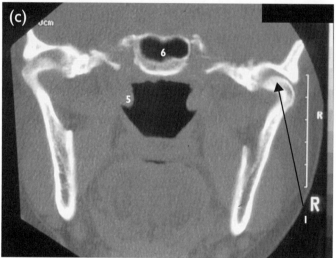

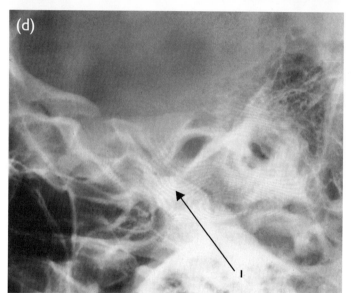

Fig. 2.9 The condylar process of the mandible (1) forms the temporomandibular joint (TMJ) (arrow). (a) Axial CT; (b) sagittal CT; (c) coronal CT; (e,f) plain films of the TMJ with the mouth open and closed. The condylar process of the mandible is seen in the mandibular fossa of the temporal bone (1). External auditory canal (2), mastoid air cells (3), jugular foramen (4), torus tubarius (5) and sphenoid sinus (6).

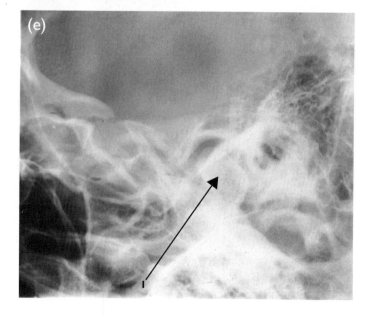

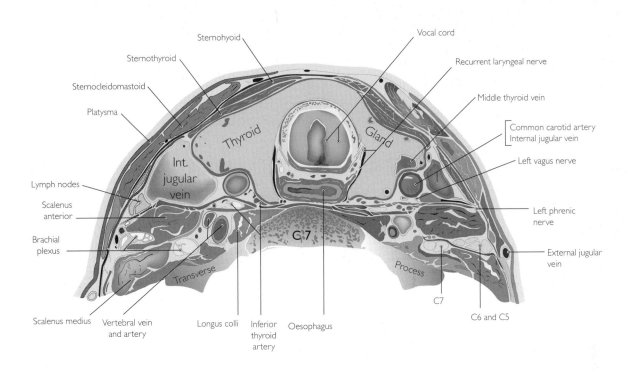

Fig. 2.10 Diagram of the thyroid gland.

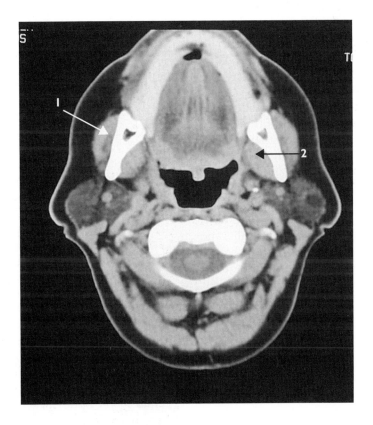

Fig. 2.11 CT: axial CT shows the masseter (1); lateral pterygoid (2).

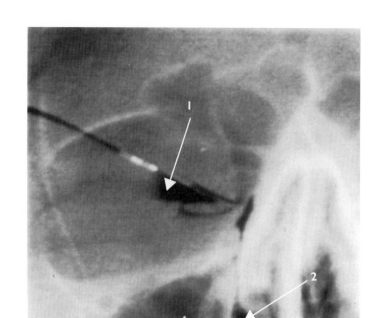

Fig. 2.12 Dacrocystogram: contrast filling the eyelid (1), draining via the lacrimal sac into the nasolacrimal duct (2) and the inferior meatus (3).

The orbits

- The bony orbit is a pyramid-shaped cavity made up of the greater and lesser wings of sphenoid. The lamina papyracea or lacrimal bone, maxilla and ethmoid form the medial border of the orbit and the lateral border is formed by the zygomatic bone anteriorly and the greater wing of sphenoid posterolaterally. Superiorly is the frontal bone.
- The orbit contains the globe and its muscles, the optic nerve, the lacrimal gland, which lies superolaterally, and fat (Fig. 2.13).
- The globe is spherical and has three layers: outermost is the tough sclera and the transparent cornea anteriorly; the middle layer is the choroid posteriorly and the ciliary body and iris anteriorly; innermost is the retina and optic disc.
- The globe is divided into two segments by the lens. Posterior to the lens is the posterior segment containing vitreous humour. Anterior to the lens are two chambers separated by the cornea that interconnect through the pupil. The anterior segment contains aqueous humour.
- The superior, inferior, medial and lateral rectus muscles converge within the orbit. Abnormalities occurring within the ring of muscles are described as being 'intraconal' and those outside the muscular ring as 'extraconal'. These are important anatomical distinctions to make helping in the differential pathology. The rectus muscles can become hypertrophied in Graves' disease.
- The optic nerve is cranial nerve II and enters the orbit through the optic foramen accompanied by the ophthalmic artery.
- The superior ophthalmic vein, which is a sigmoid shape entering the superior aspect of the orbit, may be confused with the optic nerve (Fig. 2.14, onaxid images).
- The optic nerves receive information from both the temporal and nasal fields with some crossover of information occurring posteriorly within the field pathways, which gives us stereotactic vision. The optic nerve has a sleeve of meninges and is surrounded by cerebrospinal fluid (CSF). It is about 4 mm in diameter.
- The optic chiasma is found above the pituitary fossa. The optic nerves run posteriorly through the optic nerve foramina to join, forming the optic chiasma. From the chiasma the optic tracts run posteriorly to lateral geniculate body and then the occipital lobe. The optic nerves, chiasma and tracts are well seen on MRI on T1- and T2-weighted imaging, particularly in the coronal plane.

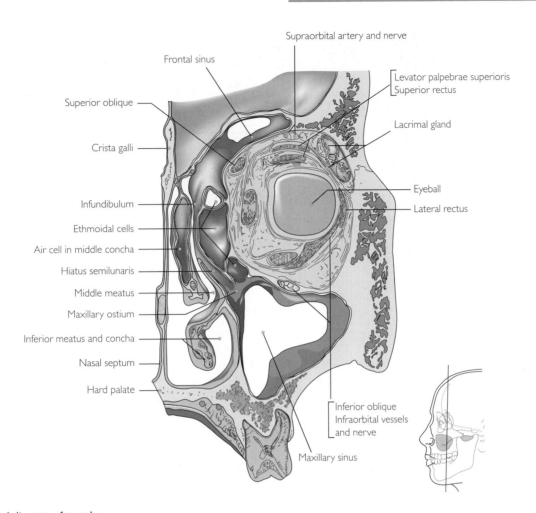

Supraorbital artery and nerve

Frontal sinus

Superior oblique

Crista galli

Levator palpebrae superioris
Superior rectus

Lacrimal gland

Infundibulum

Ethmoidal cells

Air cell in middle concha

Hiatus semilunaris

Middle meatus

Maxillary ostium

Inferior meatus and concha

Nasal septum

Hard palate

Eyeball

Lateral rectus

Inferior oblique
Infraorbital vessels
and nerve

Maxillary sinus

Fig. 2.13 Orbital diagram of muscles.

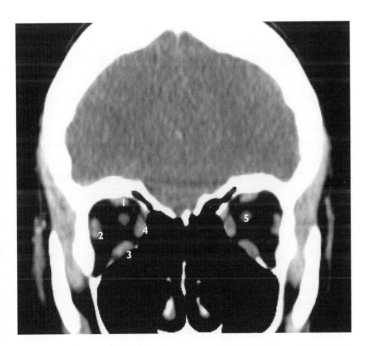

Fig. 2.14 CT of the orbit. Superior rectus (1), lateral rectus (2), inferior rectus (3), medial rectus (4), optic nerve (5) and superior ophthalmic vein.

The optic chiasma may be compressed by a pituitary mass or an abnormality within the sella. In addition demyelination may affect the optic nerves and chiasma (Fig. 2.15).

The superior orbital fissure (Fig. 2.16)

- Lies between the greater and lesser wings of the sphenoid bone.
- Communicates with the middle cranial fossa and the cavernous sinus via the superior and inferior ophthalmic veins.
- The third, fourth, sixth and lacrimal, frontal and nasociliary branches of the ophthalmic division of the trigeminal nerve pass through the fissure and the ophthalmic veins.
- A mnemonic to remember the nerves is 'Luscious French Toads Sit Naughtily In Anticipation' (Lacrimal, Frontal, Trochlea, Superior division of III, Nasociliary, Inferior division of III, Abducens).

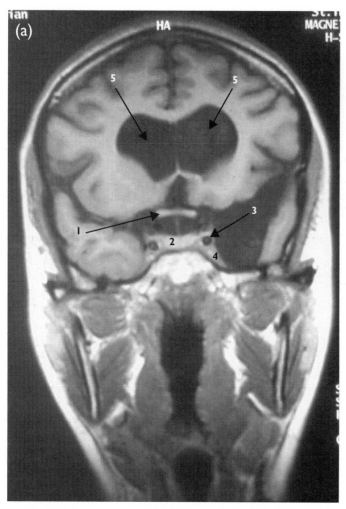

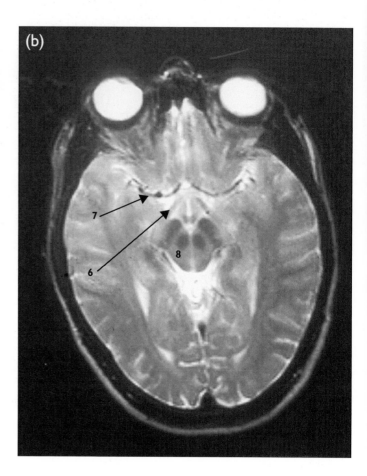

Fig. 2.15 (a) Coronal T1-weighted MRI, optic chiasma (1). Pituitary gland (2), internal carotid artery signal void (3), cavernous sinus (4) and frontal horn of lateral ventricles (5). (b) Axial T2-weighted MR image. The optic tracts are well seen (6). The middle cerebral artery (7) and midbrain (8).

The nose and paranasal sinuses (Fig. 2.17)

- The nasal septum usually lies within the midline. Deviations may lead to obstruction of sinus drainage or spurs that are bony projections from the septum.
- There are three pairs of bony conchae also called turbinates when including the mucosa in the nasal cavity: the superior, middle and inferior. The middle turbinates may be excessively pneumatized, called the concha bullosa. This may obstruct the ostiomeatal complex.
- The paranasal sinuses drain via the ethmoid infundibulum, a key anatomical area between the uncinate process and the bulla ethmoidalis. The bulla ethmoidalis is the air cell adjacent to the opening into the maxillary antrum, which can be excessively large leading to obstruction. This area and the ostia of the frontal sinuses form the ostiomeatal complexes.
- There are paired frontal sinuses in the frontal bone that appear at age 2 years and enlarge until puberty.

- The ethmoid sinuses are grouped into anterior, middle and posterior. The lateral wall of the ethmoid sinuses is formed by a very thin plate of bone, which is easily fractured and borders the orbit, called the lamina papyracea.
- The sphenoid sinuses are paired and lie within the sphenoid bone below the pituitary fossa. They appear at age 3 years, enlarging considerably in adolescence.
- The maxillary sinus is lateral to the nasal cavity. In the roof is the inferior orbital foramen which communicates with the orbit and also the foramen rotundum, carrying the maxillary division of the trigeminal nerve.
- The lateral wall of the antra may show a defect due to the vessels.
- Openings of the sinuses:
  - the sphenoid sinus opens into the sphenoethmoidal recess
  - the posterior ethmoid air cells open into the superior meatus.

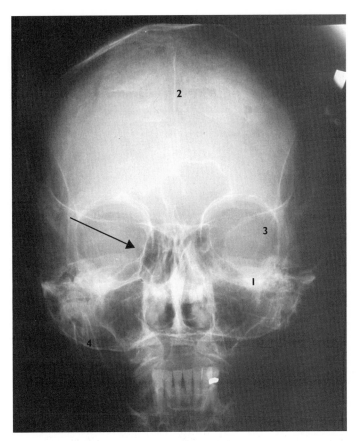

Fig. 2.16 A PA20 skull radiograph shows the superior orbital fissure (black arrow). Petrous apex (1), calcification of falx (2), innominate line (3) and basiocciput (4).

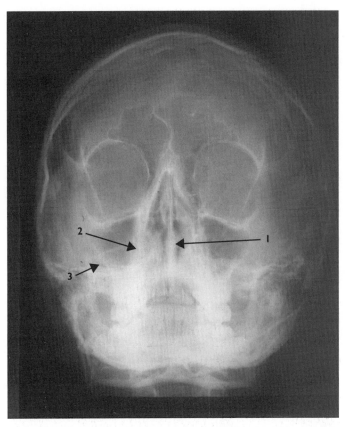

Fig. 2.17 Occipitomental (OM) view shows the paranasal sinuses. The petrous apex (2) should be projected at the floor of the maxillary antra (3) in order to visualise the sinuses correctly. Inferior orbital foramen (1).

– the frontal sinuses, middle and anterior ethmoid air cells and the maxillary antra open into the middle meatus (Fig. 2.18).
- The nasolacrimal duct opens into the inferior meatus.
- The olfactory nerve enters the nose through the cribriform plate.

The ear

The ear is divided into external ear, the middle-ear cavity and the inner ear.

External ear

- The tympanic membrane divides the external ear and middle ear. The membrane attaches superiorly to a bony spur called the scutum (Fig. 2.19). This can be seen on coronal CT and should be sharp and pointed. It can be eroded in cholesteatoma.
- The external ear is more caudad than the inner and middle ear and internal auditory canal. The external auditory canal is therefore seen on more inferior sections than the middle and inner ear.
- The TMJ lies anterior to the external auditory canal.

- The external canal is about 3 cm long, being half bony and half cartilaginous.
- The drum attaches at an oblique angle.

Middle ear

- The middle ear is a cube-shaped chamber lying between the drum and the inner ear.
- The tympanic membrane marks the opening of the middle ear. Part of the middle-ear chamber extends above the tympanic membrane and is called the epitympanic recess. The incudomalleolar complex lies in the recess (Fig. 2.20).
- The recess narrows posteriorly and then widens to open into the mastoid air cells. This has an hour-glass shape and is called the aditus or opening to the mastoid air cells.
- The middle-ear cavity contains the ossicular chain of incus, malleus and stapes.
- The malleus articulates with the tympanic membrane and the incus.
- The incudomalleolar complex sits in the epitympanic recess.
- The stapes is attached to the oval window by a ligament and the incus at its other end.

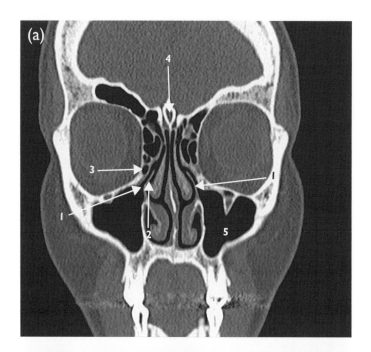

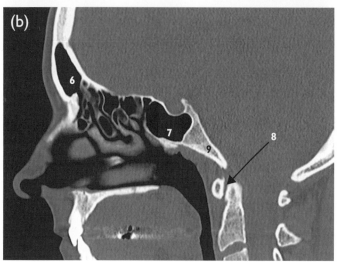

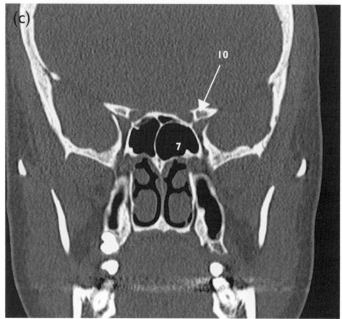

Fig. 2.18 CT of the paranasal sinuses. (a) Coronal CT: the ostiomeatal complex is seen (1) formed between the infundibulum (2) and the bulla ethmoidalis (3); crista galli (4) and maxillary antra (5). (b) Sagittal CT: frontal sinus (6), sphenoid sinus (7), atlantoaxial joint (8) and clivus (9). (c) Coronal CT: anterior clinoid processes (10) and sphenoid sinus (7).

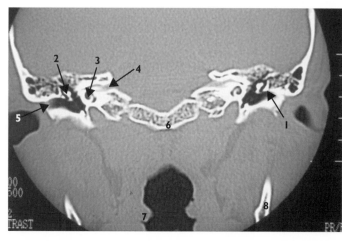

Fig. 2.19 Coronal CT of petrous bone. The scutum is seen bilaterally, which should be sharp and pointed (1). Incudomalleolar complex (2), cochlea (3), internal auditory canal (4), external auditory canal (5), clivus (6), torus tubarius (7) and mandible (8).

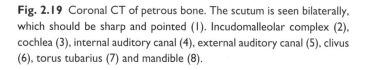

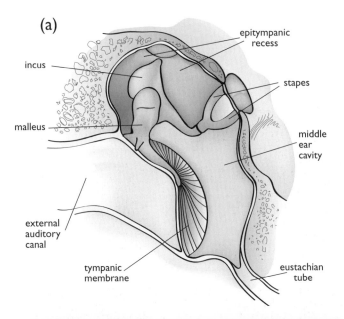

(a)

incus

malleus

external
auditory
canal

tympanic
membrane

epitympanic
recess

stapes

middle
ear
cavity

eustachian
tube

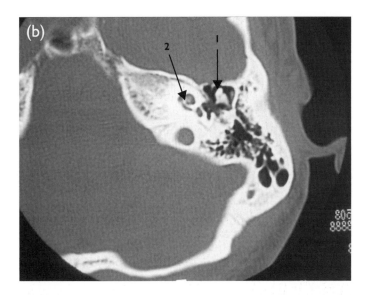

(b)

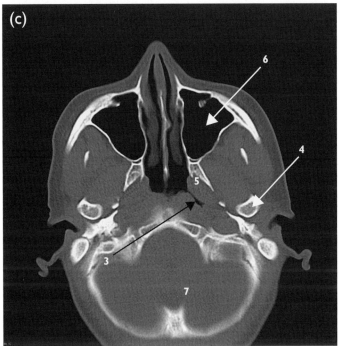

(c)

Fig. 2.20 (a) Diagram of the middle ear: (b) Axial CT of middle ear. The incudomalleolar complex is seen in the epitympanic recess (1). Cochlea (2). (c) Axial CT shows the opening of the eustachian tube in the nasopharynx (3). Condylar process of mandible (4), pterygoid plates (5), maxillary antra (6) and posterior fossa (7).

- The eustachian tube (Fig. 2.20c) arises from the anterior wall of the middle ear and runs inferiorly and medially to the nasopharynx.
- The roof of the middle-ear cavity and mastoid air cells is called the tegmen tympani and is commonly very thin; pathology in the middle ear can erode into the cranium through this thin bone.
- A branch of the facial nerve, the chorda tympani, runs around the malleus through the middle ear.
- The space in the epitympanic recess which is invisible to the otoscope lies deep to the ossicular chain and is called Prussak's space.

Inner ear

- The inner ear comprises the cochlea, vestibule and semi-circular canals, which contain endolymph. These are a series of connecting tubes (Fig. 2.21).
- The cochlea lies anteriorly medially and inferiorly to the vestibule. The cochlea normally has two and a half turns.
- The internal auditory canal lies in the petrous bone. Cranial nerves VII and VIII run in the canal.
- Nerve VII runs through the IAM (internal auditory meatus) and posterior to the cochlea, to the geniculate ganglion; it then makes a sharp bend at the genu, runs

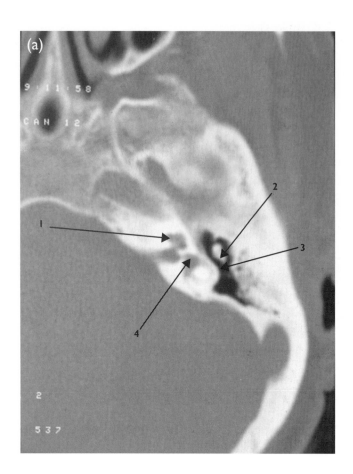

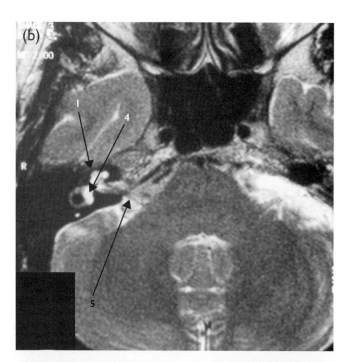

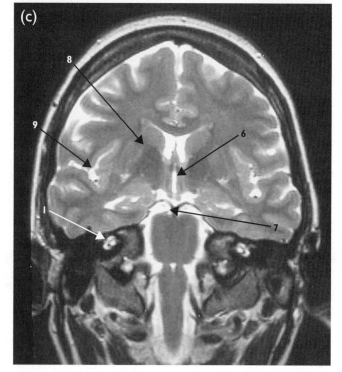

Fig. 2.21 Axial and coronal petrous bone. (a) Axial CT shows the basal turn of the cochlea (1). The incudomalleolar complex in the epitympanic recess (2); aditus or opening to the mastoid air cells (3); vestibule with horizontal semicircular canal (4). (b) Axial T2-weighted MRI: basal turn of cochlea (1). Nerves VII and VIII in internal auditory canal (5). (c) Coronal T2-weighted MRI: cochlea (1), third ventricle (6), basilar artery (7), internal capsule (8) and insula (9). (d) Diagram of the inner and middle ear.

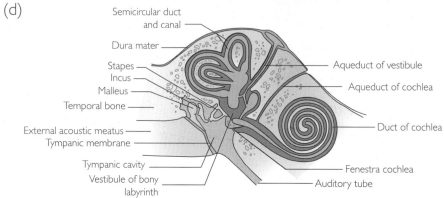

Semicircular duct and canal

Dura mater

Stapes

Incus

Malleus

Temporal bone

External acoustic meatus

Tympanic membrane

Tympanic cavity

Vestibule of bony labyrinth

Aqueduct of vestibule

Aqueduct of cochlea

Duct of cochlea

Fenestra cochlea

Auditory tube

posteriorly, descends in the posterior wall and exits through the stylomastoid foramen.

- The geniculate ganglion, i.e. the nerve VII ganglion, lies on the medial wall of the epitympanic recess and can be eroded by cholesteatoma (Fig. 2.22).
- The three semicircular canals can be seen opening into the vestibule.
- The internal carotid artery and the jugular vein run close to the middle-ear cavity (Fig. 2.23).
- The inner ear has a different embryological development from the middle and external ear.

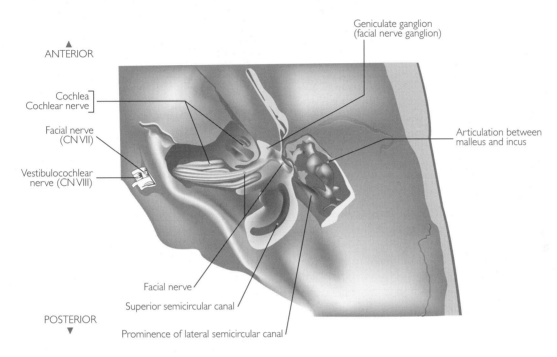

Fig. 2.22 Diagram of the geniculate ganglion.

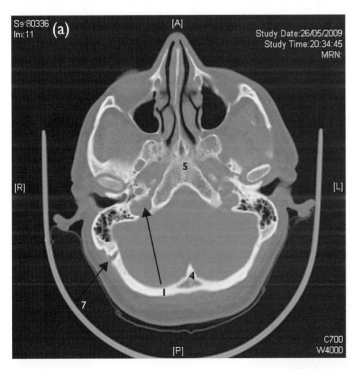 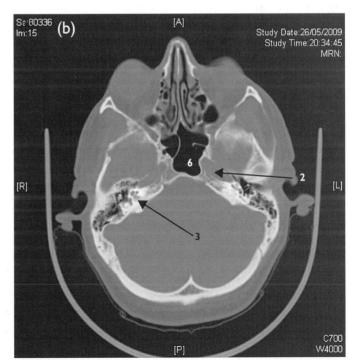

Fig. 2.23 Axial CT: (a) jugular foramen (1). (b) Foramen lacerum for the internal carotid artery (2). Internal auditory canal (3), internal occipital protuberance (4), clivus (5), sphenoid sinus (6) and lambdoid suture (7).

IMAGING

Imaging of the neck

CT and MRI of the neck

Indication
MRI shows similar anatomy to CT; the bony structures are, however, less apparent. Head and neck cancers, lymphadenopathy and thyroid masses are among the many indications.

Technique
Images with MR are usually taken in the axial and coronal planes, with a mixture of T2-weighted, T1-weighted and STIR (short tau, inversion recovery) images. CT images are taken axially with multiplanar reformatting.

Findings

Landmarks in the neck
- The vallecullae and epiglottis lie at the tongue base with the typical appearance of two small crescents with a midline fold (Fig. 2.24).
- At C3 the hyoid bone is a U shape. The submandibular glands are seen on either side of the hyoid bone. The carotid artery divides into external and internal carotids at the C3 level. There can be marked asymmetry in the jugular veins, with one appearing much larger as a normal finding (Fig. 2.25).
- At C4 is the V-shaped thyroid cartilage. At C4 lie the true vocal folds (Fig. 2.26).
- The true vocal folds have a boat or triangular shape (Fig. 2.27). Anterior to the true vocal folds is the anterior com-

missure. This should not measure more than 2 mm in thickness. It is important to assess the anterior commissure for spread of cancer. A small amount of piriform fossae may be left at this level. The strap muscles lie anterior to the thyroid cartilage.
- Below the true vocal folds is the subglottic region which has an oval shape (Fig. 2.28). The airway assumes an oval shape in the subglottic region. The management of subglottic carcinoma is different to glottic carcinoma.
- At C6 there is a signet-ring shape due to the cricoid cartilage (Fig. 2.29). The cricoid is broader posteriorly.
- The arytenoid cartilages lie above the cricoid and the true vocal folds attach to them.
- At C6 the trachea and the oesophagus start and the vertebral arteries enter the foramen transversarium.
- The trachea is horse-shoe shaped (Fig. 2.30). When a horse-shoe shape is seen the airway has become the trachea. The thyroid gland is closely related to the trachea and lies anteriorly. The carotid artery and jugular vein lie lateral to this.
- The scalene muscles are seen posterior to the trachea arising from the spine. The brachial plexus emerges between the scalene muscles.
- Dental amalgam artefact causes a double-ring shadow on MRI and streak artefact on CT (Fig. 2.31).

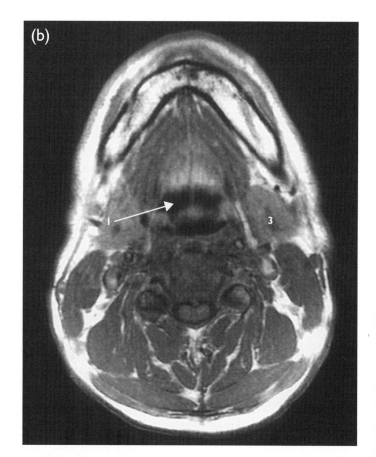

Fig. 2.24 Axial CT and MRI of the valleculae (1): epiglottis (2), submandibular glands (3), hyoid bone (4) and sternomastoid muscle (5).

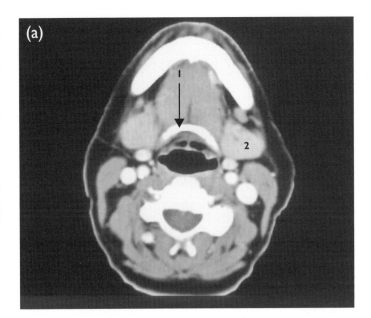

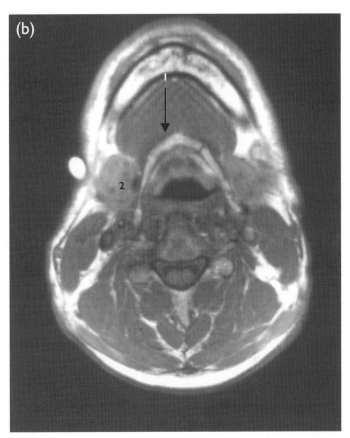

Fig. 2.25 (a) Axial CT of the C3 hyoid bone (1). This is a U-shaped structure which helps identify it. The submandibular glands (2) are seen on either side of the hyoid bone. (b) Axial MR of the hyoid bone. Hyoid (1), submandibular gland (2).

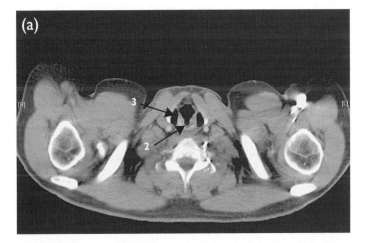

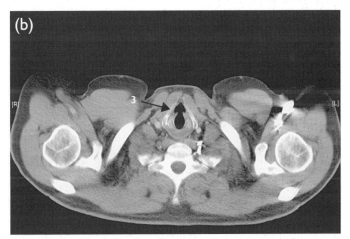

Fig. 2.26 Four examples of axial CT all showing the slightly different appearance at the level (1) of the V-shaped thyroid cartilage of the true vocal folds. Cricoid cartilage (2) can be seen posteriorly, piriform fossa (3). (a) Level of the thyroid cartilage, (b) level of the true cords, (c) level of the true cords and (d) further level of the true cords.

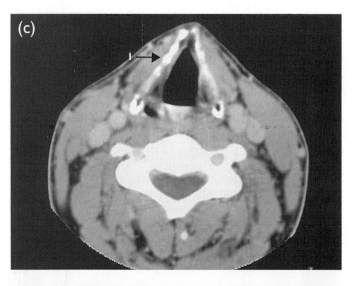

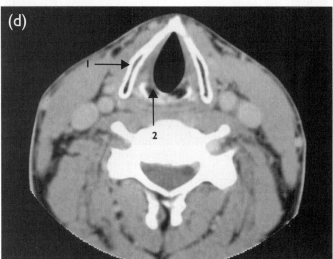

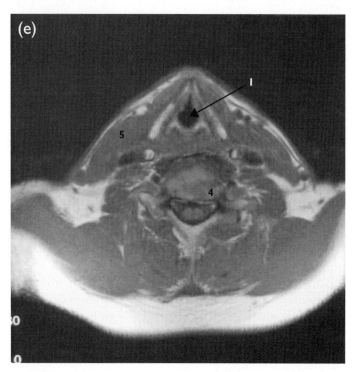

Fig. 2.26e Axial T1-weighted MRI. Thyroid cartilage again seen at the level of the true vocal folds (3). Vertebral body (4) and sternomastoid (5).

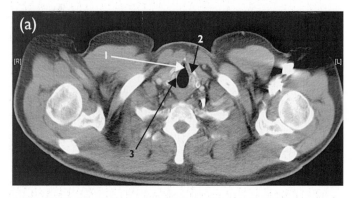

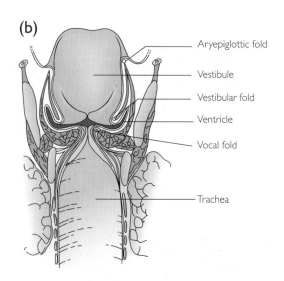

Fig. 2.27 (a) CT of the larynx; (b) diagram of the larynx. The true vocal folds attach to the arytenoid cartilages posteriorly with the anterior commissure (1) anteriorly. The true vocal folds have a characteristic boat shape. The anterior commissure should not measure more than 2 mm thick. Thyroid cartilage (2) and cricoid cartilage (3).

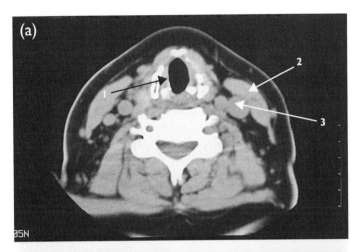

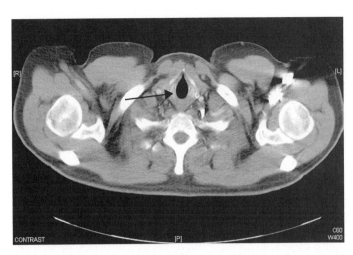

Fig. 2.29 CT of the true vocal folds at the level of the cricoid cartilage C6, which is shaped like a reverse signet ring seen at the level of the larynx (black arrow).

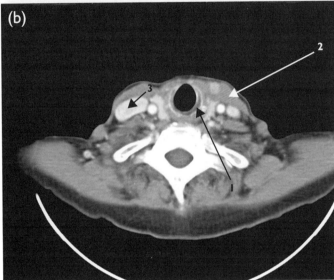

Fig. 2.28 (a,b) Two examples in different patients showing CT of axial subglottic region (1), which has a characteristic oval shape seen at the level of the cricoid cartilage. Sternomastoid muscle (2) and internal jugular vein (3).

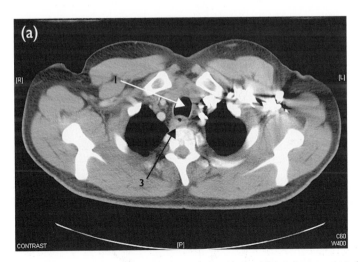

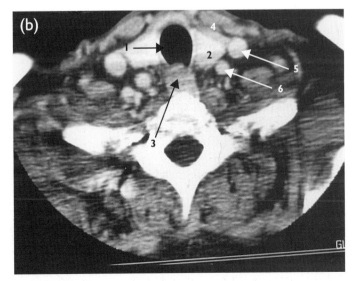

Fig. 2.30 (a,b) Two patients showing the trachea with its characteristic horseshoe shape (1). The thyroid gland is related to the tracheal cartilages (2). Oesophagus (3), strap muscles of the neck (4), internal jugular vein (5) and common carotid artery (6).

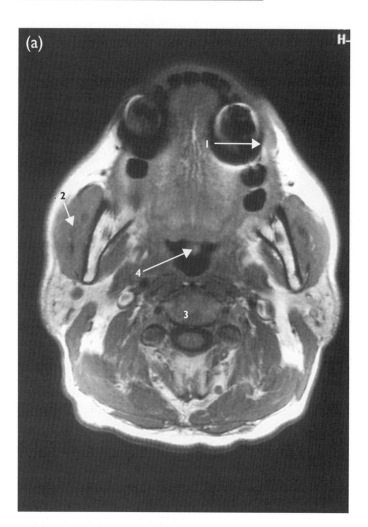

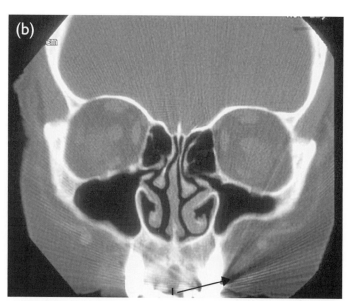

Fig. 2.31 Dental amalgam causes a characteristic black-and-white ring artefact on MRI. (a) T1-weighted MRI. (b) Coronal CT with dental amalgam artefact (1). Masseter (2), vertebral body (3) and uvula (4).

Imaging the salivary glands

CT, MRI and ultrasound of the salivary glands

Indications

Lesions of the gland parenchyma are best shown with cross-sectional imaging using CT/MRI/ultrasound. Ultrasound can detect most lesions in the salivary glands, but cannot see the deeper structures and relations.

Technique

Linear-array high-resolution probes are used for ultrasound. CT and MRI are useful for assessing deeper structures and the remaining neck and relations.

Findings (Fig. 2.32)

* Ultrasound may not adequately visualize the deep lobe of the parotid gland. The submandibular glands are well seen with ultrasound.
* The parotid glands are normally homogeneous on CT and fine ducts can be seen in the gland, as well as the facial nerve in 30% of individuals. The retromandibular vein and external carotid artery can normally be seen in the parotid on ultrasound. Small nodes can normally be seen in the parotid.

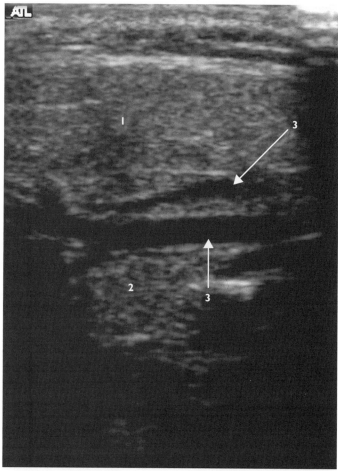

Fig. 2.32 Ultrasound of the paroid gland. Superficial lobe (1), deep lobe (2), paroid ducts (3).

Sialography

Indications
Imaging of the salivary ducts, i.e. Wharton's (Fig. 2.33) and Stensen's ducts: strictures, calculi, sialectasis.

Technique
- A plain preliminary film should be taken to look for calculi before contrast injection.
- A 30-gauge fine catheter is used such as a Rabinoff. Contraindications would be infection or allergy to contrast or sialadenitis.
- Local anaesthetic is used.
- A sialogue is given to stimulate salivation before catheter insertion. A vitamin C tablet may be adequate.
- Initially 0.5 ml of contrast is used with a maximum of 2 ml.
- The patient is instructed to raise the arm if the procedure becomes painful.

Findings
- The parotid gland ducts are best seen on an anteroposterior (AP) projection and Stensen's duct is well seen on a lateral view. The submandibular gland duct system may be seen on the lateral projection. Ducts of the sublingual gland are not amenable to canalization.
- Delayed films are taken to look for sialectasis; continued presence of contrast in the ducts at 10 min indicates obstruction.

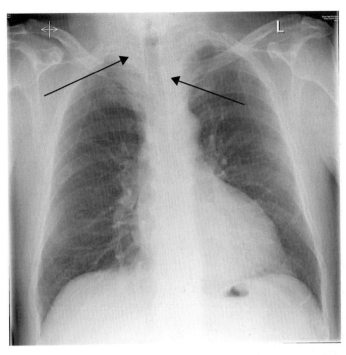

Fig. 2.34 PA chest radiograph: a thyroid goitre may be seen on a chest radiograph (arrows showing both sides of goitre). This is seen as a superior mediastinal mass and may cause deviation of the trachea.

Imaging of the thyroid gland

Chest radiograph

The thyroid gland may be seen as a superior mediastinal mass with a displacement of the trachea when enlarged due to goitre (Fig. 2.34).

Ultrasound

Indication
Ultrasound is the first-line investigation of the thyroid because it shows both lobes clearly and then the presence and extent of an abnormality.

Technique
A linear-array high-frequency transducer provides excellent detail. The thyroid gland is well visualized with ultrasound and should be scanned in both the axial and sagittal planes. The isthmus of the thyroid can then be measured.

Findings
Cysts, colloid cysts and solitary nodules can be identified easily within the thyroid gland itself. Nodules are amenable to percutaneous sampling. The thyroid has a thin, slightly reflective capsule and the gland is normally homogeneous in reflectivity (Fig. 2.35).

On ultrasound the trachea causes reverberation artefact.

The isthmus of the thyroid gland should measure less than 3 mm.

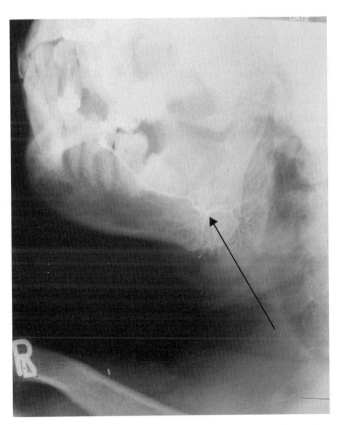

Fig. 2.33 Submandibular sialogram with Wharton's duct shown (arrow).

The thyroid lobes vary in size but should measure less than 2 cm in thickness, i.e. AP diameter each. The right lobe is usually larger than the left lobe.

CT of the thyroid gland

Technique
On CT the thyroid gland has natural contrast due to iodine being present (Fig. 2.36). It can be assessed for retrosternal extension and pure compression with CT. Care is needed when giving intravenous iodine-based contrast media if the patient is to undergo any treatment with radioactive iodine.

Nuclear medicine

Indication and technique
Isotope scanning provides functional anatomy using technetium-99m, i.e. pertechnetate, or iodide (123 I) using a

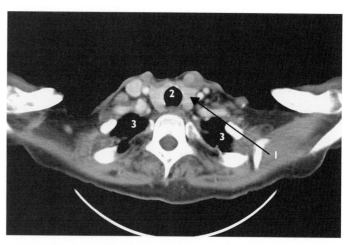

Fig. 2.36 CT of the thyroid gland. The left lobe of the thyroid (1). Trachea (2) and lung apices (3).

gamma camera with a pinhole. Radioactive labelling of iodine (131 I) may be used to treat thyroid nodules.

Findings
Ectopic thyroid tissue can occur anywhere along the line of the thyroglossal duct from the tongue base to the lower neck, and there may be no functioning tissue in the normal site, i.e. there may be a lingual thyroid. Nuclear medicine can be useful to detect this.

The parathyroid glands

Ultrasound and nuclear medicine

Indications
Hyperparathyroidism. These small endocrine glands are posterior to the thyroid glands in most cases. There are usually four glands altogether. The parathyroid glands may be hard to identify using imaging.

Technique
Ultrasound. Nuclear medicine studies may help to identify them using a thallium-201 or sestamibi scan and a technetium-99m thyroid scan using subtraction; CT and MRI or venous sampling is also used for parathyroid detection.

Findings
On ultrasound they appear as echo-poor structures behind the thyroid glands. They can, however, lie anywhere between the thyroid glands and the posteromediastinum.

The orbit

Orbit plain X–ray

Indications
Plain films may be performed before MRI to look for shrapnel of foreign bodies that would contraindicate MRI.

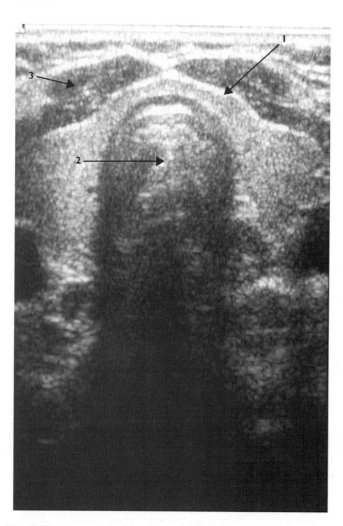

Fig. 2.35 Ultrasound of the thyroid gland: the isthmus runs anterior to the tracheal rings (1). The reverberation artefact of trachea (2) and strap muscles (3).

CT orbits (Fig. 2.37)

This shows the orbit but causes radiation to the lens which should be avoided. CT is indicated to assess bony trauma to the orbit and blow-out fractures to the floor. The medial wall of the orbit is vulnerable to trauma as a result of its thin nature. High-resolution images are required to assess the fractures. It can be used to show carotid–cavernous fistulas.

Ultrasound orbits

This is very useful for assessing the globe, retina and vitreous, for ocular tumours and the lens.

MRI orbits

This has become the investigation of choice for suspected neurological optic lesions because it assesses the optic nerve and the chiasma (Fig. 2.38), and the orbit itself, in a multiplanar non-ionizing way. It can also assess trauma but requires more patient cooperation, resulting in CT being the first-line investigation in bony trauma.

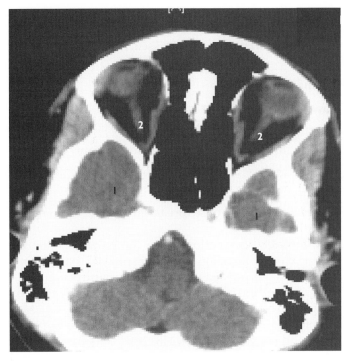

Fig. 2.37 CT scan of the orbits: middle cranial fossa (1) and optic nerve (2).

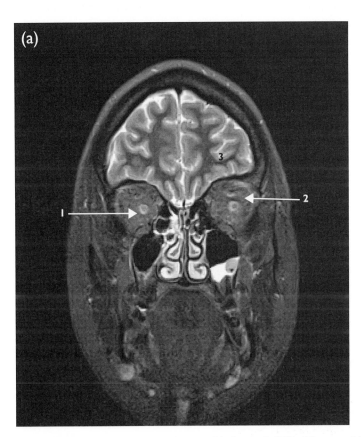

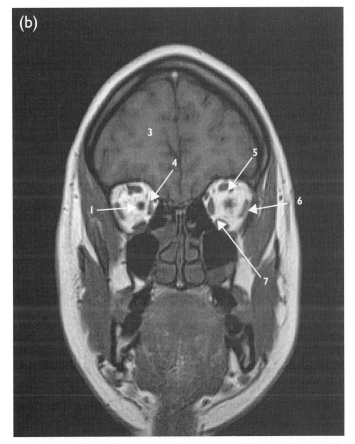

Fig. 2.38 MRI of the orbit and chiasma. (a) Coronal, STIR; (b) coronal T1. (a) On the coronal STIR image, the optic nerves are seen as the low-signal dot within a sheath of high-signal CSF, which lies within a sleeve of meninges. The intraconal fat has been suppressed (2). On (b), coronal T1-weighted image of the nerve root, the optic nerve and the CFS cannot be differentiated. Optic nerve (1), intracoral fat (2), frontal lobe (3), medial rectus (4), superior rectus (5), lateral rectus (6) and inferior rectus (7).

Findings

On MRI the anatomy is seen well on T1-weighted and pathology on STIR or fat-suppressed T2-weighted images.

Paranasal sinuses

Plain films and CT/MRI

Indication

Sinusitis, nasal obstruction, suspected tumour. CT before functional endoscopic sinus surgery (FESS).

Technique

* Plain films of the sinuses are taken in the occipitomental (OM) position.
* CT formerly was performed in the prone position for direct coronal imaging, but, using spiral CT axial supine, scans can be obtained with coronal reconstruction. With **m**ulti**p**lanar **r**econstruction (MPR), it can be performed supine. The anatomy is identical on MRI to CT. MRI avoids ionizing radiation. CT gives a better view of cartilage and bony destruction. MRI is used for assessing the soft-tissue extent of malignancy and complex infection.

Finding

* Plain films can show mucosal thickening, bony destruction and fluid levels, and is useful in the clinic setting.
* The ostiomeatal complex should be reviewed with the uncinate process on the coronal images (Fig. 2.39).
* Variants such as pneumatization of the middle turbinate may lead to compromise of the ostiomeatal complex. Likewise a note should be made of a large bulla ethmoidalis, the air cell adjacent to the infundibulum.
* Spurs may project from the nasal septum and lead to nasal obstruction.
* CT can falsely show bony defects in areas of thin bone resulting from partial volume averaging. This is common in the lamina papyracea and medial wall of the maxillary antra.
* MRI may have difficulty differentiating tumour from surrounding oedema on T2-weighted images and gadolinium with T1-weighted images can help.

Dacrocystography

Indication

This is an investigation performed to look at the nasolacrimal duct. The nasolacrimal duct runs from the inferior punctum of the eyelid down to the inferior meatus. There are several natural narrowings within the nasolacrimal duct. This investigation studies the duct and assesses for strictures.

Technique

* An OM view is used.
* Fine catheter, i.e. Rabinoff 30G.
* The lacrimal sac is massaged which lies inferiorly and medially.

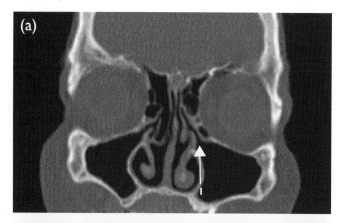

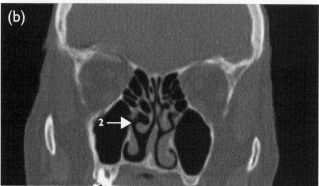

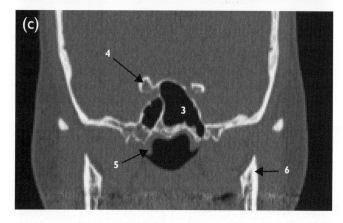

Fig. 2.39 CT of the paranasal sinuses and nasopharynx. (a) coronal CT showing the ostiomeatal complex (1); (b) coronal CT of the paranasal sinuses: (2) shows apparent defect in medial wall of maxillary antrum due to partial volume averaging as a result of the thin bone. (c) Coronal CT of the sphenoid sinus (3), anterior clinoid processes (4), torus tubarius and fossa of Rosenmüller (5) and mandible (6).

* The inferior punctum is cannulated.
* Note that the lacrimal gland lies superolaterally.
* Subtraction radiography and macroradiography are both used.

Findings

The duct has several normal narrowings in its course (Fig. 2.40).

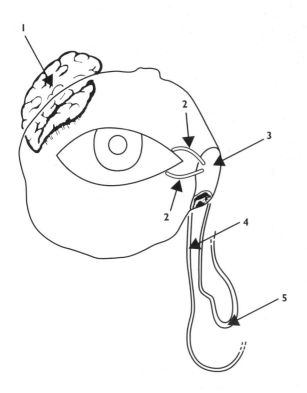

Fig. 2.40 Diagram of the nasolacrimal duct. Lacrimal gland (1), canaliculus (2), lacrimal sac (3), nasolacrimal duct (4), inferior meatus (5).

The ear

CT

Indications
CT is the mode of choice for visualization of the bony structures of the ear and bony destruction.

MRI is superior at the internal auditory canal and nerves VII and VIII. It shows nerve VII throughout its pathway and can visualize the labyrinth and cochlea.

Technique
Fine CT cuts in both planes, axially and coronally, show the bony structures and ossicles. On MRI, fast-spin T2 echo or HASTE (**h**alf-Fourier **a**cquisition **s**ingle-shot **t**urbo spin-**e**cho) shows the nerves. Gadolinium-enhanced images may be required for suspected intracanalicular masses.

Findings (Fig. 2.41)
- The incus and malleus are well seen on CT of the petrous bone in both the axial and coronal positions. Together they form the incudomalleolar complex. These lie within the middle-ear cavity in the epitympanic recess. Just lateral to the incudomalleolar complex is Prussak's space.
- The incudomalleolar complex has the appearance of an ice-cream cone in the epitympanic recess on axial images.

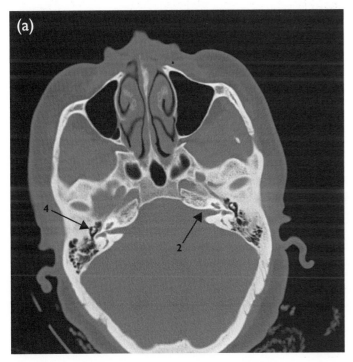

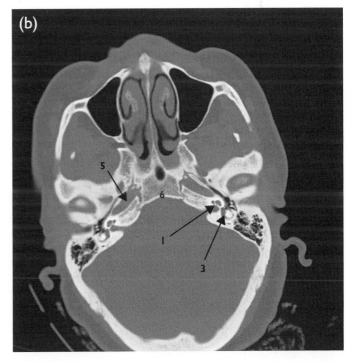

Fig. 2.41 Axial CT scans of the petrous bone and middle and inner ear: (a) more cranial and (b) more caudal showing the vestibule (3) lying posterior and lateral to the cochlea (1). Internal auditory canal (2), incudomalleolar complex (4), foramen lacerum (5), clivus (6).

- The scutum is best seen on coronal CT. The tympanic membrane attaches to the scutum. The scutum should be sharp and pointed and symmetrical with the opposite side.
- The cochlea lies anterior medial and inferior to the vestibule. When assessing for middle-ear or inner-ear disease observe the following structures (Fig. 2.42):
  - scutum on coronal view
  - incudomalleolar complex on axial view
  - Prussak's space adjacent to the incudomalleolar complex.
  - the vestibule with the three semicircular canals posteriorly and the cochlea anteriorly
  - the facial nerve course, i.e. geniculate fossa medial to the cochlea and the course posteriorly.

- The mastoid air cells should be aerated. Fluid in the mastoids may indicate blood in the context of trauma or mastoiditis. Absence of pneumatization of the mastoid may impede cochlear implants.
- The course of the jugular and carotid arteries may be aberrant. The jugular bulb may be dehiscent with no bony wall separating it from the middle-ear cavity. The carotid artery can lie in an ectopic position in the middle ear.

The epitympanic recess and the opening into the mastoid air cells, i.e. the aditus to the mastoid air cells, should have an 'hour-glass' or 'figure-of-eight' shape.

On axial T2-weighted images nerves VII and VIII are demonstrated in the IAMs (Fig. 2.43).

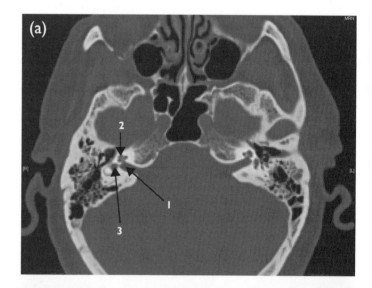

Fig. 2.42 CT scan of the ear: (a) axial: internal auditory canal (1), cochlea (2) and vestibule (3). (b) Coronal plane: external auditory canal (1), cochlea (2), scutum seen on coronal plane (3), incudomalleolar complex (4), tegmen tympani or arcuate eminence (5).

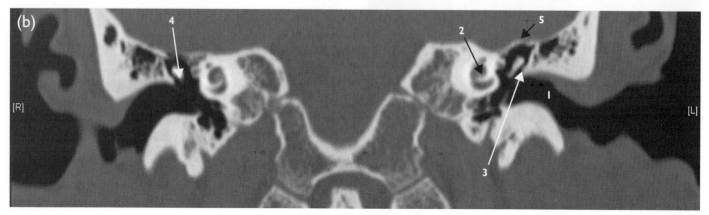

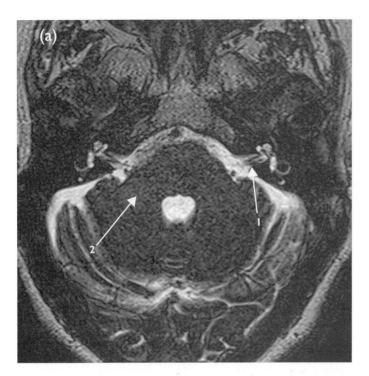 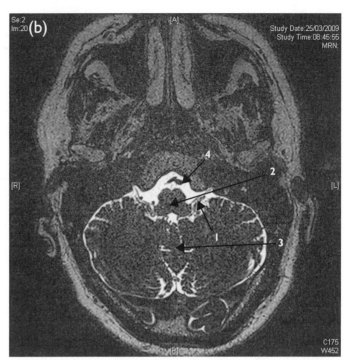

Fig. 2.43 MRI of the internal auditory meatus: (a) T2-weighted MRI axial. (b) HASTE heavily weighted T2 axial images. (a) is more cranial than (b). Nerves VII and VIII are well seen entering internal acoustic canal (1). The vertebral arteries are seen in the prepontine cistern converging from the basilar artery (4). The medulla with the characteristic anterior medial sulcus (2) and cerebellar vermis (3).

CASES

Case 2.1

A patient presents to A&E after being hit in the left eye. Initially a facial series of plain films is performed, followed by a CT.

Findings

On the OM soft-tissue swelling is seen over the left orbit and there is some air seen under the left eyelid and in what appears to be the orbit itself. No definite blow-out fracture is seen. The normal side can be used to compare for subtle pathology.

The CT shows proptosis of the left eye. There is a fracture of the medial wall of the left orbit and air is seen in the orbit intraconally and around the eyelid. The images would need to be reviewed in the coronal plane to look for a blow-out fracture.

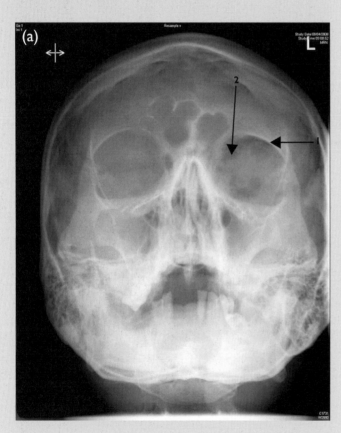
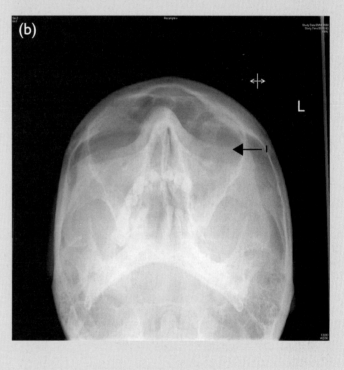

Fig. 2.44 (a) Occipitomental (OM) and (b) OM30 facial views; (b) soft-tissue swelling of the left orbit (1) and (a) abnormal air (2) within the left globe. (c,d) Axial soft-tissue windows through orbit show a fracture of the medial wall (3) of the orbit with intraconal and preseptal air and proptosis. (e–g) Axial CT of the orbit bony windows showing the air preseptally (4); intraconal air is better seen on bony windows.

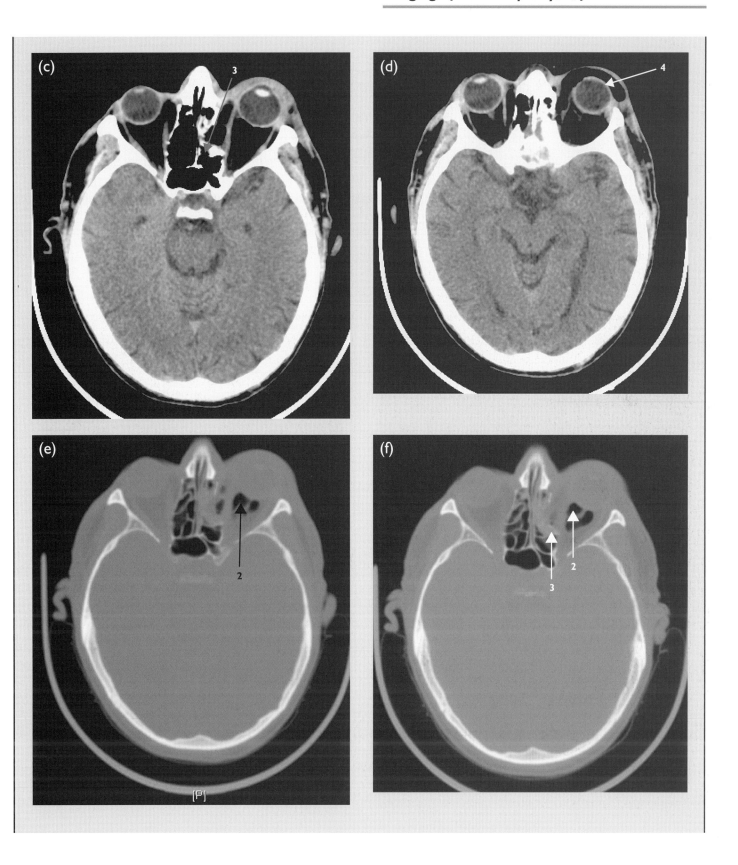

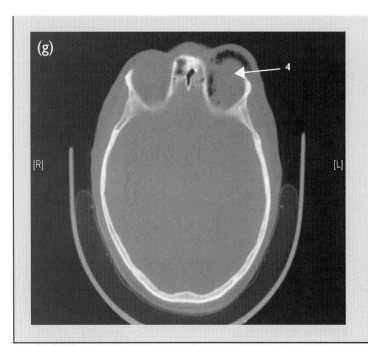

Review areas

Look within the brain itself for any contusions or haemorrhage.

Diagnosis

Fracture of the medial wall of the left orbit.

Case 2.2

A patient presents with swelling of the neck anteriorly.

A chest radiograph shows a soft tissue mass at the sternal inlet. An unenhanced CT is performed to look for retrosternal extension of the thyroid.

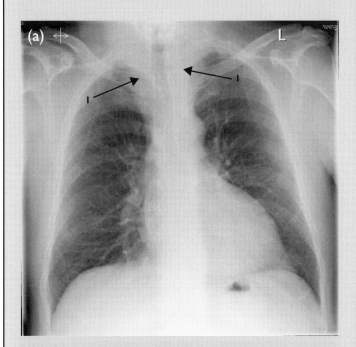

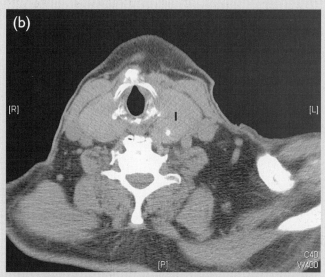

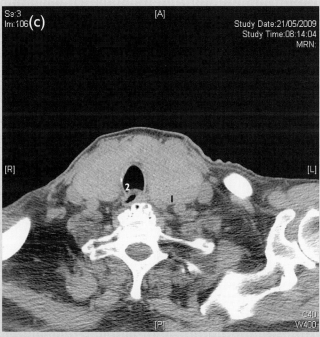

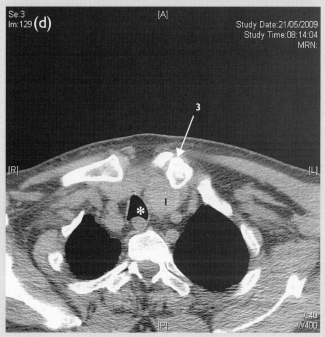

Fig. 2.45 (a) Chest radiograph: a superior mediastinal mass consistent with goitre (1). (b) Axial unenhanced CT at level of vocal folds: axial CT at level of trachea; (c) axial CT at level of great vessels: retrosternally shows the goitre with some retrosternal extension, but no significant tracheal stenosis. Thyroid (1), trachea (2), sternoclavicular joint (3).

Findings

The idealized report reads:

> There is a thyroid goitre which extends retrosternally but stops at the level of the great vessels. No significant tracheal compromise is seen.

Case 2.3

A patient presents with sinusitis. CT is performed before FESS. The images are taken in the axial plane and reviewed in both coronal and sagittal planes.

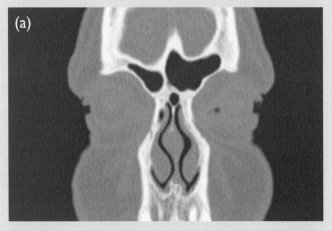

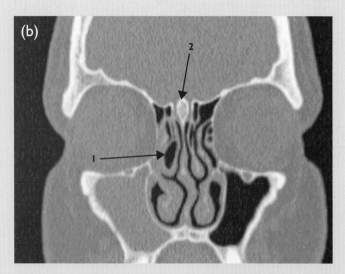

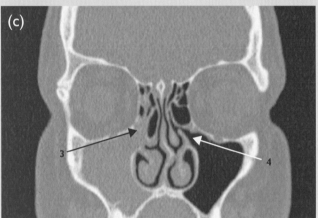

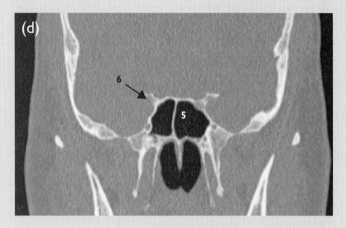

Fig. 2.46 CT scan of the paranasal sinuses (a–c) shows opacification of the right maxillary antra with obstruction of the right ostiomeatal complex (3). There is a right concha bullosa abnormality (1). The left ostiomeatal complex is patent (4). Crista galli (2). (d) Level sphenoid sinus (5). anterior clinoid process (6).

Findings

The nasal septum is displaced to the left inferiorly:
- Conchae: there is pneumatization of the right middle turbinate – called a concha bullosa, which can contribute to narrowing of the ostiomeatal complex.
- Sinuses: are all patent other than opacification of the right maxillary antrum and ethmoid air cells.
- Ostiomeatal complex: patent on left, obstructed on right.

The idealized report reads:

> There is opacification of the right maxillary antrum with obstruction of the right ostiomeatal complex, There is a concha bullosa of the right middle turbinate contributing to compromise of the right ostiomeatal complex. The remaining sinuses are clear. The nasal septum is deviated to the left.

3 Chest imaging

RADIOLOGICAL ANATOMY

Chest wall: the ribs

- There are 12 pairs of ribs and costal cartilages. The upper seven ribs are true ribs and attach to the sternum. Ribs 8–10 are false ribs joining to the rib above and not to the sternum. Ribs 11 and 12 are floating ribs.
- A typical rib has a head with two facets for articulating with its corresponding vertebra and the one above.
- On the undersurface of the rib lies the costal groove containing the neurovascular bundle. Hypertrophy of the structures in the groove leads to rib notching, found on the undersurface of the rib in conditions such as neurofibromatosis with neurofibromas or vascular hypertrophy in coarctation of the aorta. The costal groove itself has a flange causing apparent loss of cortex in the mid and posterior lower ribs on a chest radiograph. This is a normal finding which can be mistaken for rib erosion or malignancy (Fig. 3.1).
- A prominent first costochondral junction can be mistaken for a mass on a chest radiograph or CT due to partial volume averaging (Fig. 3.2).
- Prominent first and second ribs and cervical ribs in the supraclavicular fossa can mimic a clinical mass.
- Cervical ribs occur in 1–2% of the population and commonly are bilateral although asymmetrical. They arise from C7. They can be distinguished from normal thoracic ribs by looking at the transverse processes: thoracic transverse processes point upwards as opposed to cervical transverse processes which point downwards. If the

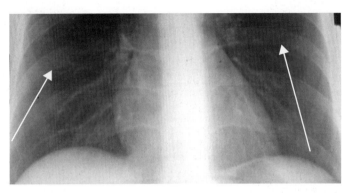

Fig. 3.1 PA chest radiograph: the flange lies on the inferior aspect or undersurface of the rib (arrows) and causes loss of the sharp cortex. This is a normal finding.

rib arises from a vertebra with a downward-pointing transverse process it is cervical (Fig. 3.3).
- Ribs may be bifid or splayed congenitally and of no clinical significance, but occasionally are part of a wider abnormality such as Klippel–Feil syndrome with Sprengel shoulder.

The sternum

This is made up of three parts: the manubrium, the body and the xiphoid process.
- The manubrium (see Fig. 3.3a) is the most superior part, lying at T3–4, forming the sternal notch, and is a

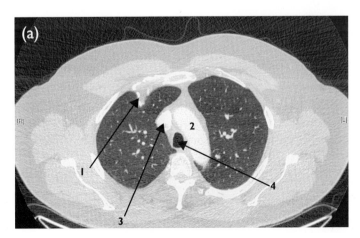
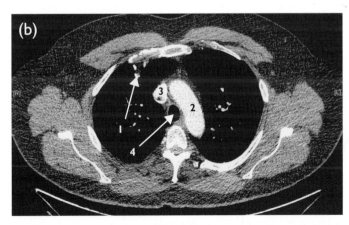

Fig. 3.2 Axial CT: the first rib (1) on CT due to partial volume averaging can give the impression of a mass on the lung windows. Contiguous images clearly show this is part of the first rib when scrolling through the images. (a) Axial CT lung windows and (b) soft tissue mediastinal windows. Aortic arch (2), superior vena cava (3) and trachea (4).

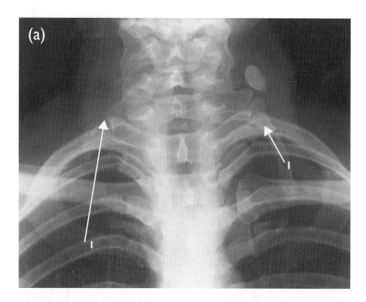

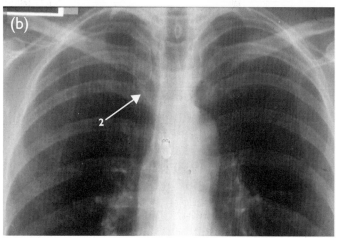

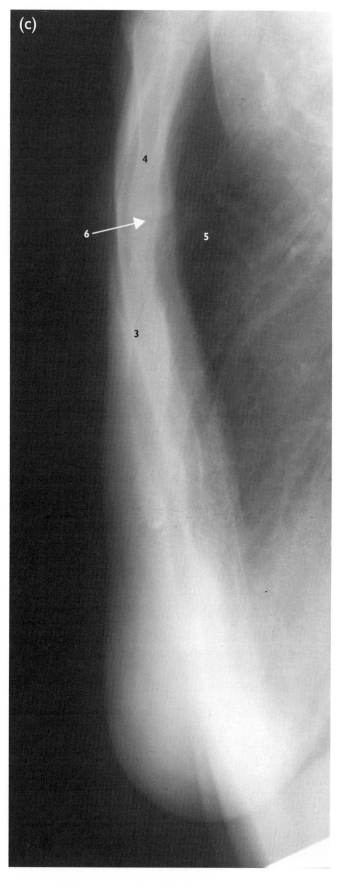

Fig. 3.3 (a) Radiograph of thoracic inlet. Cervical ribs arise from down pointing cervical transverse processes (1). Thoracic ribs arise from upwards pointing thoracic transverse processes. (b) Chest radiograph: the manubrium sternae can mimic a right paratracheal mass (2). (c) Lateral sternal view: the sternum (3) is shown articulating with the manubrium (4) and the retrosternal fat space (5). Manubriosternal joint (6).

triangular bone that can simulate a soft-tissue mass in the mediastinum on a chest radiograph.

- The sternal body originates from sternebrae, sternal ossification centres that develop in utero. The sternebrae fuse from age 15 to 25 years. Sternebrae can mimic healing fractures in a child (see Fig. 3.3b).
- The angle between the sternal body and the manubrium is called the sternal angle of Louis and lies at T4–5.
- The xiphoid process usually lies at T10. The xiphisternal joint can be confused with a fracture. Fusion to the sternal body occurs at age 40 years.
- Oblique sternal views show the sternum, but have mainly been superseded by CT.
- A depressed sternum is known as pectus excavatum.

The clavicle

- The medial ends of the clavicles are used to assess for rotation of a chest radiograph. The distance between the spinous processes and the medial end of the clavicle on each side should be the same.
- The clavicle is the first bone in the body to appear in utero by endomembranous ossification at age 5–6 weeks.
- The secondary ossification centre develops at the medial end of the clavicle at age 15 years and fuses at age 25.
- A lordotic or apical view projects the clavicles off the lungs to enable a better view of the lung apices.
- The clavicle has a slight irregularity as a normal variant inferomedially, the rhomboid fossa, which may simulate an apical cavity on a chest radiograph.
- The conoid tubercle arises from the inferior surface of the clavicle just above the coracoid process and gives rise to the attachment of the coracoclavicular ligament.
- The clavicle has a line of soft tissue above it on a chest radiograph called the companion shadow. Supraclavicular masses can be detected by looking for widening of the shadow (Fig. 3.4).
- The clavicle may be hypoplastic, particularly laterally, in a number of syndromes including cleidocranial dysostosis.

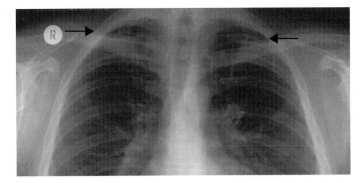

Fig. 3.4 PA chest radiograph: zoomed view. Soft tissue overlying the clavicle causes the companion shadow (arrows).

Intercostal space
- Three muscle layers: external, internal intercostals and innermost intercostals.
- Intercostals nerves run in the rib flange, hence in neurofibromatosis rib notching occurs due to neurofibromas eroding the rib.
- Intercostal arteries: in coarctation of the aorta the collateral vessels hypertrophy and erode the ribs.

The thoracic spine (see Chapter 7)

Can be seen on a chest radiograph and CT.

Bronchial tree

- The trachea starts at the lower border of the cricoid cartilage at C6 and is 9–12 cm long. The trachea and bronchi are made up of 'C'-shaped rings of hyaline cartilage which are deficient posteriorly. The characteristic shape of the rings helps recognition of the trachea on CT (Fig. 3.5). In the lower neck, the region below the true vocal folds, called the subglottic region, has an 'oval' shape on an axial CT section. The shape of the airway changes at the start of the trachea to become a 'horse-shoe' shape.
- The trachea is 2 cm wide The normal range for transverse diameter of the trachea is 13–26 mm in men and 10–22 mm in women.
- The tracheal rings can calcify after the age of 40 years.
- As the trachea enters the thorax it inclines slightly to the right side.
- The bifurcation of the trachea, the carina, lies at the level of T4–5. It can be seen on a chest radiograph. The left atrium lies under the carina and when enlarged can cause upward splaying of the carina.
- The angle of the carina is normally 55–80°. Left atrial hypertrophy pushes cranially and compresses the carina, leading to splaying or widening of the angle. An increase in the angle. >90° is considered pathological (Fig. 3.6).
- The right main bronchus, also known as the eparterial bronchus, is wider, shorter and more vertical, hence foreign bodies tend to go down the right bronchus. After 3 cm the right main bronchus terminates in three main bronchi: the upper, middle and lower lobes. The right upper lobe bronchus arises before the hilum and the main bronchus continues as bronchus intermedius. Bronchus intermedius then divides into the right middle and lower lobe bronchi. A mass or obstruction of bronchus intermedius will therefore lead to collapse/consolidation in both the middle and lower lobes (Fig. 3.6b).
- The apical segment bronchus of the right lower lobe arises at the same level as the middle lobe bronchus.
- The left main bronchus or hyparterial bronchus is longer, being 5 cm long. It passes under the aortic arch. It divides into only two main bronchi: the upper lobe which also supplies the lingula and the lower lobe bronchus. In

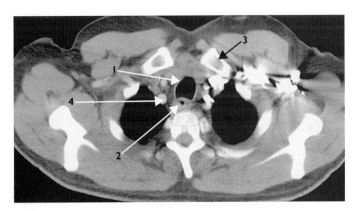

Fig. 3.5 Axial enhanced CT at thoracic inlet. The trachea has a characteristic horse-shoe shape on CT (1). Oesophagus (2), clavicle (3) and right subclavian artery (4).

the left upper lobe there is a common apicoposterior segment to the upper lobe and no medial basal segment in the lower lobe.

- There are 10 bronchopulmonary segments on the right and 8 on the left. Each segment is pyramidal with its apex directed to the lung root and base at the pleural surface. Each segment is surgically separable, containing a vein, artery and tertiary bronchus.

The pleura

- The pleura have two layers: the visceral layer, which closely adheres to the lung and invests the fissures, and the parietal layer. The pleural cavity lies in between. There may be up to 15 ml fluid in the normal pleural cavity.
- The fissures divide the lung into lobes and usually there are three lobes on the right and two on the left (Fig. 3.7a). The left lung is smaller, with the cardiac notch lying anteriorly. A thin slither of lung extends down over the heart anteriorly, called the lingula. Collapse or consolidation in the lingula therefore gives rise to a veil over the heart on a chest radiograph (Fig. 3.65a).
- The oblique fissure extends from T4–5 down to the sixth costal cartilage anteriorly. On a posteroanterior (PA) chest radiograph consolidation in the apical segment of the lower lobe can be seen up to the level of T4.
- On a lateral chest radiograph the left oblique fissure is more vertical.
- The horizontal fissure extends from the oblique fissure to the fourth rib anteriorly on a lateral chest radiograph. On a PA chest radiograph the horizontal fissure extends laterally to the sixth rib in the axillary line.

Variations in lobes

- An extra fissure may occasionally divide a lung. It is important to know this radiologically so as not to confuse lines on a chest radiograph with a pneumothorax. In the azygos lobe, seen in 1% of people, the azygos vein arches over the lung apex, not the hilum, and isolates the medial part of the lung. This has four layers of pleura and the course of the azygos vein through the lung can be seen on CT. Just as the vein is about to pierce the superior vena cava (SVC) the vein may mimic a soft-tissue chest nodule (Fig. 3.8).
- Other fissures that are uncommon are:
  - inferior accessory fissure – separation of medial basal segment
  - left horizontal fissure – separation of the lingula from the left upper lobe
  - superior accessory fissure – separation of the apical segment of the lower lobe.

The pulmonary vessels

- The pulmonary trunk arises from the right ventricle. At the sternal angle the main pulmonary artery or trunk divides into the longer right and shorter left pulmonary arteries. The main pulmonary artery is called the conus just before its division and is of variable size in young people.
- Each lung is supplied by a single artery and two pulmonary veins on the left and three on the right. The right pulmonary artery is longer than the left (Fig. 3.9).
- The bronchial arteries supply the supporting structures of the lungs. The left bronchial artery arises from the

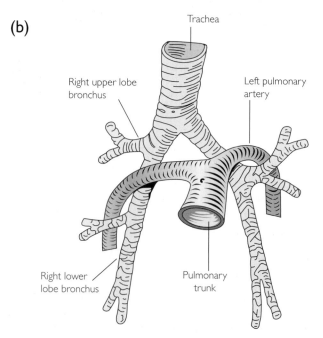

Fig. 3.6 (a) PA chest radiograph: zoomed view. The carina can be seen on a chest radiograph (arrow). Left atrial enlargement can cause splaying of the carina. (b) Diagram of the bronchi.

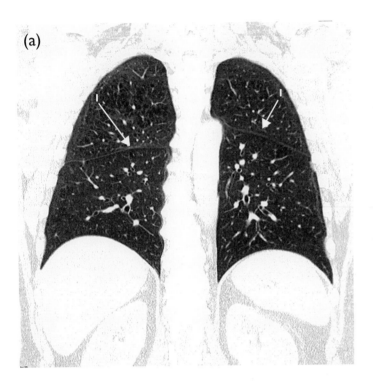

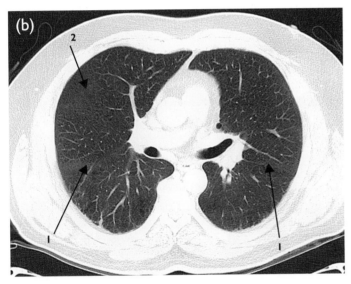

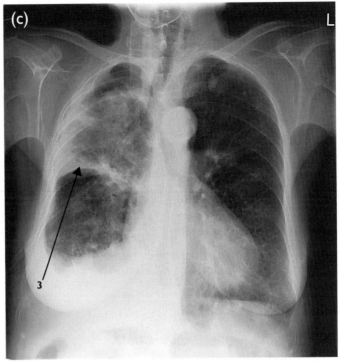

Fig. 3.7 (a) Coronal and (b) axial CT lung windows showing the fissures: The fissures of the lung are well seen on CT. The oblique fissures (1). The horizontal fissure is recognized by a bare area on the axial images (2). (c) PA chest radiograph. In this patient with consolidation in the right upper lobe the horizontal fissure clearly demarcates the upper lobe from the middle lobe (3).

descending aorta and the right artery arises from the superior posterior intercostals.

- The left pulmonary artery is attached to the aortic arch concavity by the ligamentum arteriosum.
- The aortopulmonary window lies between the aortic arch and the pulmonary trunk.

The mediastinum

This is the central compartment of the thorax and is divided into four sections. Knowledge of the normal anatomy aids in differential diagnosis of the pathology (Fig. 3.10):

- Superior: extends from the thoracic inlet to a plane at T4 at the level of the sternal angle. It contains the SVC, aortic arch, thymus, great vessels, trachea, oesophagus and thoracic duct.
- Anterior: the smallest division lying between the sternal body and the fibrous pericardium of the heart. It is continuous with the superior mediastinum. Inferiorly it is limited by the diaphragm. It contains fat, nodes and the thymus in children, and may contain thyroid tissue.
- Posterior: contains the thoracic duct, the oesophagus, aorta, lymph nodes, azygos and hemiazygos, and nerves. It lies between the vertebral bodies and the fibrous pericardium.
- Middle: the heart, pericardium, roots of great vessels, ascending aorta, SVC, pulmonary trunk, azygos and main bronchi, lymph nodes.

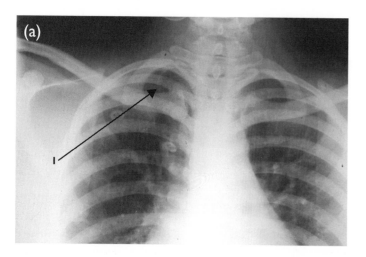

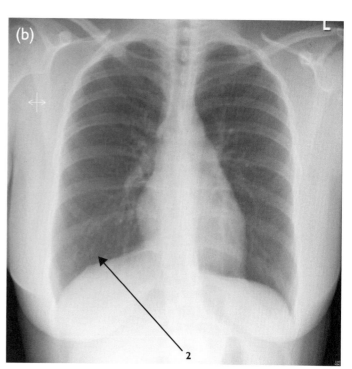

Fig. 3.8 (a) PA chest radiograph: the azygos fissure is marked by (1). (b) PA chest radiograph: the inferior accessory fissure is marked by (2).

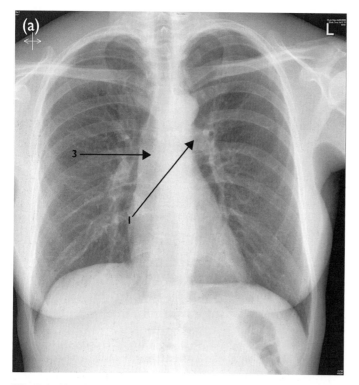

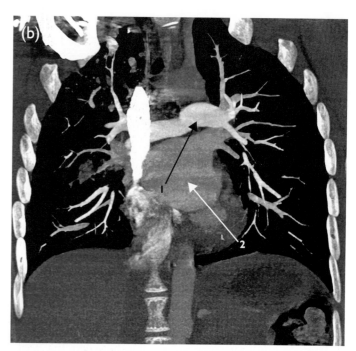

Fig. 3.9 (a) PA chest radiograph: the main pulmonary artery is called the conus and runs in this direction and is shown on the chest radiograph; (b) CTPA (1): left atrium (2) and ascending aorta (3).

- The mediastinum should ideally be assessed on a PA chest radiograph on full inspiration. An expiratory or supine film can cause apparent mediastinal widening, leading to erroneous investigations for aortic rupture, etc. (Fig. 3.11).

- Loss of the silhouette of structures helps place a mass into one of the mediastinal compartments (Fig. 3.11b).

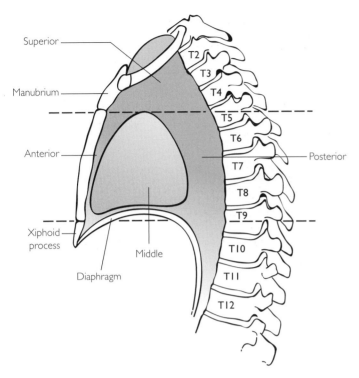

Fig. 3.10 labels: Superior, Manubrium, Anterior, Xiphoid process, Diaphragm, Middle, Posterior, T2, T3, T4, T5, T6, T7, T8, T9, T10, T11, T12

Fig. 3.10 Mediastinal divisions: the dotted line divides the mediastinum into superior and inferior divisions.

The heart

- The four chambers of the heart can be identified on the cardiac silhouette on a chest radiograph. The axis of the heart is rotated in the chest, on a PA chest radiograph (Fig. 3.12). This means that the chambers of the heart are not seen enface, but the long axis is tilted pointing towards the left apex.
- The right atrium forms the right heart border. It receives blood from the inferior vena cava (IVC) and SVC returning deoxygenated blood to the heart in addition to the cardiac veins from the coronary sinus.
- The IVC can simulate a paracardiac mass as it drains into the right atrium (Fig. 3.13).
- The left ventricle forms the left heart border.
- The left atrium receives the pulmonary veins. The left atrium lies posteriorly and is best seen on a lateral chest radiograph (Fig. 3.14.)
- The left atrial appendage forms part of the left heart border on a PA chest radiograph. In left atrial enlargement a prominent left atrial appendage can be seen and a double right heart border where the atrium enlarges posteriorly.

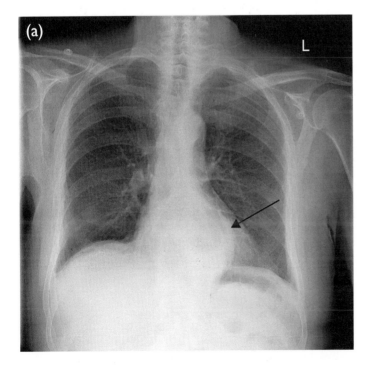

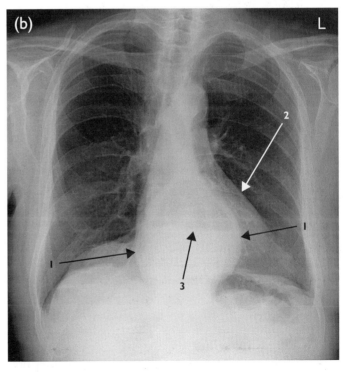

Fig. 3.11 (a) PA chest radiograph with a mass in the posterior mediastinum (1). The left heart border which is situated anteriorly is seen clearly and separately from the mass. (b) PA chest radiograph with a posterior mediastinal mass (1) separate from the left heart border (2). The mass has a fluid level (3) commonly seen on an erect chest radiograph in a hiatus hernia.

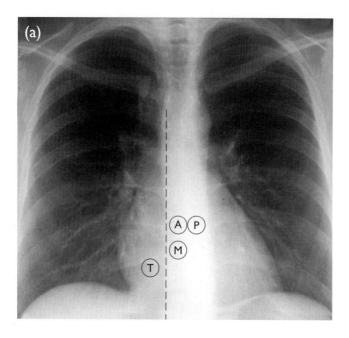

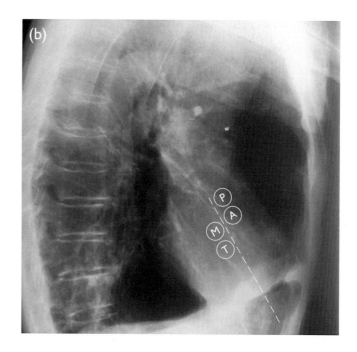

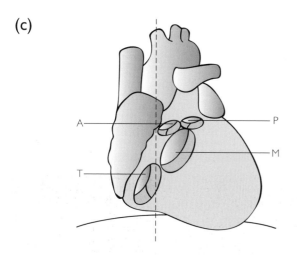

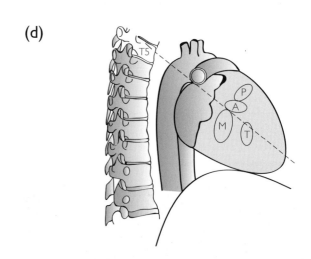

Fig. 3.12 (a,b) PA chest radiograph and (c,d) lateral chest radiograph with the valve positions drawn on.

- The right ventricle lies mainly anteriorly but also inferiorly. Hypertrophy causes elevation of the heart, best seen on a lateral chest radiograph. Trabeculae, which are irregular muscular elevations, lie inside. The pulmonary artery arises from the top of the right ventricle.
- The tricuspid valve lies on the right between the right atrium and the right ventricle. The valve has three cusps.
- The mitral valve lies on the left between the left atrium and the left ventricle. The mitral valve is normally bicuspid.
- The pericardium has two layers forming a sac. Subpericardial fat may mimic a pneumothorax.

- Around the heart surface lies epicardial fat, which can simulate a soft-tissue mass on a lateral or PA chest radiograph (Fig. 3.14b).

The aorta and coronary arteries

- The aortic arch lies at T4. The junction of the aortic arch and descending aorta is known as the isthmus. The aortic arch is usually on the left side of the chest.
- The aortic valve has three cusps, i.e. it is tricuspid.
- Aortic cusps: above each cusp is a small dilatation called a sinus of Valsalva, from which the coronary arteries

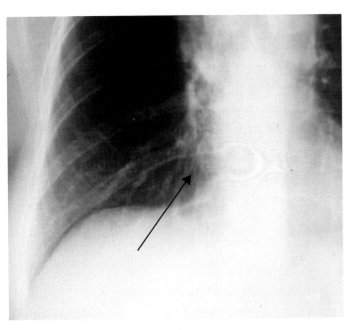

Fig. 3.13 PA chest radiograph – zoomed view. The inferior vena cava (arrow) can give the impression of a paracardiac mass on chest radiograph.

arise. The sinuses must be located to perform a coronary angiogram.

- The right coronary arises from the right aortic sinus, which is to the right and anterior, and the left coronary from the left sinus, which is slightly posterior and on the left. The third sinus is redundant – non-coronary.
- The branches of the right coronary artery (Fig. 3.15):
  - sinoatrial (SA) node branch in 60%
  - right marginal
  - atrioventricular (AV) node branch in 80%
  - posterior interventricular branch.
- It is common for arrhythmias to occur during a right coronary angiogram. The right coronary artery can be recognized on a coronary angiogram by its classic shape of passing to the right descending vertically, then passing medially and ascending again.
- The left coronary artery has a short main stem and then divides into the circumflex (Cx) and left anterior descending (LAD) arteries.
- The LAD gives off diagonal branches supplying the interventricular septum and descends in the anterior interventricular groove. The LAD can be recognized

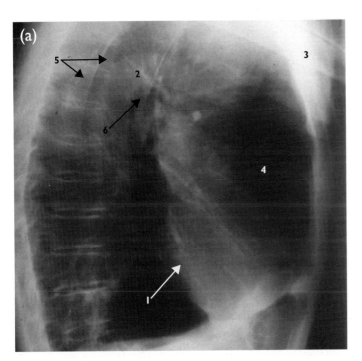

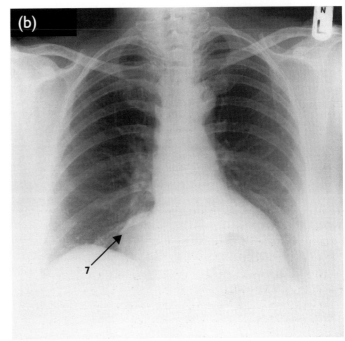

Fig. 3.14 (a) Lateral chest radiograph. The left atrium is the most posterior chamber of the heart (1). Aortic arch (2), humerus (3), retrosternal space (4), blades of scapulae (5) and aortopulmonary window (6). (b) PA chest radiograph: an opaque cardiac fat pad can simulate a paracardiac or pericardial mass (7). The low density and the presence of vessels visible through the mass aid the diagnosis.

on a coronary angiogram by its characteristic anterior position on a near lateral view where it is concave posteriorly.

- The circumflex gives off obtuse marginal branches and passes backwards and leftwards.
- It may give off an SA nodal branch that supplies the anterior two-thirds of the interventricular septum.
- In coronary dominance, the dominant vessel supplies the left ventricle mainly. In left coronary dominance the left coronary artery supplies the left ventricle. Coronary dominance indicates the coronary artery that supplies the posterior descending branch to the inferior surface of the heart. Right dominance is most common.

The aorta congenital variants

- After the origin of the left subclavian artery, the aorta narrows forming the isthmus.

- Three great vessels arise from the aortic arch: the brachiocephalic, left common carotid and left subclavian in 65%.
- In 27% the left common carotid and the brachiocephalic arteries arise from a common trunk (Fig. 3.16).

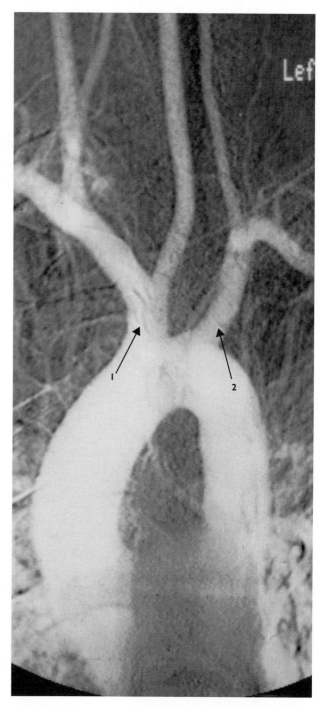

Fig. 3.16 Thoracic aortogram showing a variant of the origin of the great vessels. The left common carotid artery is arising with the brachiocephalic artery (1) with only two trunks arising from the aorta. The second trunk is the left subclavian artery (2) giving origin to the left vertebral arteries.

Fig. 3.15 Conventional thoracic aortogram showing the origin of the left common coronary artery (1) and the right coronary artery (2). Left ventricle (3), ascending aorta (4), brachiocephalic artery (5), left common carotid (6) and left subclavian (7).

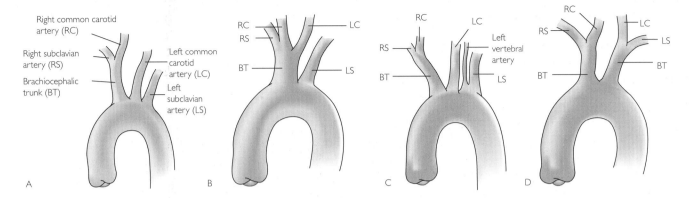

Fig. 3.17 Diagram of variants of great vessel origin from aortic arch.

- In 2.5% four vessels may originate independently, with separate left vertebral artery.
- In 1.2% there may be two brachiocephalic trunks (Fig. 3.17).
- Double aortic arch and retroaortic right subclavian artery are all variants.
- A right-sided aortic arch is associated with congenital heart disease in 50%. It may form part of a vascular ring with a patent ductus arteriosus. On a chest radiograph the left hilum looks exposed and the right arch becomes apparent if searched for. It is a review area.

Azygos vein

- The azygos venous system is important if there is obstruction to the vena cavae to ensure venous return to the heart (Fig. 3.18).
- The azygos venous system arises at L1 L2 from anastomoses with the IVC, the left renal vein in 60% and the ascending lumbar veins. The paired veins – azygos and hemiazygos – run up through the aortic hiatus at T12 and the azygos ascends on the right of T4–8.
- The azygos arches over the root of the right lung, over the right main stem bronchus and drains into the back of the SVC at T4–5, forming an important venous collateral anastomosis. It runs up on the right.
- The hemiazygos runs up on the left and crosses the midline to join the azygos at T9 or higher. The veins receive the intercostal veins and drain the posterior walls of chest and abdomen plus the mediastinal organs (Figs 3.19 and 3.20).
- It can be normal to see contrast reflux into the azygos on a CT due to force of injection rather than SVC obstruction.

Thoracic duct

- This originates from the cisterna chyli behind the right diaphragmatic crus at L1–2. It conveys most of the body's lymph to the venous system. An injury can lead to a chylothorax which looks like a pleural effusion on a chest radiograph (see Fig. 3.18).
- It lies in the posterior mediastinum, having ascended through the aortic opening at T12. It initially runs up on the right but crosses to the left at T4–6.
- The duct drains into the left internal jugular vein, left subclavian or left brachiocephalic vein.

Thymus

- This is found within the superior/anterior mediastinum, behind the manubrium. It extends into the aortopulmonary window.
- The thymus has two lobes with the left being larger than the right.
- Thymic size is variable until age 20 years. In young adults it is usually arrowhead shaped (62%) or has two separate lobes (32%).
- After puberty and between age 20 and 60 it undergoes fatty involution. In adults it becomes completely involuted and fatty replaced, and fat is seen on CT only in the mediastinum.
- The maximum thickness of each lobe is up to 15 mm on CT between age 20 and 50.
- On a PA chest radiograph in children the thymus is visible as a mediastinal soft-tissue mass.
- The thymus is identified by certain criteria (Fig. 3.21):
  – the edges gradually fade
  – it does not displace other structures
  – it is larger on expiration than inspiration
  – it appears within 24 hours of birth (Fig. 3.22)
  – it involutes at age 2 years and is rarely seen on a chest radiograph after age 8 years
  – it shrinks with steroids
  – it is largest at age 20, but more apparent in infancy.

The vagus nerves

- These are cranial nerve X arising from medulla.
- They run through the jugular foramen with nerves IX and XI.

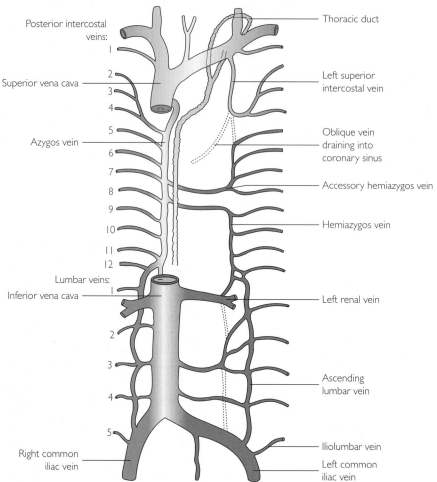

Fig. 3.18 Azygos diagram.

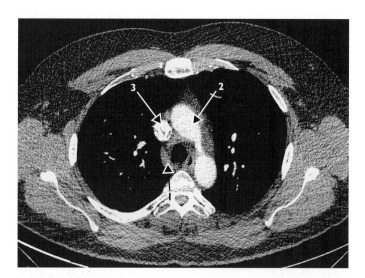

Fig. 3.19 Axial CT aortic arch level: azygos on CT. The azygos can be seen on axial CT draining into the posterior aspect of the superior vena cava (1). Ascending aorta (2) and superior vena cava (3).

- They run through the neck within the carotid sheath.
- They give off the recurrent laryngeal nerve, which on the left lies in the aortopulmonary window.
- They pass through diaphragm at T10 with the oesophagus.

The phrenic nerves

- Right phrenic passes through diaphragm with the IVC at T8.

Paediatric anatomy

- The same criteria for heart size on a chest radiograph cannot be applied in children. Up to 60% can be used for cardiothoracic ratio in a normal neonate.
- A relatively large normal thymus can simulate cardiomegaly in a child.
- Skin folds can mimic a pneumothorax.
- The trachea can narrow and buckle physiologically in the lateral and anterior position in a child up to age 5 years.
- Bulging intercostal spaces can be normal in a child on a chest radiograph.

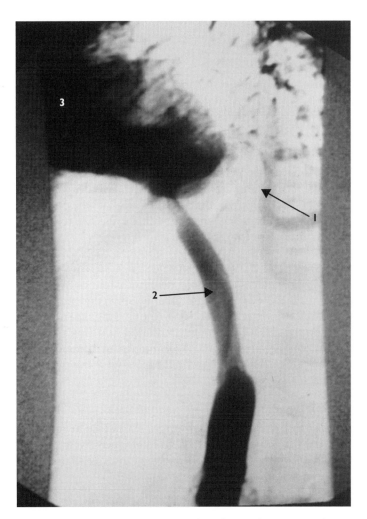

Fig. 3.20 Inferior vena cavogram: this abnormal cavogram due to Budd–Chiari disease shows reflux into the azygos, demonstrated through the azygos venous system (1). Inferior vena cava, with stenosis (2), and liver (3).

Openings of the diaphragm

There are three openings in the diaphragm:

- T8: the IVC and right phrenic nerve pierce the right dome of the diaphragm.
- T10: oesophagus and vagus nerves and left gastric vessels.
- T12: aorta, thoracic duct and ayzgos veins pass through the crura which lie posteriorly (Fig. 3.23).
- 'C 3, 4, 5 keeps the diaphragm alive'.
- The gas bubble under the left hemidiaphragm helps in recognition of the left hemidiaphragm. It is important to establish what is the diaphragm in lower lobe pathology in case there is a diaphragmatic hernia, etc.

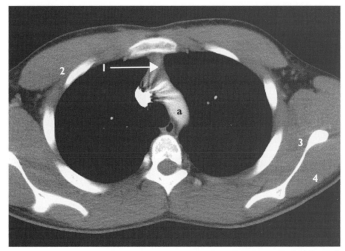

Fig. 3.22 Post-contrast CT of the chest showing the thymus (1): shows its characteristic shape which can normally be seen in children or young adults. Pectoralis major muscle (2), subscapularis (3), infraspinatus muscle (4). a = aortic arch.

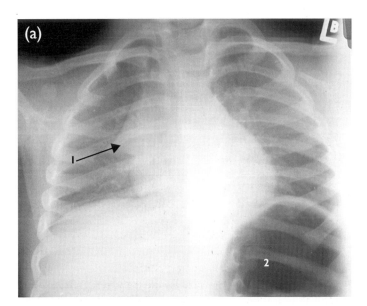

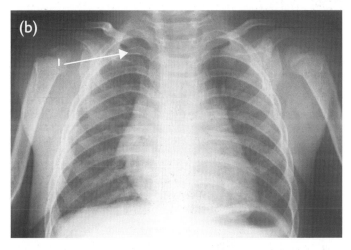

Fig. 3.21 Chest radiographs: two different infants with the infantile thymus causing a variety of shadows in the infant on chest radiograph. (a) Sail sign. Thymus (1). Stomach bubble (2), which may be very large in infants when crying. (b) Widened superior mediastinum.

- The normal diaphragm is 2–3 mm thick. When the lungs are hyperinflated, the diaphragmatic slips can be seen passing upwards, and can simulate a small pleural effusion.
- Each hemidiaphragm has a large centrally placed tendon which the IVC pierces to the right slightly anteriorly.

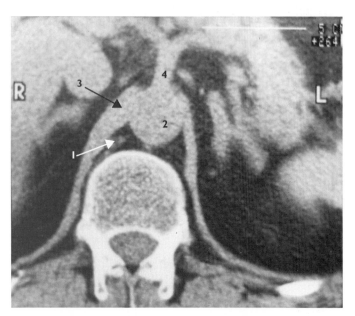

Fig. 3.23 CT of the upper abdomen post-contrast showing the aortic hiatus at T12 with the azygos running through (1). Aorta (2), crural (3) and coeliac (4).

IMAGING

Imaging of the chest

The chest radiograph

The standard views are PA, lateral, anteroposterior (AP) and supine.

PA chest radiograph (Fig. 3.24)
This is the standard view taken in the erect position on full inspiration. Poor inspiratory effort or an expiratory film can simulate a basal pneumonitis. The scapulae are projected away from the lungs by abducting the arms. The following are the important things to assess for.

Centring
The spinous processes should lie equidistant between the clavicles. If there is a greater distance between the spinous processes and medial clavicle on one side, then this is the side to which the patient is rotated and this side will appear more transradiant. A difference in transradiancy could wrongly be called without assessing if the patient is rotated.

Adequate inspiration
In most individuals the diaphragm should lie at or lower than the fifth or sixth anterior rib interspace. Poor inspiration creates false abnormalities in the lung vasculature and false consolidation.

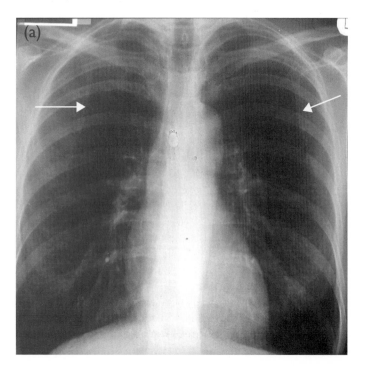

Fig. 3.24 (a) Standard PA chest radiograph: the scapulae are projected off the lung fields (arrows). Rotation is assessed by looking at the medial end of the clavicles and the spinous process. There is no rotation in this case.

Heart size

The heart size reflects the position of the left ventricular apex. The cardiothoracic ratio (CTR) is used to assess heart size on a PA chest radiograph (Fig. 3.24). The CTR is around 50% in most individuals, although it can be difficult to assess if there is large cardiac fat pad or a poor inspiratory effort. In black and Asian individuals it can be up to 55%.

The hila

The hilum is made up of the upper lobe vein and the lower lobe artery (Fig. 3.25). The following rules help interpret abnormality and aid detection of volume loss/collapse:
- The left hilum is never lower than the right hilum.
- The left hilum can be up to 2 cm higher than the right hilum or the same height as the right hilum.
- The hilar angle is approximately 120°. This may be altered in lobar collapse.
- The hila are important to assess for shape, contour and density for masses, and for position to assess volume loss. The hila should be equally dense and of approximately equal size.
- The transverse diameter of the pulmonary vessels can be used to assess for plethora and pulmonary hypertension.
- The transverse diameter of the lower lobe artery 1 cm below the hilar point should be 15 mm or less in a female and 16 mm or less in a male.

Stripes

Within the mediastinum various stripes can be detected that aid detection of lymphadenopathy or masses (Fig. 3.26):

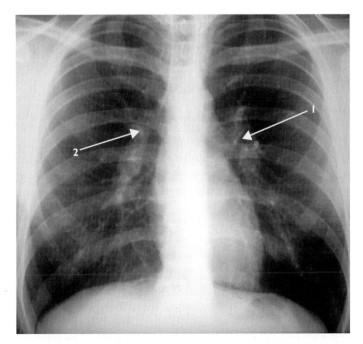

Fig. 3.25 PA chest radiograph: the hilum. The left hilum is marked by (1). In this case it lies at the same height as the right hilum (2). The left hilum should never be lower than the right hilum.

- Right paratracheal stripe: a thin line of soft tissue adjacent to the right side of the trachea. This should be <5 mm.
- Right and left paravertebral stripes: found towards the lower chest adjacent to the vertebra. The left stripe is <10 mm and the right <2 mm. The left is usually wider due to the presence of the descending thoracic aorta. This can be widened by an ectatic aorta, excess fat or a hypertrophic psoas muscle (Fig. 3.26b).
- Azygo-oesophageal line: created by the right lung abutting the azygos vein and oesophagus. Posterior mediastinal lymphadenopathy can be detected by a change in contour of this stripe. This usually has a concave or straight shape as it ascends cranially to the right. A bulge or convexity in the contour would imply pathology/lymphadenopathy, left atrial enlargement (Fig. 3.26b).

Diaphragm

The position of the diaphragm will be affected by volume loss due to lobar collapse. This may lead to an elevation of the diaphragm whereas consolidation will cause a loss of the silhouette of the diaphragm.
- Pleural fluid will blunt the cardiophrenic and costophrenic angles.
- The highest point on the diaphragm should be just medial to the lung midline. A subpulmonary effusion causes 'lateral tenting' with the highest point displaced laterally.
- The diaphragm can be normally lobulated, called a dromedary hump (Fig. 3.27).

Rules

- The right hemidiaphragm can be up to 3 cm higher than the left.
- The left can be same height as the right (9%).
- The left can be up to 1.5 cm higher than the right, but never more (3%).
- Hyperinflation of the lungs will lead to flattening of the diaphragms. A line drawn across the dome of the diaphragmatic insertions at the costophrenic and cardiophrenic angles on a PA chest radiograph, with a perpendicular dropped from its midpoint, will show flattening if this measures <1.5 cm.

Fissures

- The horizontal or transverse fissure can be viewed on the PA chest radiograph and the oblique fissure can be viewed on the lateral chest radiograph.
- Normally the horizontal fissure arises 1 cm below the hilar point. For a fissure to be visualized on a radiograph it has to be tangential to the beam. The position of the fissure can aid in the detection of volume loss or collapse in the lung. An elevated horizontal fissure is seen in right upper lobe collapse.
- Azygos fissure: commonly seen as made up of four layers of pleura, it is seen in 1% of postmortem examinations (Fig. 3.28) and its presence is not pathological.

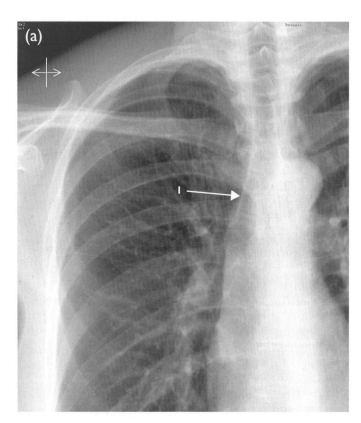

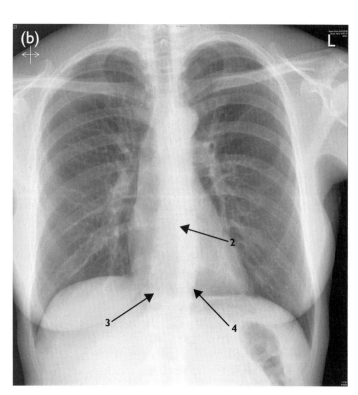

Fig. 3.26 PA chest radiograph – zoomed view. The right paratracheal stripe is demonstrated, which should measure no more than 3 mm (1). The vascular markings of the superior vena cava gradually fade into the distance and are not to be confused with the right paratracheal stripe. (b) PA chest radiograph: the azygo-oesophageal line (2) can be seen behind the heart as the azygos curves up towards the superior vena cava. The paravertebral stripes are demonstrated, measuring up to 2 mm on the right (3) and 10 mm on the left (4).

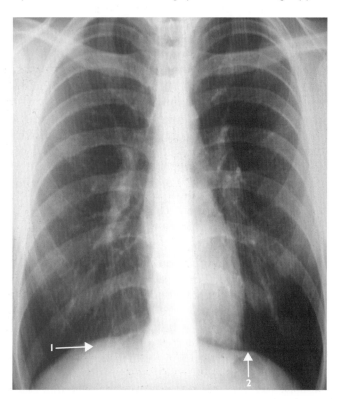

Fig. 3.27 PA chest radiograph: the diaphragm. The right (1) can be higher than the left (2) and the left can be higher than the right by only up to 1.5 cm.

Bones

The ribs and clavicles should be assessed for erosion, particularly the distal ends of the clavicles. The flange of the rib in which the neurovascular bundle passes inferiorly may appear irregular, but the ribs generally all have the same appearance on the undersurface. The thoracic spine can be seen through the mediastinum. Cervical ribs may be present.

Mediastinal nodes

- The right paratracheal stripe, hila, subcarinal region and paravertebral regions, and aortopulmonary window/recess are all potential sites for lymphadenopathy.
- Subcarinal nodes will splay the carina; hilar nodes will increase the hilar density and give a lobulated contour. Different distribution of abnormal nodes alters the differential diagnosis, e.g. sarcoidosis causes bilateral hilar symmetrical lymphadenopathy and right paratracheal adenopathy (Fig. 3.28b).

Transradiancy

- To detect volume loss, look at hila position, diaphragm height, transradiancy, position of fissures and silhouette sign (Fig. 3.29). Difference in transradiancy can be seen in volume loss, but can also be seen in many other causes. The two lungs should normally be of equal transradiancy.

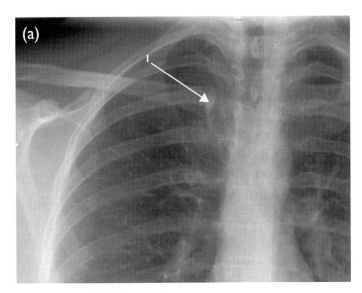

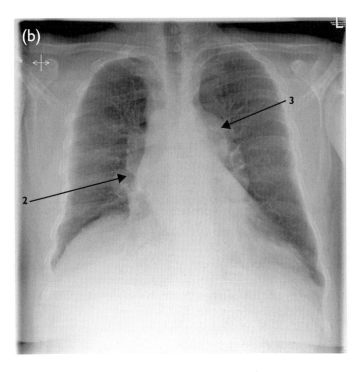

Fig. 3.28 (a) PA chest radiograph: the azygos (1) can cause a knob giving the impression of a soft-tissue density. This should measure <1 cm. (b) PA chest radiograph: bilateral hilar lymphadenopathy causing a dense lobulated appearance to the hila with loss of the normal hilar angle. Right hilum (2) and left hilum (3).

- If there is difference in transradiancy for no apparent cause, an expiratory film may show air trapping.
- It helps to view the chest anatomically from the chest wall to the pleura then lungs, thinking of all that can affect each anatomical area.
- Some causes of difference in transradiancy of the lungs:
  – outside the lungs: Poland's syndrome – absent pectoralis, mastectomy, breast implant, chest wall mass
  – pleural abnormality: pneumothorax, pleural fluid or mass
  – vascular pulmonary atresia/small pulmonary artery
  – lungs: air trapping – Macleod's syndrome.

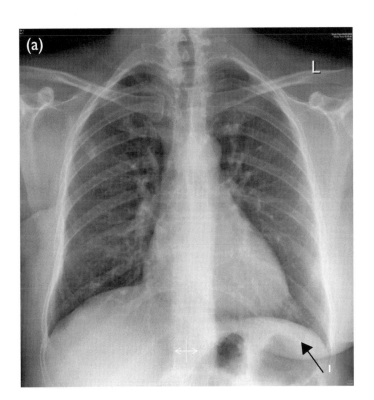

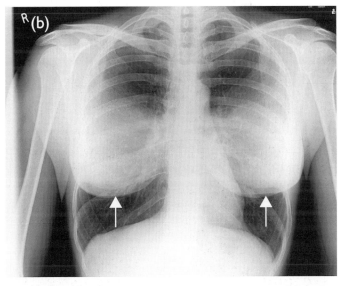

Fig. 3.29 PA chest radiograph: difference in transradiancy of the lungs. (a) The right lung is more transradiant than the left lung due to the right mastectomy. Left breast (1). This is one cause of a difference in transradiancy. (b) Chest radiograph of bilateral breast implants: cause bilateral increased density. A unilateral implant can cause abnormal unilateral transradiancy.

Normal variants that mimic pathology

- The normal thymus in neonates (Fig. 3.30).
- A pectus excavatum where the sternum is depressed causing:
  - the heart to be displaced to the left
  - right heart border obscuration, mimicking RML pathology
  - vertical anterior ribs
  - horizontal posterior ribs (Fig. 3.31)
  - clear visualization of the thoracic spine.
- A right-sided aortic arch:
  - may be a normal variant or associated with congenital heart disease
  - its absence on the left causes a prominent left hilum (Fig. 3.32).
- A cardiophrenic fat pad:
  - the fat pads lie in the cardiophrenic recesses
  - can look like an eventration of the diaphragm or pathology adjacent to the heart
  - on a lateral chest radiograph the cardiac incisura or fat pad is well seen
  - the IVC can be seen passing through the right hemidiaphragm into the right atrium.
- High kilovoltage/low kilovoltage: with digital radiographs this factor can be overcome by manipulating the image to see the mediastinum. Traditionally high-kilovoltage images lost bony and calcified detail while visualizing the mediastinum to greater advantage.

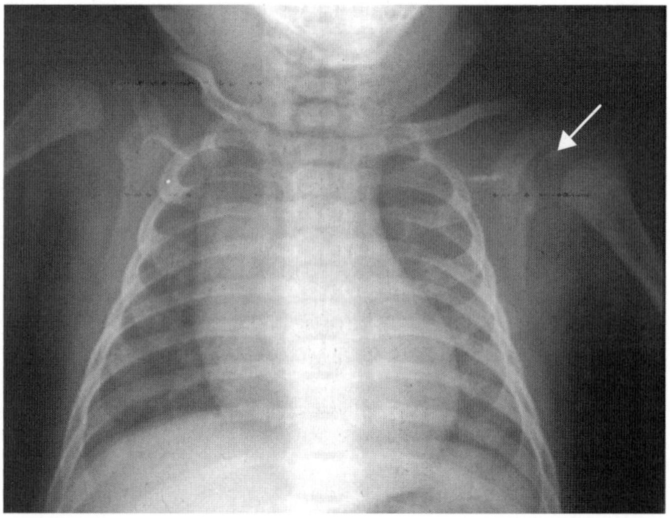

Interpretation of the chest radiograph

- Is there an anatomical marker?
- Is the film rotated?
- Is there any adequate inspiratory effort?
- Assess heart size.

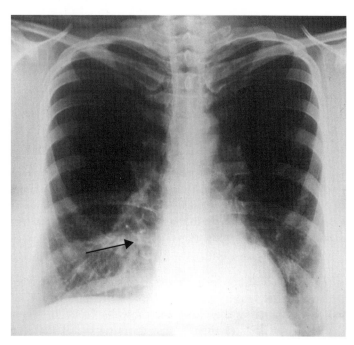

Fig. 3.31 Chest radiograph: pectus excavatum. Note the very vertical anterior ribs and horizontal posterior ribs. There is an obscured right heart border (arrow) mimicking right middle lobe collapse/consolidation.

Fig. 3.30 Chest radiograph of an infant. There is an apparent increase in heart size. The cardiothoracic ratio can be up to 0.6 in an infant. The humeral head ossification centre is noted, which should appear by the age of 1 year (arrow).

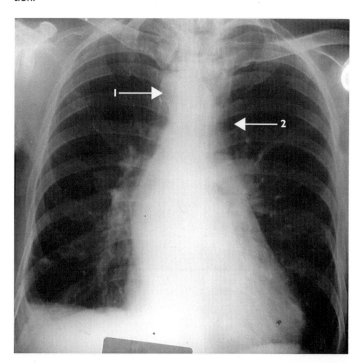

Fig. 3.32 PA chest radiograph: the right-sided aortic arch (1) causes an unusual appearance to the left hilum, which appears prominent (2).

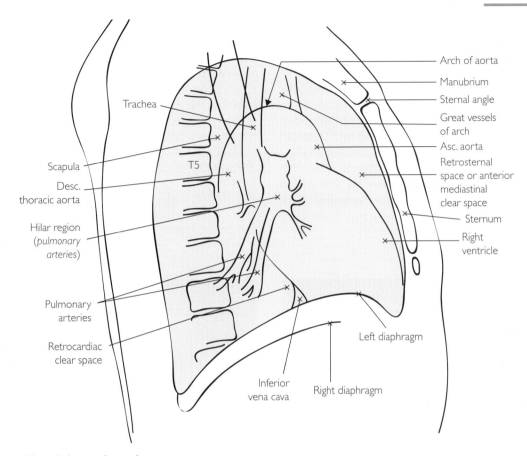

Fig. 3.33 Diagram of lateral chest radiograph.

- Look at the lungs. Use the silhouette sign, which is the interface between the lung and the mediastinal soft tissue. If the air at interface is removed due to collapse or a mass, the silhouette will be lost. However, if the interface is overlapped by a remote opacity the silhouette will still be seen.
- Are there cervical ribs? Look at the transverse processes.
- Bones and chest wall: rib variants and look at the undersurface of the ribs; the flange can look irregular.

Lung lesions

These can be simulated by:
- hair braid-calcified costal cartilages
- breast implants
- prominent transverse processes
- nipple shadows
- pulmonary vessels end on
- Skin folds and starched sheets can mimic pneumothorax.

Lateral chest radiograph

This is useful for quick evaluation of suspected pathology on a PA chest radiograph but has largely been superseded by CT (Fig. 3.33):
- The lateral chest radiograph is taken with the arms raised anteriorly, which can be seen running across the top of the image. It has a considerable radiation dose compared with a PA chest radiograph (Fig. 3.34).

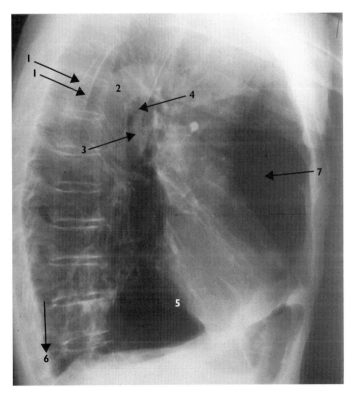

Fig. 3.34 Lateral chest radiograph: blades of scapulae (1), aortic arch (2), left pulmonary artery (3), aortopulmonary window (4) and left atrium (5). Increased transradiancy as one descends down the thoracic spine (6) and retrosternal fat space (7).

- The ascending aorta can be seen extending into the aortic arch. The descending aorta disappears as it descends on the image.
- The aortopulmonary window: this lies in between the arch of the aorta and the left pulmonary artery and conus. The contents are ligamentum arteriosum, lymph nodes, left vagus nerve, left bronchial artery and fat. These all begin with 'l' except fat.
- The retrosternal space is seen behind the sternum: this should normally be lucent and is a review site for an anterior mediastinal mass. This lies anterior to the heart.

- The trachea forms lucency towards the top of the image and the two bronchi can be seen end on as ring-like lucencies; the left pulmonary artery can be seen hooking over the left main bronchus. The left main bronchus is below the right main bronchus.
- There should normally be an increase in transradiancy inferiorly over the thoracic spine. If an increase in opacity is seen on descending down the thoracic spine on a lateral chest radiograph, collapse or a mass may be present.

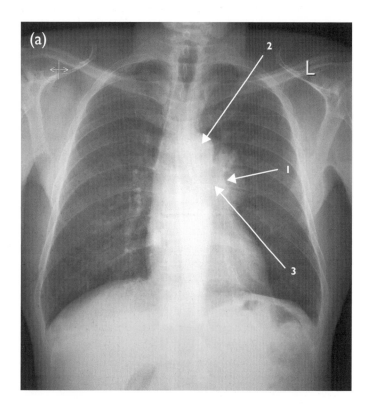
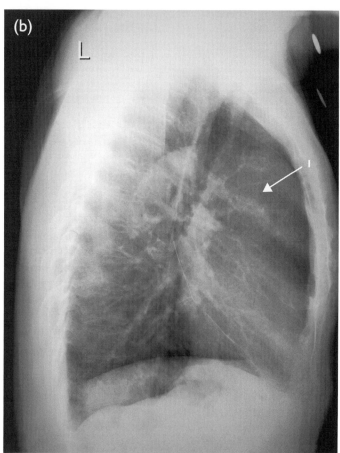

Fig. 3.35 (a) PA chest radiograph: large soft mass (1) at the left hilum. The aortic knuckle (2) and left hilar vessel (3) can be seen clearly separate, indicating an anterior mass. (b) The lateral chest radiograph confirms an anterior mass (1).

Rules and lines on a lateral chest radiograph
- Retrosternal line 3 mm: this is a line taken along the posterior aspect of the sternum. Pathology in the sternum, e.g. metastasis, may increase the soft tissues.
- Parasternal line <7.5 mm: this is the wavy line alongside the sternum, which may be increased due to lymphadenopathy in the nodes around.
- Retrosternal lucency. (Fig. 3.35).
- There should be an increase in transradiancy as one descends the chest on a lateral chest radiograph.

Sternal views
- High radiation dose and now largely superseded by CT. Note retrosternal and parasternal lines. There is a high probability of mediastinal trauma if there is a sternal fracture (Fig. 3.36).

CT of the chest

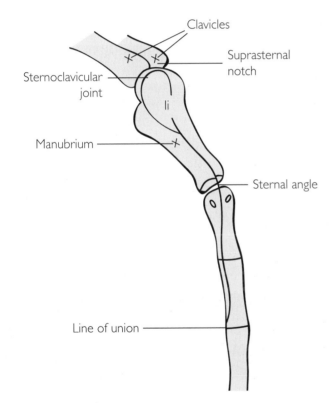

Clavicles

Suprasternal notch

Sternoclavicular joint

li

Manubrium

Sternal angle

Line of union

Fig. 3.36 Sternal diagram.

Indications
CT is the most sensitive mode for evaluating the lung parenchyma, the airways, for tumour staging, diagnosis and follow-up of pulmonary and mediastinal lesions, and detection of occult thoracic lesions.
- CT pulmonary angiography is now a routine investigation.
- High-resolution thin-section CT (HRCT) evaluates the lung parenchyma.

- CT can be useful in identifying the presence of fat or feeding vessels to a lung mass.

Technique
The technique depends on whether the whole lung is to be examined or part of it as in HRCT, when a disseminated process can be evaluated by discontinuous scans.
- Oral contrast is not given unless oesophageal malignancy is suspected.
- Intravenous contrast should always be used for investigation of mediastinal, pleural and focal intrapulmonary lesions, and for all vascular studies.
- The patient lies supine with arms elevated. Scans are taken on full inspiration. The prone position is used to differentiate subpleural gravitational change in the lung bases from subpleural fibrosis on HRCT. Expiratory scans are performed in HRCT if there is variation in lung parenchymal density to exaggerate air trapping. Multislice CT has meant that the whole chest including the adrenals in most individuals can be scanned on a single breath-hold.
- Images are taken from the thoracic inlet to the posterior pleural space or lower, to include the adrenal glands in suspected thoracic malignancy.
- The window settings: the chest must always be reviewed on the two standard window settings: 40/400 or 60/400 for the mediastinum and between −350/1000 and −650/1500 for lung parenchyma. Without using both windows and relying solely on the mediastinal windows, lung pathology will be missed. The slices can be thickened to look for lung nodules using maximum intensity projection (MIP) (Fig. 3.37).
- An example of a possible intravenous protocol in the chest is a 25- to 30-s delay: 100 ml of contrast at 2–3 ml/s. Bolus tracking can estimate the ideal contrast delay in CT pulmonary angiography (CTPA) or in patients with poor cardiac function.
- Low-dose CT is used for screening of bronchogenic cancer in some centres.
- Virtual bronchoscopy is a three-dimensional visualization technique of the bronchial tree requiring various interactive tools using a high-resolution data-set.

Cross-sectional anatomy and findings
The anatomy is the same but the axial appearance different, and can be discussed at each anatomical level.

Standard anatomical section 1 (Fig. 3.38)
- At the level of the sternal notch at T2 the great vessels arising from the aorta can be seen. Remember that CT is reviewed as if looking from the end of the bed, hence the brachiocephalic artery lies on the right, then left common carotid and left subclavian artery.
- The right paratracheal stripe is the bare area adjacent to the trachea and is a review area for abnormal soft tissue.
- The brachiocephalic veins can be seen anteriorly. Only one is opacified, which is the side of the arm used for

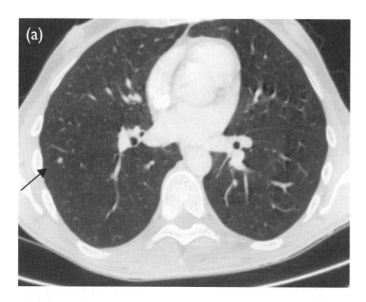

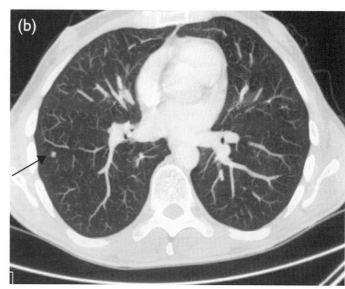

Fig. 3.37 Axial CT of the chest: lung windows using (a) normal slices and (b) maximum intensity projection (MIP) of three slices showing the difference in the lung parenchyma. On the MIP images in (a) nodules and lines are easier to see. Luna nodule (arrow).

intravenous contrast. The left brachiocephalic vein looks like a banana anteriorly.

- Normal thymus may be present in the anterior mediastinum (see Fig. 3.22).

Standard section 2 (Fig. 3.39)

- At the level of T4 the aortic arch is visible and the SVC. Filling defects may be apparent in the SVC due to mixing of unopacified blood from one arm with opacified blood from the other arm; this may appear as a low-density area.

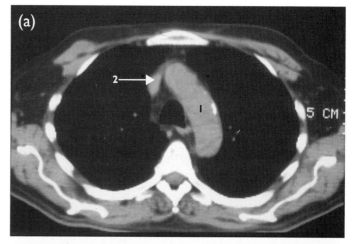

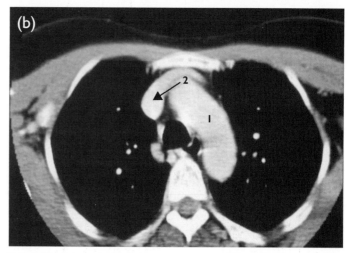

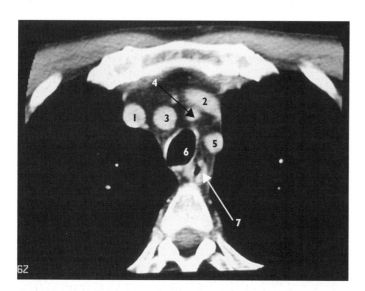

Fig. 3.38 Axial CT of the chest, standard section 1. Great vessels: Left brachiocephalic vein (1), right brachiocephalic vein (2), brachiocephalic artery (3), left common carotid artery (4), subclavian artery (5), trachea (6) and oesophagus (7).

Fig. 3.39 CT of the aortic arch: (a) pre- and (b) post-contrast aortic arch (1). Superior vena cava (2).

Standard section 3: CT aortopulmonary window (Fig. 3.40)

- Just below the aortic arch and above the pulmonary artery lies the aortopulmonary window, an important review area for lymphadenopathy.
- The azygos vein can be seen draining into the back of the SVC at this level. It is normal to have backflow of intravenous contrast into the azygos vein; it does not imply SVC obstruction unless there are other signs to support this such as a mass obstructing the SVC.
- There may be a pretracheal node at this level measuring up to 1 cm in short axis diameter. Nodes are measured in their shortest diameter; in the chest, other than retrocrural nodes with a normal short axis of 6 mm, the normal short axis diameter of nodes is 1 cm in all regions.
- The superior pericardial recess is a superior extension of the pericardium which can almost reach the right para-

tracheal region that lies behind the ascending aorta and causes confusion with pathology. It has the CT number of fluid (Fig. 3.41).

Standard section 4 (Fig. 3.42)
There are important differences between the hila.

Right hilum
The relationship from anterior to posterior is vein, artery, bronchus (VAB) – the right pulmonary artery runs in front of the bronchus and so there should be no soft tissue behind bronchus intermedius. Careful review of this area is necessary.

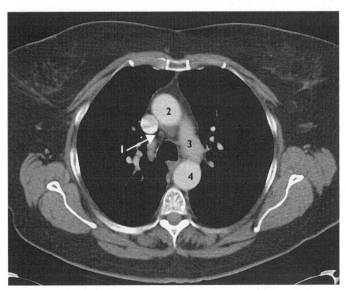

Fig. 3.41 CT post-contrast of the chest: the superior pericardial recess lies behind the ascending aorta, is of fluid density and can mimic lymphadenopathy (1). Ascending aorta (2), descending aorta (3) and pulmonary artery (4).

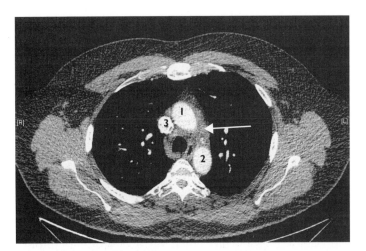

Fig. 3.40 CT post-intravenous contrast of aortopulmonary window. Ascending aorta (1), descending aorta (2) and superior vena cava (3). White arrow marks the aortopulmonary window.

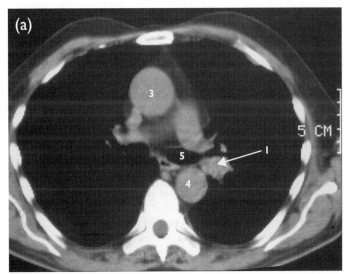

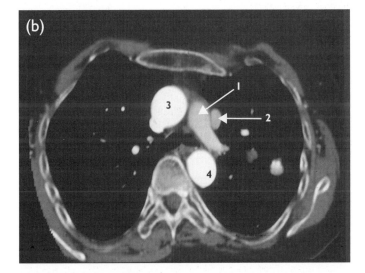

Fig. 3.42 CT scan: (a) pre- and (b) post-contrast of the left hilum; shows the left pulmonary artery (1) hooking over the left main bronchus. Left pulmonary vein (2). Ascending aorta (3), descending aorta (4) and left main bronchus (5).

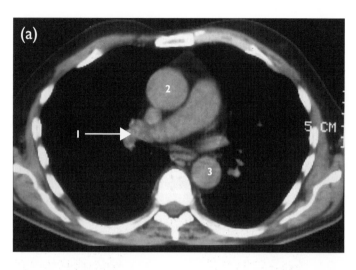

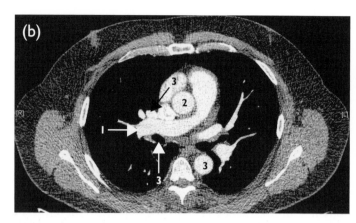

Fig. 3.43 (a) Pre- and (b) post-contrast CT of the right hilum shows the right pulmonary artery (1) running anteriorly to the right bronchus (b). Ascending aorta (2), descending aorta (3) and right pulmonary cein (4).

Left hilum

The relationship from anterior to posterior is vein, bronchus, artery (VBA) – the left pulmonary artery hooks over the left main bronchus, so the artery is seen behind the bronchus on axial CT. The left pulmonary artery hooks over left main bronchus to run posteriorly.

Standard section 5 (Fig. 4.43)

- At the level of right pulmonary artery running in front of right bronchus intermedius. There should be a bare area behind the right bronchus intermedius, i.e. no soft tissue should be visible. The right pulmonary vein lies anteriorly. At this level the descending left pulmonary artery is visible behind the left bronchus.
- The subcarinal region can be reviewed for lymphadenopathy. The oesophagus is seen tucked in between the descending aorta and the azygos vein.
- The pulmonary arteries can be well seen to look for filling defects but care must be taken not to confuse with the pulmonary veins (Fig. 3.44).

Standard section 6 (Fig. 3.45)

The left atrium is seen posteriorly with the pulmonary veins draining into it. The left ventricle forms the left heart border and the myocardium can be visualized due to its thickness. The pericardium is visible as a thin dense line on CT separated from the heart by epicardial fat.

Lung windows

- Normal bronchi: standard CT can define fourth-order bronchi (3 mm), while HRCT can define eighth-order bronchi (1–2 mm). CT relies on detection of the normal bronchial wall. CT cannot usually resolve bronchi in the lung periphery within 2–3 cm of the subpleural space. The presence of visible bronchi in the lung periphery implies abnormality. The bronchi are not normally bigger than the corresponding vessel. If dilated the bronchus gives an appearance of a reverse signet ring next to a vessel (Fig. 3.46).
- Lung parenchyma on HRCT: the smallest anatomical unit that can be identified on HRCT is the secondary

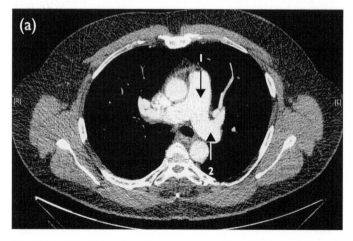

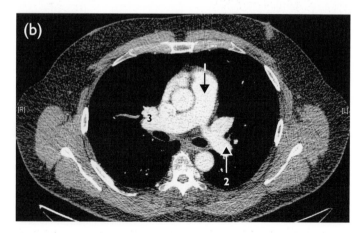

Fig. 3.44 CT of (a) main pulmonary artery (1) and (b) two different levels. The left pulmonary artery (2) and the pulmonary veins (3).

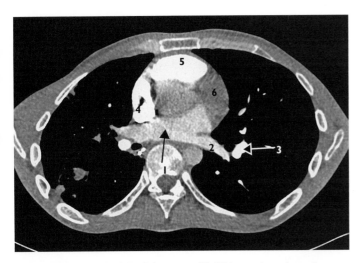

Fig. 3.45 CT level of the left atrium (1). This receives the pulmonary veins (2), which should not be confused with pulmonary arteries (3) when looking at a CT pulmonary angiogram. Right atrium (4), right ventricle (5), left ventricle (6).

lobule which has a characteristic polygonal shape with an edge length of 1–2.5 cm. It has a central arteriole and bronchiole.

- The fissures are normally seen only on lung windows. The horizontal fissure on axial images is a bare area in the centre of the left lung as the fissure runs parallel to the axial slice. The oblique fissure can be seen running from posterior to anterior on HRCT.
- The lung window is used to look for interstitial lung disease (Fig. 3.47), for metastases, to look for a pneumothorax and to measure the size of lung masses (Fig. 3.48).

Interpretation of CT of the chest

Develop a system to follow when reporting CT and adhere to it on every occasion because this makes an area of review less likely to be forgotten and, second, an individual reporting pattern develops which enables recognition of an individual's reports from the style used.

1. Mediastinum: assess for nodes, vascular rings, aortic calibre, mediastinal masses, pulmonary emboli.
2. Look for nodes in the anterior mediastinum: anterior to ascending aorta, right paratracheal region, aorto-

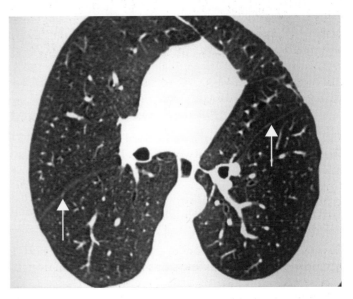

Fig. 3.47 CT chest lung windows showing the fissures (arrows) clearly. Any difference in lung density, such as increase or decrease, should be observed.

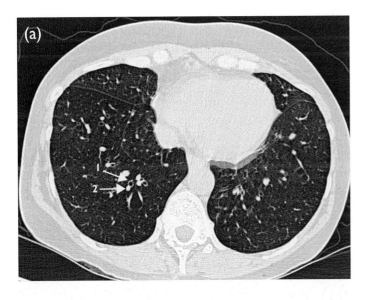

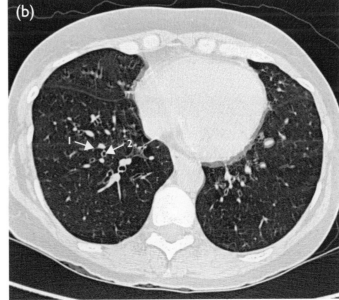

Fig. 3.46 CT chest lung windows: (a,b) two different levels showing the bronchi. The bronchi (1) should not be wider in diameter on CT than their corresponding artery (2). If the bronchus is bigger than the artery this would implicate bronchiectasis.

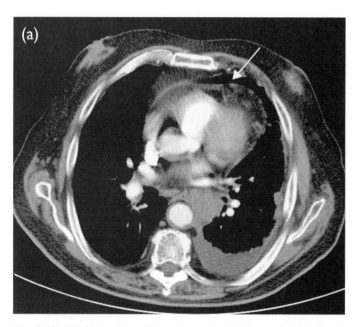

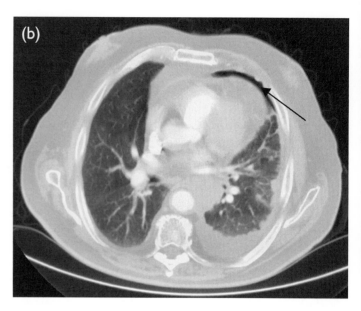

Fig. 3.48 CT of the chest: (a) mediastinal and (b) lung windows. The lung windows are required in order to detect a pneumothorax (arrow). This may not be seen on mediastinal windows.

pulmonary recess, hila, posterior mediastinum and retrocrural.

Review lung windows on every occasion. With HRCT decide if prone or expiration scans are required.

Interstitial lung disease

Checklist
This can be helpful when first reporting HRCT to help focus on possible pathology:
- Is there bronchiectasis? Are the bronchi bigger than vessels? Signet ring?

- Are there lines subpleurally or honeycombing? Fibrosis?
- Are there bullae or air trapping? Emphysema?
- Are there nodules?
- Is lung density normal? Too black/transradiant? Air trapping?
- Is the parenchyma too dense, which can occur in ground-glass shadowing, or too 'black' in air trapping?
- Do any nodules have haloes that can indicate fungal infection?

Pitfalls
- Pseudo-tumours: the hemidiaphragms on a single cut can mimic a parenchymal mass, especially if the patient

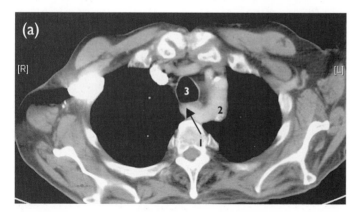

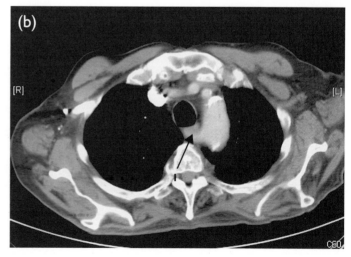

Fig. 3.49 CT of the chest: an anomalous right subclavian artery (1) is demonstrated running posterior to the trachea at two different levels. (a) Just above the arch and (b) at the level of the arch. This creates a vascular ring that can cause dysphagia and tracheal stenosis. Aortic arch (2) and trachea (3).

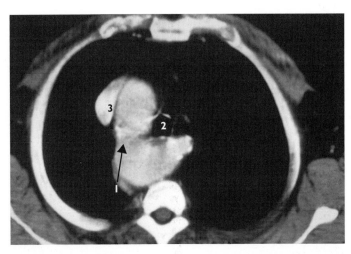

Fig. 3.50 CT of right-sided aortic arch. A right-sided aortic arch (1) is demonstrated with a vascular ring around the trachea (2). Superior vena cava (3).

has breathed during the scan. Use scrolling to go up and down through the chest to assess what is a normal anatomical structure. The first rib can mimic a mass.

- Variants – vascular anomalies, such as right arch, vascular rings, high aortic arch, which may be seen in coarctation of the aorta, a right-sided aortic arch often associated with a vascular ring running behind the trachea and oesophagus such as an anomalous subclavian (Figs 3.49 and 3.50).

CT pulmonary angiography

- Catheter pulmonary angiography, due to its invasive nature, has been superseded by CTPA and nuclear medicine ventilation–perfusion scans.
- Nuclear medicine ventilation–perfusion scans provide a probability estimate of acute pulmonary embolism (PE). The best results are obtained in previously healthy patients with a normal chest radiograph. Poor results are obtained with ventilation–perfusion imaging in patients with an abnormal chest radiograph or known cardiopulmonary disease. In this population CTPA is the investigation of choice for acute PE.

Indication
CTPA is the first-line investigation in evaluating stable patients with suspected PE with an abnormal chest radiograph or cardiac or pulmonary lung disease.

Technique
- Multislice CT enables thin section imaging with good intravascular contrast medium opacification.
- Bolus tracking is used to optimize pulmonary arterial enhancement. High-contrast flow rates greater than 3 ml/s optimize enhancement. Thin-slab MIP can be helpful in evaluating peripheral emboli (Fig. 3.51).

Findings
- These are intraluminal filling defects or lack of enhancement of an artery. Emboli get trapped at bifurcations or in vessels of smaller calibre than the embolus.
- False-positive findings: breathing and pulsation artefact, partial volume effects, hilar lymph nodes, unenhanced pulmonary veins, differential enhancement of arteries. The veins are medial to the lower lobe arteries and separate from the bronchi.
- False-negative findings: breathing and pulsation artefact, high-contrast artefact, poor vascular enhancement, partial volume effects.

Imaging of the heart

Cardiac CT

Multi-detector row CT has developed as a non-invasive imaging technique for the heart. It can morphologically image the heart, perform calcium scoring and detect coronary artery disease with CT angiography (CTA). ECG synchronization of data is used to capture the heart in a relatively motionless phase.

Calcium scoring

Indications
The rationale behind calcium scoring is that calcium in coronary vessels can be easily seen due to the high CT number (in HU) of calcium. Atherosclerotic plaques in the coronary arterial wall begin much earlier than luminal stenosis and frequently calcify; CT calcium scoring is designed to detect these plaques.

Technique
Multislice CT is performed unenhanced with ECG gating. The heart rate may be slowed medically to 65 beats/min to improve image acquisition. Total calcium load in the coronary arteries is quantified using a calcium-scoring algorithm. A threshold of 90–130 HU is applied to the whole image set and tissues with a CT number equal or higher than the set threshold are identified as calcified lesions (Fig. 3.52).

CT coronary angiography

Indications
This is a non-invasive technique for assessing coronary artery stenosis.

Technique
Intravenous contrast is used with bolus tracking similar to CTPA. A suggested regimen is 100 ml of contrast at 5 ml/s. A continuous spiral scan is acquired with ECG recording. Oversampling is used with a low pitch so that data are acquired from each part of the cardiac cycle. The heart is therefore scanned more than once.

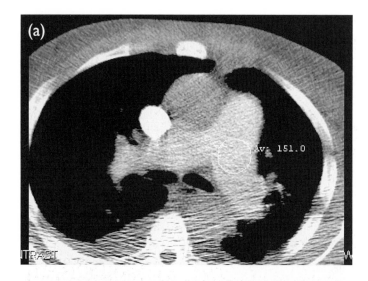

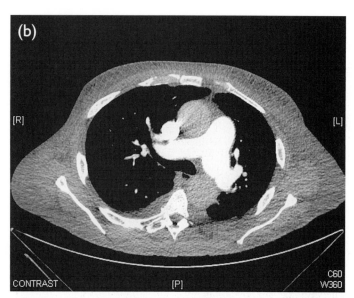

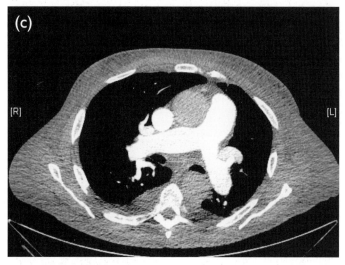

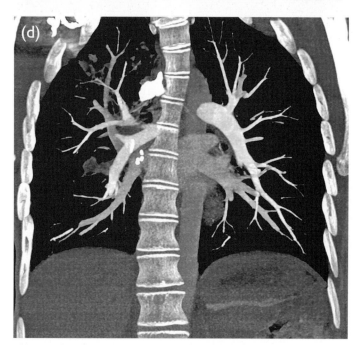

Fig. 3.51 CT pulmonary angiogram. (a) Bolus tracking that aids optimal opacification of the pulmonary arteries; (b,c) good opacification of the pulmonary arteries; (d) maximum intensity projection (MIP) coronal images thickening the slices, showing the pulmonary arteries to advantage.

Cardiac and chest MRI

Indications

MRI is used to assess cardiac anatomy, function and flow with minimal risk to the patient. It is absolutely contraindicated in patients with a permanent pacemaker.

MRI can be used for problem-solving in thoracic malignancy to assess Pancoast's tumours (Fig. 3.53).

Left ventriculography and aortography

Indications

A thoracic aortogram may be done as part of a cardiac or head and neck study, or to evaluate the aorta itself. CT now does most of the investigation for aortic aneurysms and dissections. Aortography is still required for intervention and stent insertion.

Technique

A percutaneous femoral approach is used. A flexible-ended 'j' wire is introduced through a cutting needle:

- A pigtail catheter with six side holes is introduced over the wire for the aortogram.
- Contrast is injected using a pump injector at about 15–20 ml/s for a flush aortogram, with a pigtail catheter.
- If multiple catheter changes are expected a sheath is used. For a left ventricular angiogram the catheter is passed into the left ventricle (Figs 3.54 and 3.55).

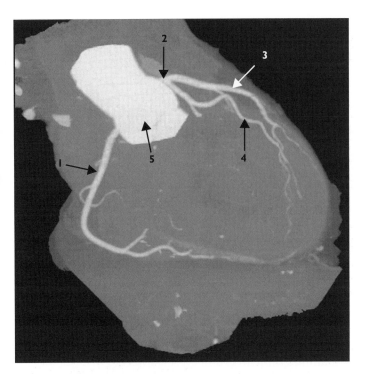

Fig. 3.52 CT coronary angiogram: (1) right coronary artery; (2) left main stem; (3) left anterior descending; (4) circumflex; and (5) ascending aorta.

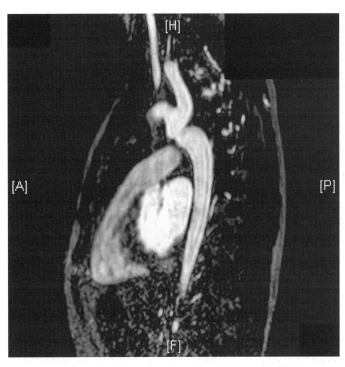

Fig. 3.53 MRI of the chest: sagittal image showing the vascular structures.

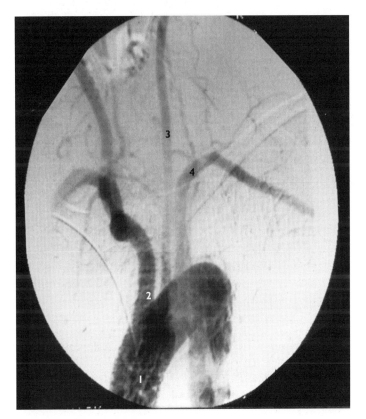

Fig. 3.54 CT aortogram: angiography can be used to look at the great vessels before performing head and neck angiography or coronary angiography. A pigtail catheter is used. Aorta (1), brachiocephalic artery (2), left common carotid artery (3) and left subclavian artery (4).

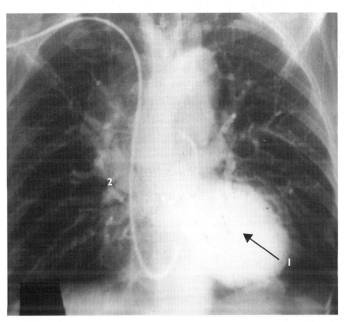

Fig. 3.55 Conventional pulmonary angiogram. This is the late venous phase of a pulmonary angiogram showing the left ventricle (1) with the pulmonary veins (2) draining into the left atrium. The catheter is in the pulmonary artery.

Findings

The aortic arch is seen on a left anterior oblique view, with the great vessels clearly seen arising from the arch.

Coronary angiography

Technique

Coronary angiography involves selective injection of contrast into the right and left coronary arteries and into the left ventricle for a left ventriculogram.

- A catheter can be introduced from the arm, the Sones' technique, using the brachial artery, or using the femoral artery in the groin.
- Disposable preshaped catheters are used which are different for each artery and the left ventricle – Judkins or Amplatz can be used. Three catheters are required for each examination.
- Each coronary artery is found at its aortic valve cusp. Hand injections are used for the coronary arteries themselves and a pump injector for the left ventriculogram phase.

Findings

- Congenital variation of coronary anatomy is common such as the circumflex can originate from the right coronary artery or rarely the LAD can arise from the circumflex. These make catheterization difficult.
- The vessel that supplies the posterior descending artery to the inferior surface of the heart is called dominant. There is usually right dominance, i.e. the right coronary artery supplies the inferior heart/posterior descending artery. The right coronary may be small when the left circumflex supplies the inferior heart, called left dominance (Fig. 3.56).

Imaging the bronchial tree

Bronchography

Indication

This investigation has been superseded by CT virtual bronchoscopy is non-invasive and can image the tracheobronchial tree, but CT cannot replace fibreoptic bronchoscopy and biopsy. Knowledge of the bronchopulmonary anatomy is required for CT to enable accurate location of the tumour (Fig. 3.57).

Technique

A thin section data-set is required as obtained with multislice CT. Perspective rendering and interactive tools are required to give the impression that the observer is moving in the data volume.

BREAST AND MAMMOGRAPHY

Breast

Anatomy

- The breast extends into the axilla as the axillary tail. Each mammary gland consists of 15–20 lobes which radiate out from the nipple. The main duct from each lobe opens separately on to the nipple. The pigmented skin around the nipple is the areola, which has small areolar glands forming tubercles on it. Fibrous septa separate the lobes.
- Within each lobe are 50–80 lobules of glandular breast tissue (Fig. 3.58).
- The breast is made up of glandular tissue, ducts and fatty tissue. Cooper's ligaments are found throughout the breast. The amount of dense glandular tissue decreases with age when the fatty tissue increases. In lactation and pregnancy the amount of glandular tissue increases. In general younger women in their 20s have dense breast and postmenopausal women tend to have fatty breast, although there are exceptions to this. In the dense breast mammography has limited sensitivity.

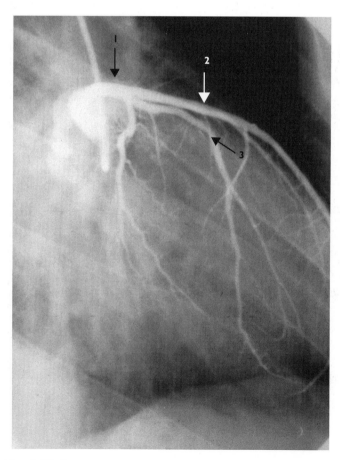

Fig. 3.56 Coronary angiogram: left main stem selective coronary angiogram showing the left main stem (1), the left anterior descending (2) and the circumflex (3).

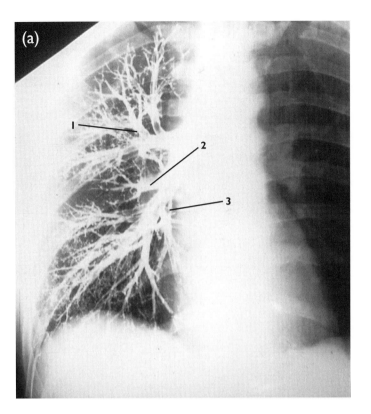

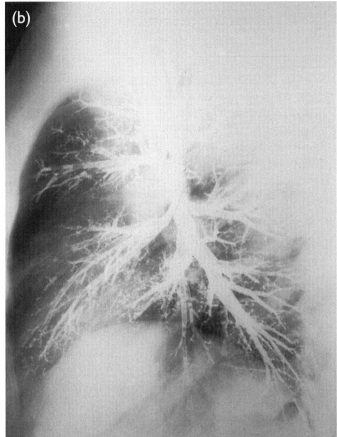

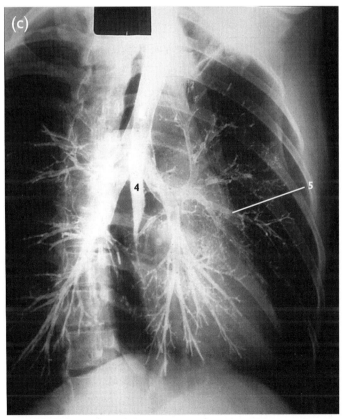

Fig. 3.57 Bronchogram: (a) AP; (b) lateral; (c) oblique. Right upper lobe bronchi posterior segment (1), middle lobe bronchi (2), lower lobe medial basal segment (3), reflux into the oesophagus (4) and superior segment of lingula (5).

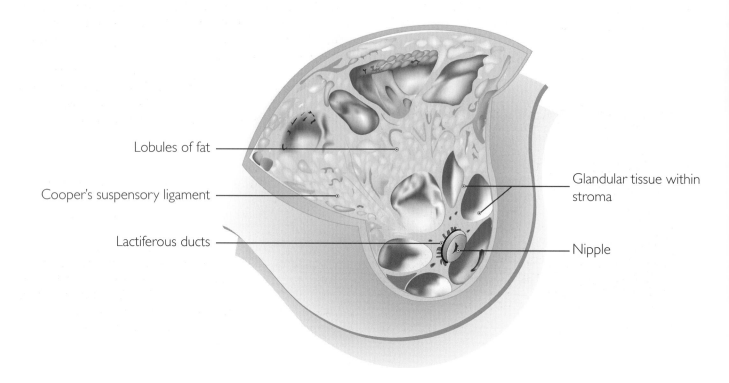

Lobules of fat

Cooper's suspensory ligament

Lactiferous ducts

Glandular tissue within stroma

Nipple

Fig. 3.58 Diagram of the breast.

Mammography

Indications

Breast imaging is divided into two populations and disciplines: breast screening that is imaging the supposedly well asymptomatic woman, aiming to detect breast cancer at an early curable stage, and symptomatic breast imaging for women with symptoms of breast pain, a breast lump, nipple discharge, etc.

Techniques

The two main techniques are mammography and ultrasound. MRI is used as a problem-solving tool and is to be introduced as a screening technique in the young women at high risk of breast cancer in 2009.

- Mammography is the mode of choice for breast screening in the 50–70 age group. The screening programme in the UK is being extended in 2009 to include 47–70 year olds. Breast screening is offered to this population every 3 years.
- Mammography is also the first-line imaging mode in the older symptomatic woman, i.e. age >35–40 years, the age cut-off depending on the individual unit. Under 35 years of age breast ultrasound is the primary mode of choice. Digital mammography is becoming the mainstay of mammography, being faster and of increased sensitivity in the dense breast than conventional mammography (Figs 3.59 and 3.60).
- Irradiation can induce carcinoma in the breast. However, the cancer induction rate from mammography is extremely low and it is impossible to predict the low dose–risk relationship. There appears to be a latent period of 15–17 years. The women most at risk form the radiation of mammography are the 20- to 34-year-old group.
- Techniques are used in mammography to ensure a low dose to the breast while providing excellent resolution and maximizing contrast between adjacent structures. The anode is changed to molybdenum with a low kilvoltage of 28 kV. A molybdenum filter may be used. Alternative anodes are tungsten or rhodium for the larger breast when a large dose is required. A monochromatic beam is used. The carbon tabletop enables a lower radiation dose to be used. Single-sided film was formerly used in conventional mammography or, in digital mammography, a selenium plate is used.
- The low kilovoltage enables very small calcium deposits to be detected.
- High resolution is needed to visualize microcalcifications and trabeculae.
- There is a long exposure time.
- There is a small anode.

- The window on the X-ray tube is made of beryllium.
- In mammography a constant potential generator is used.
- The resolution is related to the focal spot size. The smaller the spot size the better.

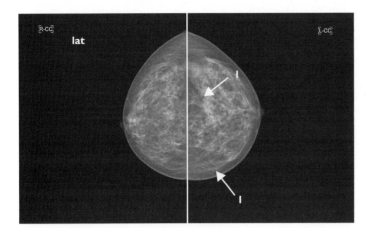

Fig. 3.59 Mammograms: craniocaudal (CC) mammograms: the anatomical marker is placed conventionally in the lateral aspect of the film. Cooper's ligaments (1), dense glandular tissue (2).

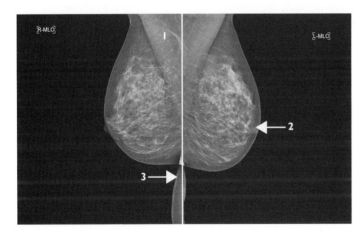

Fig. 3.60 Lateral oblique mammograms. Pectoralis muscle (1), nipple in profile (2), inframammary fold (3).

Standard mammogram views
Two views of each breast are recommended. The two standard views are the craniocaudal (CC) and the mediolateral oblique (MLO). Both breasts are imaged with mammography for comparison. Compression is applied to the breast to obtain the mammogram.

- CC or superior inferior view: to determine the orientation of the breast, the marker on the image is always sited in the lateral aspect of the breast (Fig. 3.59).
- MLO view: this should include the axillary tail of the breast and some of the pectoral muscles. The projection does not include all the upper inner quadrant of the breast and therefore two views with CC and MLO are

preferable to ensure complete coverage of the breast. A technically acceptable MLO view includes the nipple in profile, the inframammary fold and the pectoralis muscle down to the nipple level (Fig. 3.60).

- It is normal to see small lymph nodes in the axillary tail of the breast. Lymph nodes usually have a notch due to the fatty hilum, an oval shape and a low density.
- On the oblique view the Cooper's ligaments form curvilinear lines.

Supplementary views
These may be taken for further analysis of abnormalities:
- True lateral
- Extended CC concentrating on the medial or lateral aspect of the breast
- Compression views to investigate distortion
- Magnification views to investigate microcalcification taken in the true lateral and CC positions to look for layering of calcium. Benign calcium is milky calcium, which shows properties of liquids with a spherical shape en face on the CC view and a meniscus sign on a lateral view.

Breast ultrasound

Indication
Breast ultrasound is the primary imaging modality in young women aged under 35 or 40 years depending on the unit. It is an important complementary mode to mammography in older women who require further investigation of screen-detected abnormalities and breast lumps, and to aid image-guided biopsy. It can also be used to help stage the axilla. It differentiates solid from cystic lesions (Fig. 3.61).

Technique
High-resolution ultrasound is performed using a 10- to 17-MHz linear-array probe – the higher the resolution the better. Colour Doppler ultrasound can be used to assess vascularity of abnormalities. Formerly a water bath was used to improve the image. Ultrasound is of limited use in the detection of microcalcification.

Findings
- There is a wide variation in the normal density of breast tissue seen on mammography and ultrasound.
- On ultrasound the skin is clearly seen anteriorly; the pectoralis muscle should be seen at the back of the field of view to ensure complete coverage of the breast.
- Milk ducts are seen as tubular anechoic structures. The breast is scanned radially or vertically and horizontally again to ensure complete coverage.
- Abnormalities detected at ascribed positions in the breast as on a clock face with 12 o'clock being most superior and 6 o'clock being inferior.
- Ultrasound has limited use detecting microcalcifications and cannot be used for screening for this reason.
- Ultrasound is used to guide biopsy of abnormalities. It is preferable to use image-guided ultrasound biopsy for

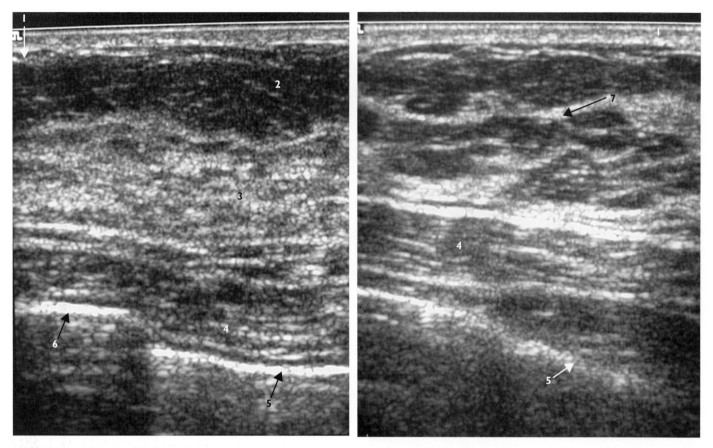

Fig. 3.61 Breast ultrasound using 17-MHz, high-resolution linear probe. Skin (1), fatty breast (2), glandular breast (3), pectoral muscles (4), pleura (5), rib (6) and Cooper's ligament (7).

accuracy, safety and comfort as it is performed with the patient supine.

- The two standard ways of performing breast biopsy are fine-needle aspiration using a 21G needle and core biopsy using an automated gun with a 14G 10-inch needle.
- Modern methods of breast biopsy use vacuum-assisted biopsy gun which takes a larger specimen, up to 10 g, while applying a vacuum that reduces the incidence of haematoma. This can be done with ultrasound or X-ray stereotactic guidance.

Stereotactic biopsy

- When lesions cannot be visualized on ultrasound and only mammography and in most cases of microcalcification, X-ray-guided biopsy is required using a stereotactic unit.
- This involves a computer added on to the mammography unit which guides position using cartesian coordinates in the x, y and z axes.
- Biopsies can be performed using the standard 14G 10-inch needles or the vacuum 10G biopsy device with lateral arm guidance (Fig. 3.62).

Needle localization biopsy

- When abnormalities are detected that are impalpable, but warrant surgical removal, localization of the abnormality is required.
- This involves marking the lesion with a wire, usually under ultrasound guidance, which is preferable as it is quicker and more comfortable, being performed in the supine position.

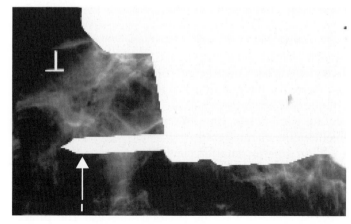

Fig. 3.62 Stereotactic pictures of the breast. showing the mammotomy biopsy needle (arrow).

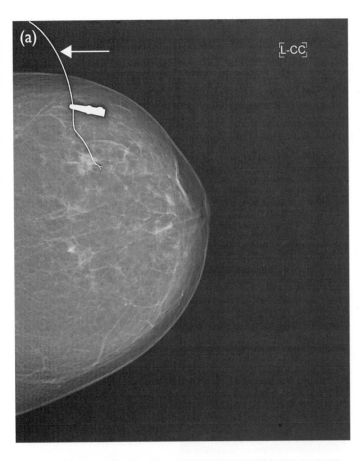

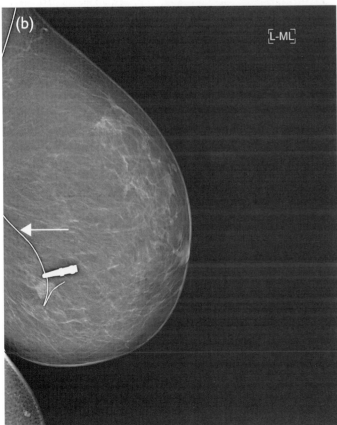

- If a lesion cannot be visualized on ultrasound then stereotactic mammography equipment has to be used. Stereotactic biopsy uses a computer attached to the mammogram machine that calculates the exact position of the lesion. The unit calculates x, y and z coordinates for precise localization of the abnormality, enabling a marker to be introduced while the patient is compressed in the mammogram unit (Fig. 3.62).
- Marker wires such as the Reidy wire or Kopan's wire are used, which are 9 cm long and either single or two piece. At the distal end of the Reidy wire is a cross-shaped tip that springs out on introduction so the wire cannot fall out.
- Localization is used for impalpable lesions.
- Localization can be ultrasound or X-ray guided.
- Following surgery specimen radiographs are taken with the Reidy wire in situ to check for adequate excision of the lesion.

Triple assessment

- Despite all the current imaging histology/cytology is still the gold standard. Correlation of the three modes of investigation – clinical examination, radiological imaging and biopsy results – is called triple assessment.
- Use of triple assessment is designed to prevent wrong conclusions being reached. A cancer can be occult on ultrasound and mammography, and only clinically palpable. If clinical findings are suspicious a biopsy should be performed regardless of the imaging.
- All three modes of triple assessment should correlate. If they do not then further investigation is warranted.

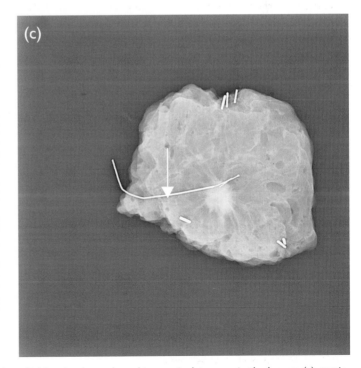

Fig. 3.63 Needle localization of the breast: Stereotactic guidance showing a Reidy wire (arrow) marking a spiculate mass in the breast: (a) cranio-caudal view; (b) lateral view; (c) specimen radiograph.

MRI of the breast

Indications

Gadolinium-enhanced MRI is used for problem-solving:

- In suspected local recurrence of breast cancer when conventional imaging is inconclusive.
- When there is discordant triple assessment.
- In some centres to assess response to chemotherapy in known breast cancer.
- It is the most sensitive technique for locoregional staging of breast cancer.
- It has recently been advocated for breast screening in high-risk women.
- The problem with MRI is its relatively poor specificity, leading to false positives.

Technique

- One recommended protocol is axial imaging with axial T2-weighted, followed by dynamic T1-weighted gadolinium-enhanced MRI. Images are acquired approximately every minute during intravenous contrast injection and for approximately 6 min afterwards.
- Curves of enhancement of any lesion are generated.
- The morphology, i.e. the shape of any abnormality, is the most important finding, but the enhancement curves provide additional information.

Findings

- Lesions that show rapid uptake of contrast and then rapid washout are suspicious for malignancy (Fig. 3.64).

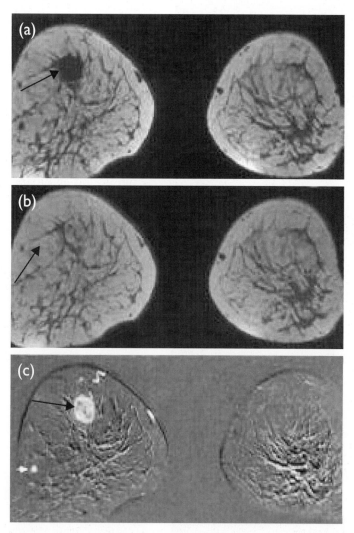

Fig. 3.64 Breast MRI showing (a) pre-T1, (b) post-T1 and (c) subtraction T1-weighted images. In the lateral aspect of the right breast there is an enhancing spiculate mass.

CASES

Case 3.1

A patient presents with a cough and haemoptysis to A&E. Initially a chest radiograph is requested.

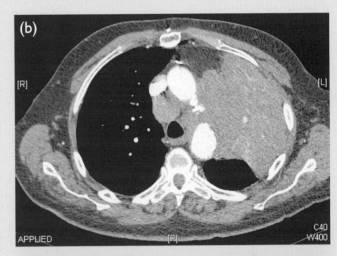

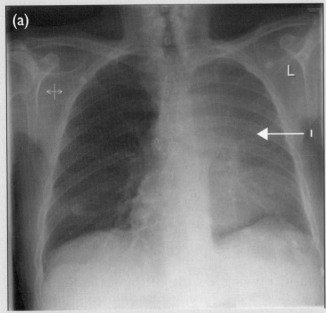

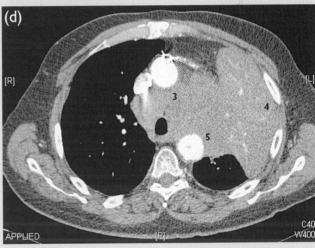

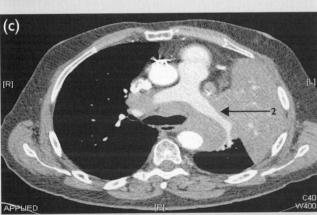

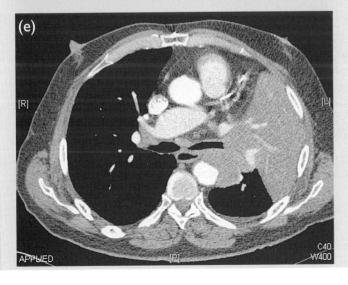

Fig. 3.65 A chest radiograph shows consolidation of the lingula with a veil over the heart (1). (b–e) Mediastinal CT windows following contrast showing a mass at the left hilum, causing narrowing of the left main pulmonary artery (2) and extension into the aortopulmonary window (3). Consolidation is seen around this, which is identified due to the presence of enhancing vessels within it (4). The vessels do not lie within the central mass (5). (f) Lung windows with a small lung nodule demonstrated.

Findings

- There has been a previous sternotomy. The patient is wearing an oxygen mask.
- Heart size: this is difficult to assess because the left heart border cannot be seen.
- Mediastinal contour: the left mediastinum and hilum have lost clarity. The trachea is displaced to the left side.
- There is a marked difference in transradiancy. To help ascertain which side is abnormal look at the diaphragms – the left is pulled up slightly. The tracheal displacement and diaphragmatic elevation point to volume loss in the left lung.
- There is a 'veil' over the heart, making it difficult to see it. This is due to pathology, i.e. consolidation or collapse of the lingula, which abuts the left heart border anteriorly. Use the silhouette sign to see if mediastinal contours or silhouette is absent.
- There is also an impression of a mass at the left hilum.
- Lungs and pleural spaces: in the right lung there is a soft-tissue nodule.
- Corners of film/review areas.

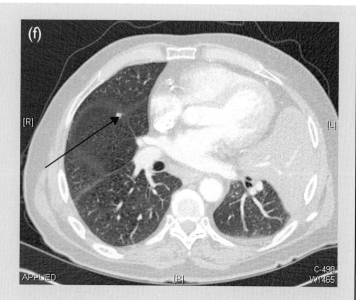

The idealized report reads: There is increased transradiancy in the left lung, elevation of the left hemidiaphragm and tracheal displacement. The veil over the heart is consistent with collapse/consolidation in the lingula. There is an impression of a mass at the left hilum and a soft-tissue nodule in the right lung. The differential would include malignancy and an urgent chest clinic referral and CT are recommended.

When reviewing the CT of the chest have a system:
- Mediastinal nodes and masses: the normal short axis limit is 10 mm. Look in pretracheal, right paratracheal and aortopulmonary windows, and hilar, subcarinal and retrocrural regions. In this case there is a large pretracheal node and right hilar node. The remaining soft tissue in the mediastinum is hard to separate from the collapsed lung. Soft tissue is seen around the descending aorta and in the aortopulmonary window.
- Pulmonary vessels and bronchi: there is abnormal soft tissue around the left pulmonary artery which is narrowing its calibre. This is evidence of vascular invasion. There is also narrowing of the left bronchus inferiorly, which again is strong evidence of malignant involvement.
- Lungs: on the mediastinal window the pulmonary vessels can be seen in consolidated lung but are absent from the tumour. This can help estimate the presence and size of a tumour.
- A lung window shows the lung parenchyma in greater detail for nodules and parenchymal disease such as emphysema. This lung window shows a nodule as seen on the chest radiograph in the right lung.
- Bones: appear normal; a bony window assesses the ribs and spines.

The idealized report should read: There is abnormal mediastinal lymphadenopathy in the pretracheal, right hilar and aortopulmonary window. There is a mass at the left hilum which is compromising the left pulmonary artery and left bronchus. There is collapse/consolidation of the lingula. There is a contralateral soft-tissue nodule in the right lung. No bony lesion seen. The CT findings are consistent with a left hilar bronchial tumour with invasion of the left bronchus and left pulmonary artery, and contralateral hilar lymphadenopathy, and a possible distant metastasis in the contralateral lung.

Diagnosis

Lingular consolidation and left bronchial carcinoma.

Case 3.2

A patient presents to the GP with a cough and night sweats. Initially a chest radiograph is performed.

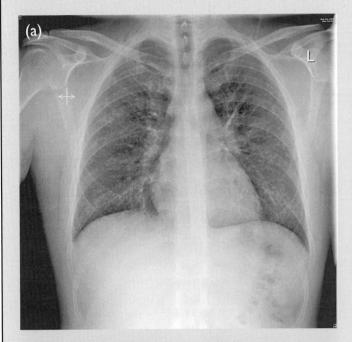

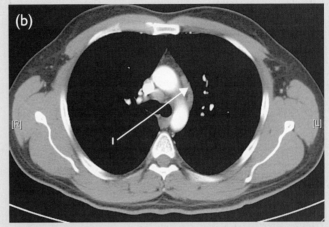

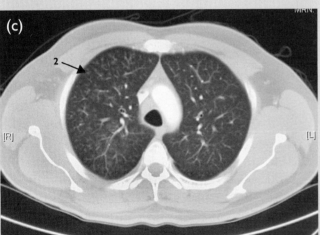

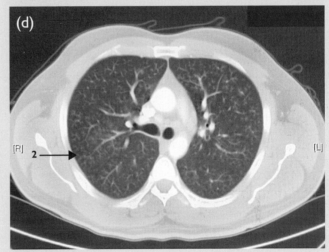

Fig. 3.66 (a) Chest radiograph shows slight prominence of the right hilum and fine nodules throughout the lungs. (b) CT showing small volume mediastinal lymphadenopathy (1). (c,d) The lung windows showing multiple small nodules (2), with a tree-in-bud appearance.

Findings

- The heart size is normal using CTR (cardiothoracic ratio).
- The hila are symmetrical and the left is the same height as the right, which is normal.
- There is no loss of silhouette and no difference in transradiancy between the two lungs. If there is nothing apparent look carefully at the lung parenchyma for interstitial diseases. This may be nodules, lines or rings. In this case the lung parenchyma is busy and contains multiple small nodules. There is a wide differential for nodules, but put into the clinical context atypical infection is a probability.

A chest clinic referral is made and a CT scan requested to look for mediastinal lymphadenopathy and help characterize the parenchymal findings.

Develop a system of reporting. Initially start with the mediastinal windows and check the sites for lymphadenopathy in order by scrolling down: right paratracheal, anterior mediastinal, aortopulmonary, pretracheal, hilar, subcarinal and retrocrural. Then review the lung windows. It can help to thicken the slices and apply the MIP if unsure.

- There are multiple enlarged mediastinal nodes.

- The lung parenchyma shows multiple tiny nodules.
- The differential includes miliary TB. CT cannot give the histology but can suggest the most likely diagnosis in the clinical context.

Diagnosis

Nodules, miliary TB.

Case 3.3

A 40-year-old patient presents with acute pleuritic chest pain. A PE was suspected. A chest radiograph is performed.

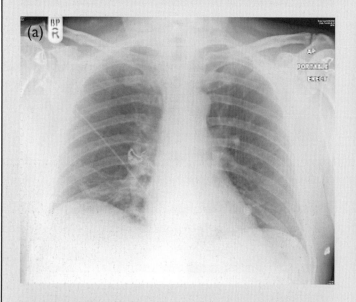

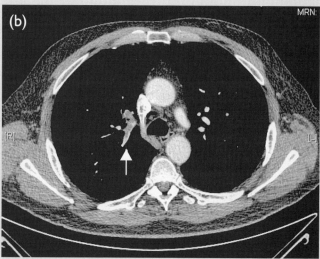

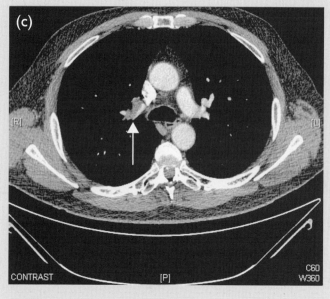

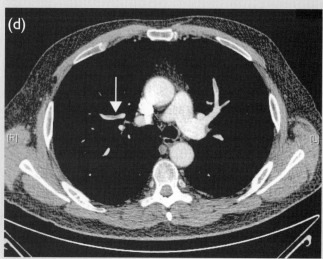

Findings

- Heart size normal
- Hila and mediastinal contours normal
- Diaphragms and fissures normal
- Lungs and pleural spaces normal
- Bones and corners of the film normal.

The D-dimers were elevated. A CTPA was performed ensuring that there was good opacification of the pulmonary arteries relative to the aorta. Used bolus tracking. A poor study may miss an embolus.

Findings

- No mediastinal lymphadenopathy is seen.
- There are multiple filling defects in the pulmonary arteries.
- On the lung windows no abnormality is seen.

Diagnosis

Pulmonary emboli.

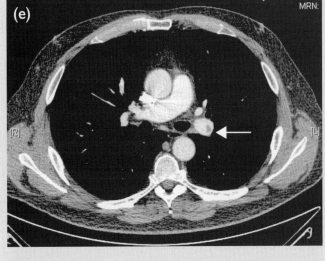

Fig. 3.67 (a) Chest radiograph: normal chest radiograph with acute chest pain. (b–e) CT pulmonary angiogram showing the presence of pulmonary emboli (arrows).

Case 3.4

A patient presented with shortness of breath. A chest radiograph was performed.
- Heart size normal.
- The hila are both elevated with evidence of volume loss in both upper lobes.
- Both hila are also dense and lobulated, suggesting lymphadenopathy.
- There is linear shadowing in both upper lobes consistent with fibrosis.
- Look at the corners of the film. Projected over the left supraclavicular fossa is a dense mass.
- The lung appearances could be due to sarcoidosis. The patient was referred for investigation of a mass in the neck. The neck findings were, however, secondary to hair braids in a pony tail, and show the importance of being aware of normal variants to prevent overcalling findings.

Diagnosis

Sarcoidosis, hair braids in neck.

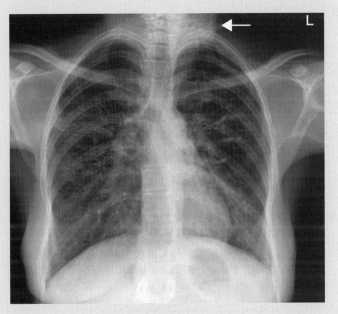

Fig. 3.68 Chest radiograph: the lung parenchyma is abnormal with some volume loss in both upper lobes. In addition there is a density in the left side of the neck (arrow). This was wrongly reported and is due to the presence of hair braids.

Case 3.5

A young adult presents with syncope. A chest radiograph is performed as part of a battery of investigations.

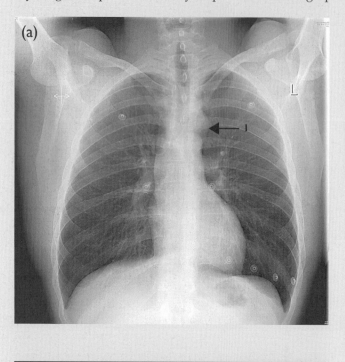

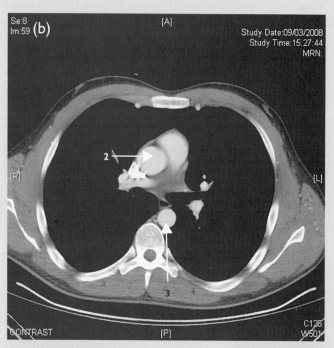

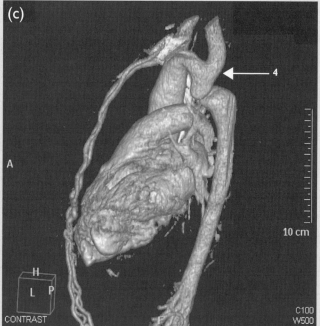

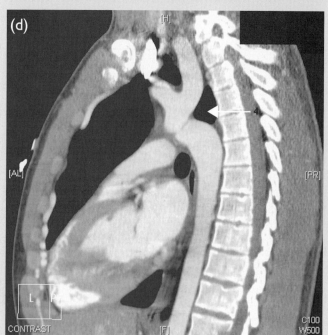

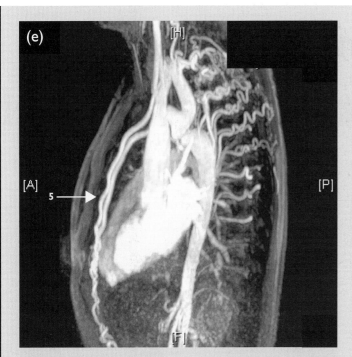
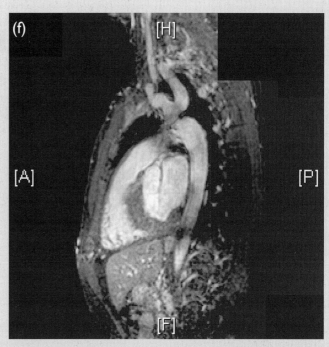

Fig. 3.69 Coarctation of aorta: (a) chest radiograph showing an abnormal appearance of the aortic knuckle and left hilum, with a high small aortic arch (1) and an indentation within it. This notching is seen on the inferior aspects of the ribs. (b) A CT scan of the chest showing the notch or reverse 3 sign in the aorta, with a marked change in calibre between the ascending and descending aorta. (c) CT volume-rendered reconstructions showing the coarct (4) and (d) sagittal CT showing the coarct (4). (e) Sagittal MRI showing with the hypertrophy collateral vessels (5) leading to the rib notching. (f) Sagittal MRI coarct.

- Heart size normal.
- Hila: are in the correct position but the left hilum looks very 'visible'.
- The mediastinal contours should be reviewed looking at hila, aortopulmonary window and aortic knuckle. In this case the aortic knuckle is on the correct side, i.e. the left side, but appears high with an indentation, i.e. two aortic bulges seen as in coarctation.
- The lungs and pleural spaces are clear.
- Associated findings can be seen on the undersurface of the third to eighth ribs with rib notching due to collateral formation via the intercostals.

A CT aortogram and MRI confirm the presence of the coarct and multiple collaterals. The stenosis and any associated valve abnormalities, collateral formation and ventricular anomalies are demonstrated non-invasively.

Diagnosis

Coarctation of the aorta.

4 Gastrointestinal imaging 1: oesophagus, stomach and bowel

RADIOLOGICAL ANATOMY

The digestive tract runs from the oral cavity to the anus. This chapter reviews the radiological anatomy relevant to the gastrointestinal (GI) tract.

The oesophagus (Fig. 4.1)

- This is a muscular tube measuring 25 cm in length. The start of the oesophagus at the cricopharyngeus lies 15 cm from the teeth at C5–6 (aboral). The gastro-oesophageal junction (GOJ) is therefore found 40 cm from the teeth. It is conventional to give the level of pathology in centimetres from the teeth.
- The oesophagus has a complex vascular supply (Fig. 4.2), which naturally divides the oesophagus into thirds; the pathology and its management differ in the upper,

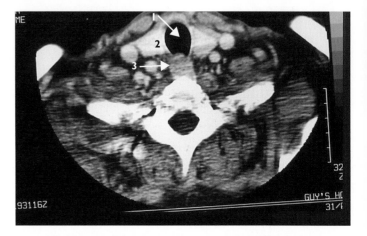

Fig. 4.1 Enhanced CT of the upper oesophagus. The trachea is recognized by the horse-shoe shape (1). Anterior to the trachea is the thyroid gland which is inherently dense (2). Oesophagus (3).

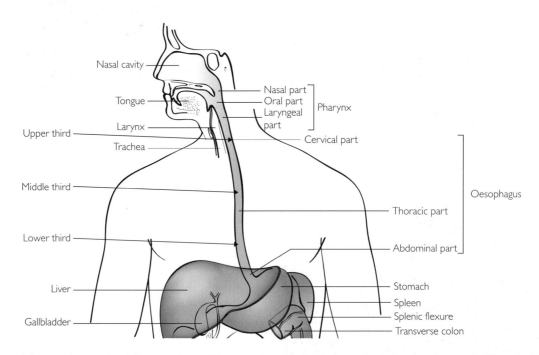

Fig. 4.2 Diagram of the vascular supply of the oesophagus. The oesophagus is divided into thirds for vascular supply. The upper third is supplied by the inferior thyroid and superior thyroid arteries. The middle third is supplied by the median aortic branches. The inferior third is supplied by the left gastric and the left inferior phrenic arteries. There are three venous drainage roots: the upper third drains to the inferior thyroid veins, the middle vein to the azygos vein and the inferior third to the left gastric drains and into the portal system.

mid and lower thirds due to histology and operable accessibility (Fig. 4.2).

- The upper oesophagus is supplied by the inferior thyroid vessels and extends from 15 cm to 25 cm aboral, i.e. the carina.
- The midoesophagus is supplied by the aortic branches and drains to the azygos vein, 25–32 cm aboral.
- The lower third is supplied by the left gastric vessels, 32–40 cm aboral. Adenocarcinomas are more common in the lower third.
- Squamous mucosa is found throughout the oesophagus, except in the inferior third where columnar epithelium is found.

The stomach

- The stomach begins at the GOJ which lies to the left of the midline at T11. The gastric cardia starts approximately 3 cm below the diaphragmatic opening for the oesophagus. This is the part of the stomach surrounding the GOJ, named the cardia due to its close proximity to the heart.

- The stomach fundus extends superolaterally above the GOJ.
- The body extends into the antrum and then into the pylorus.
- The angular incisura is a normal constriction found between the body and the antrum on the lesser curve (Fig. 4.3).
- The lesser omentum attaches to the lesser curve and continues as the important gastrohepatic ligament.
- The greater omentum attaches to the greater curve and continues as the radiologically important gastrosplenic ligament, an important site to look for abnormal nodes and peritoneal deposits (Fig. 4.4).
- The pylorus lies at L1 to the right of the midline.
- The normal gastric wall thickness is 4–10 mm depending on degree of gaseous distension.
- The lesser sac lies behind the stomach, anterior to the aorta and inferior vena cava (IVC).
- The arterial supply to the stomach is from branches of the coeliac axis: the right and left gastric and a branch of the hepatic artery proper supply the lesser curve; the

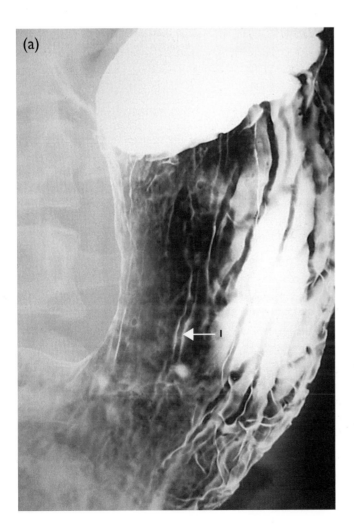

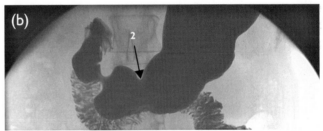

Fig. 4.3 Barium meal: two pictures from different series. (a) The gastric rugae (1) are well seen on the barium meal. (b) The angular incisura is located on the lesser curve (2).

(a)

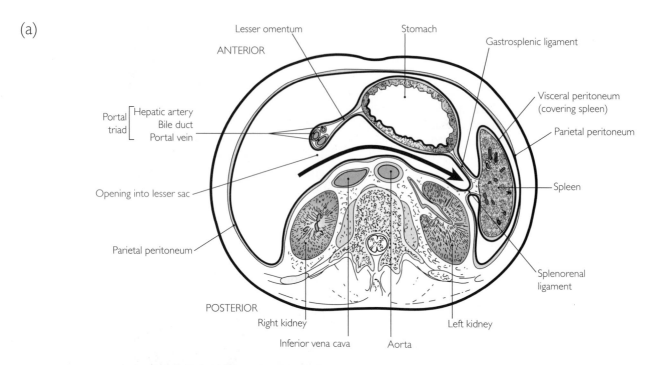

(b)

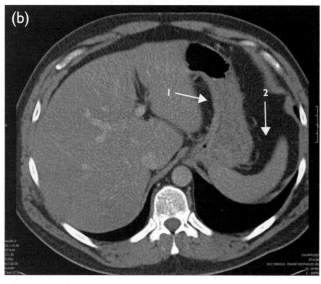

Fig. 4.4 (a) Diagram showing the stomach in an axial plain with the peritoneal reflections. The gastrosplenic ligament is shown, an important site for metastasis and the lesser omentum. The lesser omentum continues to join the liver as the gastrohepatic ligament. (b) Axial CT upper abdomen post-contrast showing the gastrohepatic ligament (1) and gastrosplenic ligament (2).

right and left gastroepiploic supply the greater curve, which are branches of the splenic and gastroduodenal branches of the coeliac (Fig. 4.5).

- The stomach is drained by the left gastric and splenic veins into the portal vein.

Small bowel: the duodenum (Fig. 4.6)

- The duodenum is divided into four anatomical parts that form an incomplete circle surrounding the head of the pancreas. The duodenum is the least mobile segment of the small bowel.

- The duodenal cap or bulb is the first part, named D1, and has some peritoneal reflection anteriorly. The folds within it are not usually visualized in a barium study due to the use of an intravenous relaxant.

- The second part of the duodenum descends vertically with the ampulla of Vater opening into the medial wall. The ampulla lies 9 cm from the pylorus. A prominent hooding fold is thrown over it and a longitudinal fold leads from it. Some 10 mm proximal to the ampulla lies the opening of the accessory duct of Santorini into the duodenal papilla, which can be seen with barium in 25%. The folds are used to locate the major and the minor papillae in endoscopy.

(a)

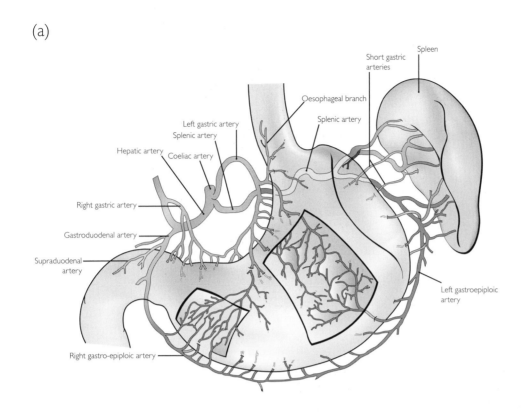

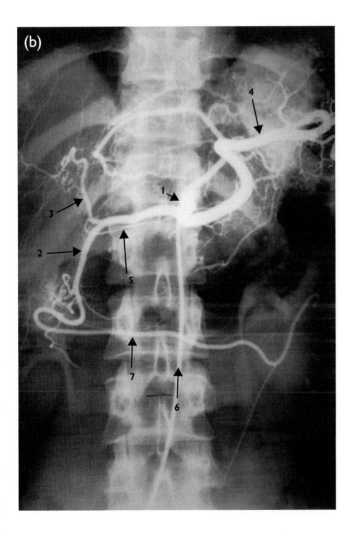

Fig. 4.5 (a) Diagram showing the vascular supply to the stomach which is from branches of the coeliac artery. (b) Conventional angiogram of the coeliac artery. Left gastric artery (1), gastroduodenal artery (2), hepatic artery proper (3), splenic artery (4), common hepatic artery (5), catheter (6) and right gastroepiploic artery (7).

- The third part of the duodenum runs horizontally under the superior mesenteric artery (SMA).
- The second and third parts have some peritoneal reflection anteriorly but not posteriorly.
- The fourth part of the duodenum ascends vertically to lie at the same anatomical level as the first part of the duodenum, where the duodenojejunal junction is fixed in position by the ligament of Treitz. The duodenum should have a curvature and, if D4 lies below D1, there may be malrotation of the small bowel and the patient is at risk of volvulus.

Small bowel: jejunum and ileum

The small bowel is made up of jejunum and ileum and is 6.5 metres long in total: two-fifths are jejunum and three-fifths ileum (Fig. 4.7).

- The duodenojejunal flexure lies 2.5 cm to the left of the midline and 1 cm below the level of the pylorus. The ligament of Trietz fixes the flexure in a constant position.

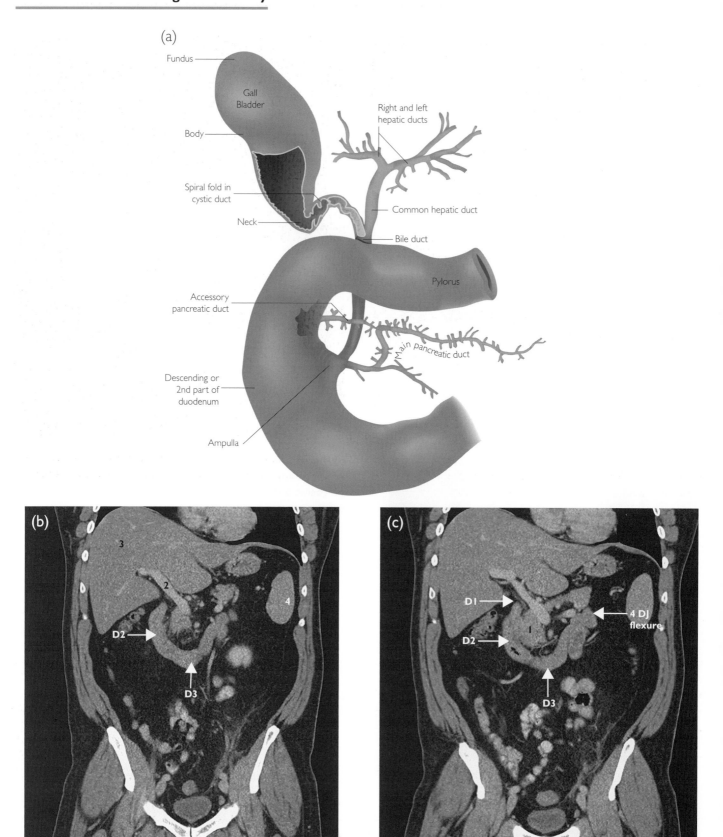

Fig. 4.6 (a) Diagram of the duodenum and pylorus showing the duodenal cap, and the second and third parts of the duodenum. The DJ flexure should lie at the same height as D1. (b,c) Coronal CT scans showing the curves of the duodenum. First part duodenum D1, second part D2, third part duodenum D3, fourth part duodenum D4, which is at the same axial level as D1. The pancreas lies within the centre of the duodenum and the portal vein runs up obliquely to the liver. Pancreas (1), portal vein (2), liver (3) and spleen (4).

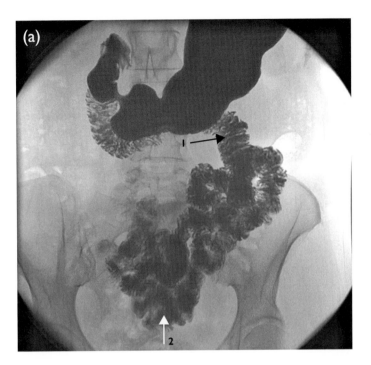
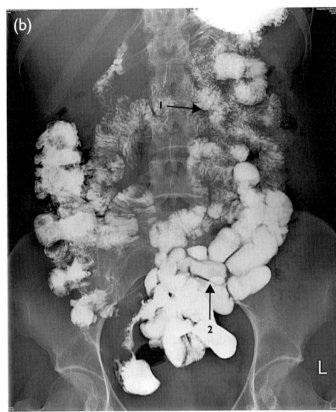

Fig. 4.7 Two images from different series from barium follow-through: (a) digital and (b) conventional. The small bowel in the left upper quadrant is jejunum (1), which has a greater calibre and more folds than the ileum. The bowel in the right lower quadrant is the ileum (2), with a smaller calibre and fewer valvulae conniventes and more Peyer's patches.

- The small bowel extends from the ligament of Treitz to the ileocaecal valve (Fig. 4.8).
- The jejunum is usually situated in the left upper quadrant and has more valvulae conniventes but fewer Peyer's patches than the ileum. The folds should measure less than 2 mm thick.
- The jejunal calibre should be less than 3.5 cm on abdominal radiograph (<4 cm when distended with barium) (Fig. 4.9).
- The ileum lies in the lower abdomen, more towards the right side and right iliac fossa.
- The ileum has a narrower calibre, with a maximum of 2.5 cm (3 cm if distended with barium).
- The ileum has more Peyer's patches/lymphoid follicles than the jejunum (Fig. 4.10).
- The small bowel is suspended by a mesentery, which has a root 20 cm long fixed between the ligament of Treitz and the ileocaecal junction.

- The ileocaecal valve can mimic a tumour due to its appearance as a soft-tissue mass in the caecum. It may contain fat submucosally which helps to identify it.
- The duodenum is supplied by branches of the coeliac artery and SMA, namely the superior and inferior pancreaticoduodenal branches, which have an important anastomosis between the coeliac artery and the SMA. The anastomosis prevents small bowel ischaemia if there is a mesenteric thrombus.
- The small bowel is supplied by jejunal and ileal branches of the SMA (Fig. 4.11).
- The venous drainage of the small bowel is to the portal vein via the splenic and superior mesenteric veins.

Large bowel/colon

- The large bowel is 150 cm long. The transverse and sigmoid colon have a mesentery.

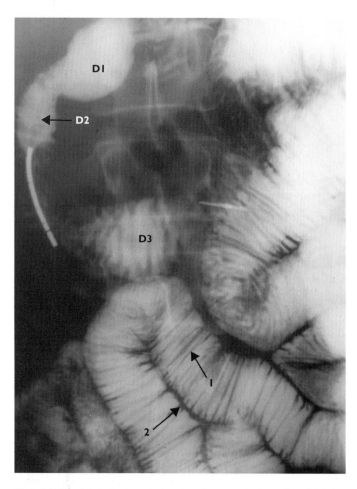

Fig. 4.8 Small bowel enema showing the introducing tube which has slipped back to lie too proximally in the second part of the duodenum. Duodenal cap D1, second part of the duodenum D2, third part D3 of duodenum. The smooth folds of the jejunum are noted, which should be <2 mm thick (1). The interspacing of the bowel loops should be even, reflecting the bowel wall thickness (2).

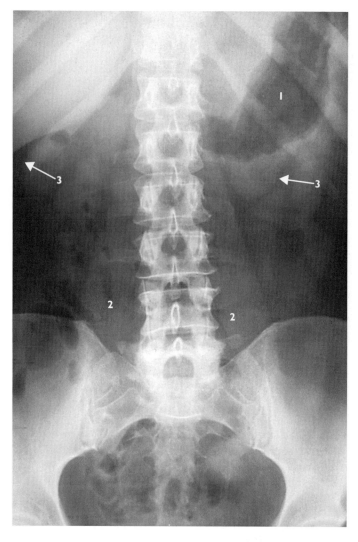

Fig. 4.9 Abdominal radiograph showing the normal stomach filled with gas and the normal bowel gas pattern. Small bowel tends to lie centrally and large bowel peripherally. Both psoas muscles are identified in this patient. Stomach gas (1), psoas muscles (2) and renal outline (3).

- The colon has three longitudinal muscle bands called taeniae coli.
- Haustral sacculations are present in the large bowel. These are crescenteric folds of the entire bowel wall thickness and lie in between the taeniae coli. Their appearance helps differentiate large bowel from small bowel on imaging (Fig. 4.12).
- The ascending colon and descending colon are partially extraperitoneal. Free fluid may be seen behind them in the paracolic gutters on CT (Fig. 4.13).
- The sigmoid colon can undergo volvulus because of its mesentery.
- The large bowel is located around the periphery of the abdominal cavity, with the small bowel lying centrally.

- The rectum is 12–15 cm long and surrounded by the perirectal fascia or mesocolon and fat. The fascia is seen as a thin line surrounding the rectum on CT.
- The rectum is mainly extraperitoneal with no posterior peritoneum.
- The posterior rectal space lies posterior to the rectum and anterior to the sacrum, measures 1 cm and can be up to 2 cm in elderly or obese people. The rectum has longitudinal folds called the valves of Houston.
- The appendix usually lies posterior to the caecum (retrocaecal) in 66% of cases.
- The appendix occupies a variable position and may be long or short. The anterior taeniae coli lead to the appendix.

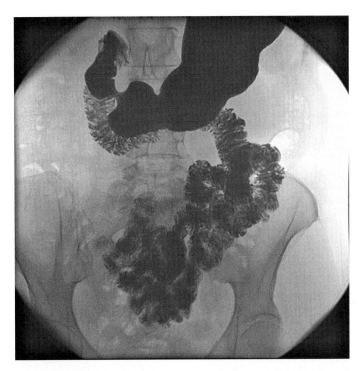

Fig. 4.10 Barium follow through showing the transit of barium through the stomach and small bowel. Note the change in calibre of the bowel and the number of folds as one descends.

- The vascular supply to the large bowel is from branches of the SMA and the inferior mesenteric artery (IMA).
- The SMA arises from the anterior aorta at L1–2 and the IMA from the anterior aorta at L3.
- The IMA is a very small branch and is hard to identify on CT. There is an important anastomosis between the portal and systemic circulations – between the superior rectal branch of the IMA and the inferior rectal arteries branches of the internal iliac artery (Fig. 4.14).
- The SMA supplies the colon proximal to the splenic flexure and the IMA the colon distal to the splenic flexure.

(a)

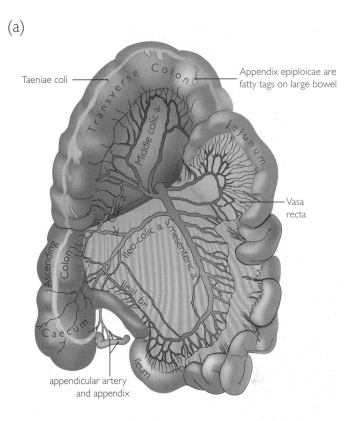

(b)

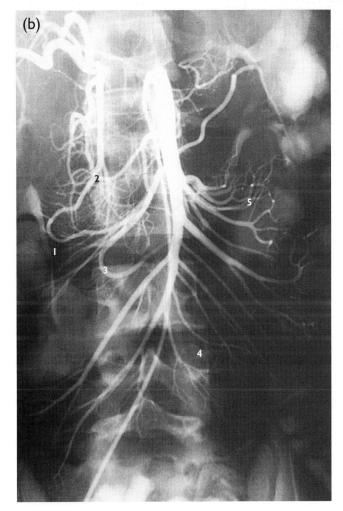

Fig. 4.11 (a) Diagram of the vascular supply to the large bowel and branches of the superior mesenteric artery. (b) A conventional superior mesenteric angiogram shows the branches: right colic (1), middle colic (2), ileocolic (3), ileal (4) and jejunal (5).

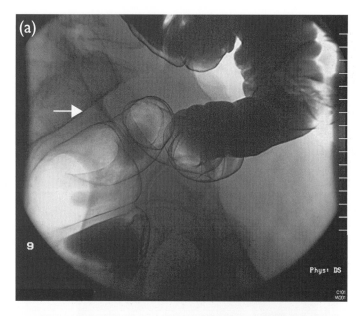

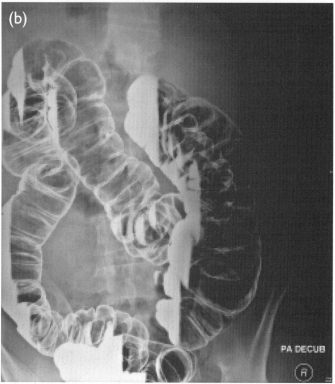

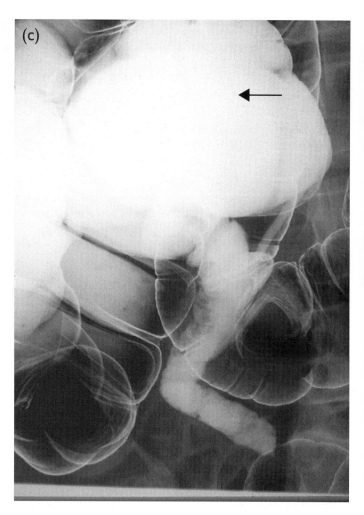

Fig. 4.12 Three images from different barium enema series: (a) lateral view of the rectum showing the presacral fat space (arrow); (b) conventional image from a lateral decubitus view of a barium enema within the right side down, showing the left colon as a double-contrast image; (c) an image of an undescended caecum and the terminal ileum.

The mesentery and omentum

- The small bowel mesentery and omenta are folds of peritoneum.
- The small bowel mesentery comprises two layers of peritoneum suspending the small bowel from the posterior abdominal wall and supplying its vascular supply.
- The small bowel mesentery is a broad fan-shaped peritoneal fold.
- The omentum comprises four layers of peritoneum and serves to limit the spread of infection.
- The greater omentum hangs from the greater curvature of the stomach and covers the transverse colon to form the transverse mesocolon.
- The lesser omentum is the same as the gastrohepatic ligament and joins the liver and the stomach. It lies anterior to the lesser sac (Fig. 4.15).

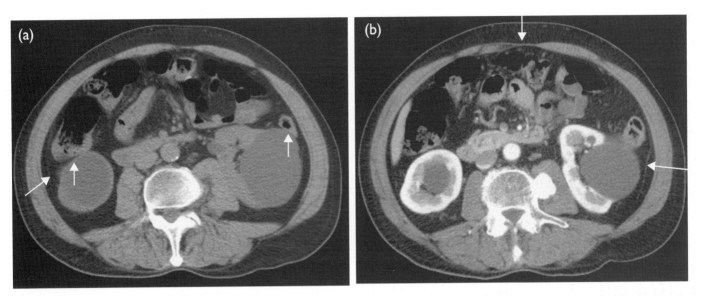

Fig. 4.13 (a, b) Axial CT abdomen showing the paracolic gutters and peritoneal reflection (arrows), which are not normally visualized unless they contain fluid.

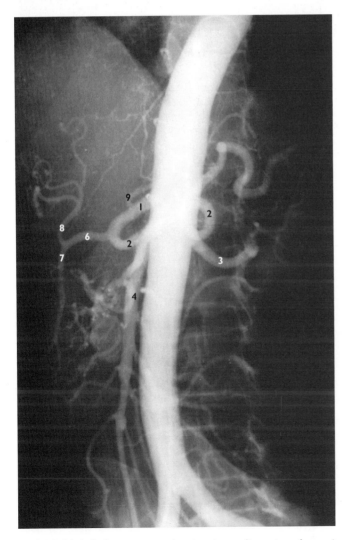

Fig. 4.14 (a) A flush aortogram showing the coeliac axis and superior mesenteric arteries arising. Coeliac axis (1), splenic artery (2), left renal artery (3), superior mesenteric artery (4), common hepatic artery (6), gastroduodenal (7), hepatic artery proper (8) and left gastric artery (9).

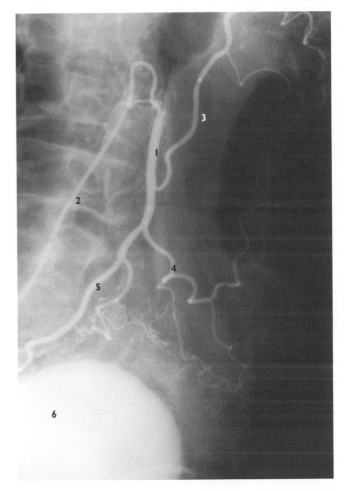

Fig. 4.15 is an inferior mesenteric artery angiogram: inferior mesenteric artery (1), catheter (2), left colic artery (3), sigmoid arteries (4), superior rectal artery (5) and full bladder (6). Ideally an inferior mesenteric artery angiogram should be performed before the bladder is full due to its origin at L3, which may be obscured by a full bladder.

IMAGING

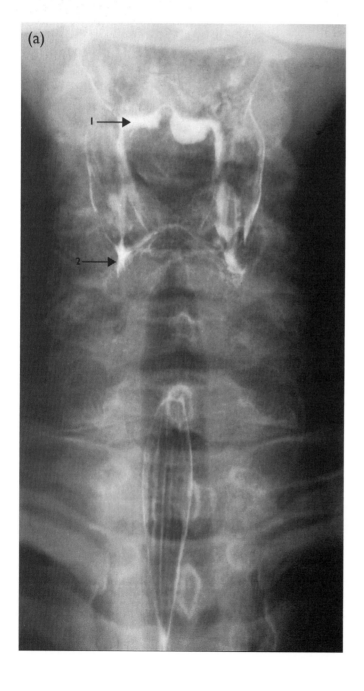

Box 4.1 Barium studies

Concentrations of barium used:
- Barium swallow 100% (weight per volume) w/v
- Barium meal – 250% w/v
- Small bowel meal – 50% w/v
- Small bowel enema – 17–19% w/v
- Barium enema polybar – 125% w/v
- High kilovoltage is used for barium examinations up to 150 kV
- In CT scanning varying oral contrasts by 3–4% is used to avoid artefact

Hypopharynx and oesophagus

Barium swallow

Indications

Dysphagia, reflux, pharyngeal pouch, to visualize the pharynx and oesophagus; should show both morphology and motility of the oesophagus. A barium swallow is still the first-line investigation for the oesophagus in dysphagia because it can show mechanical obstruction, but also abnormalities of peristalsis unlike endoscopy and CT.

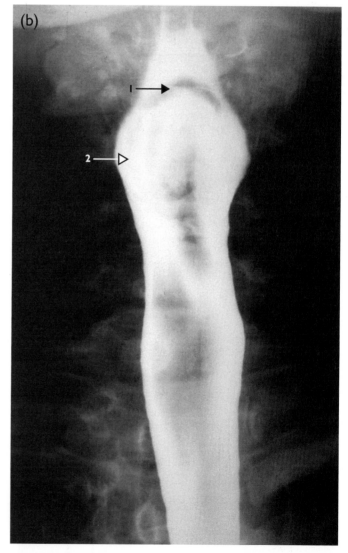

Fig. 4.16 Barium swallow AP: (a) mucosal relief view; (b) double-contrast view. (a) The valleculae (1) and the piriform fossae (2); (b) the distension of the piriform fossae with contrast (2), which then runs down the oesophagus. The epiglottis (1) is seen as a filling defect within the oral pharynx.

Technique

- In the erect position, using 50% barium, the patient ingests the barium, which contains an effervescent agent and gives double-contrast views, while fluoroscopically screening.
- The patient swallows in the anteroposterior (AP) and lateral views initially to look at the hypopharynx and cervical oesophagus. The patient is then positioned obliquely in a left posterior oblique view to throw the oesophagus outline off the thoracic spine and make it easier to see strictures in the thoracic oesophagus (Fig. 4.16).
- In a swallow both single- and double-contrast views are taken to assess the distension for strictures/extrinsic compression in the hypopharynx, oesophagus and mucosa. Ulcers or external compression may be overlooked if both contrast views are not taken. The mucosal relief view is a third view taken with the oesophagus in the collapsed state.
- The epiglottis is yellow cartilage and does not calcify on plain film. It can be seen coated in barium at the tongue base on the initial upper oesophageal lateral view (Fig. 4.17).
- The mucosal relief view may show ulcers or changes of candidiasis (Fig. 4.18).
- Longitudinal folds in the oesophagus are normally seen when collapsed and should not measure more than 3 mm in thickness. Fewer than five mucosal folds should be seen in the distal oesophagus. More than five indicate the presence of a sliding hiatus hernia.
- The GOJ is seen in the oblique view (Fig. 4.19).
- In motility disorders contrast is ingested in the erect position in the cervical region while fluoroscopically screening and using videofluoroscopy, but also in the prone position to remove the effects of gravity. This reveals abnormalities of peristalsis. A speech and language therapist may instigate the investigation and use barium-coated solid material such as bread for further analysis of peristaltic and neurological abnormalities. Single mouth swallows must be used. If multiple gulps are taken this can create a peristaltic abnormality. It is normal for secondary waves of peristalsis to be seen. Tertiary waves are usually abnormal and can cause an appearance resembling a corkscrew on a barium swallow.

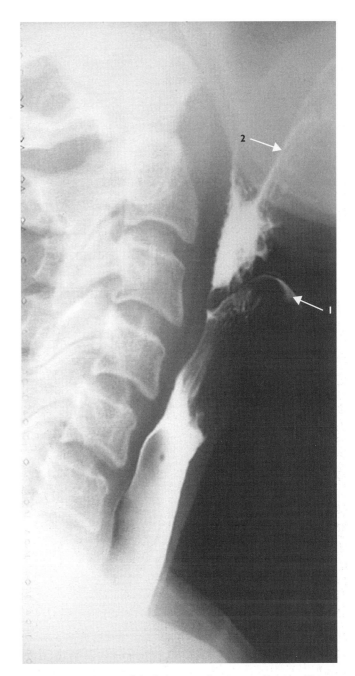

Fig. 4.17 Lateral view of the barium swallow cervical region. The outline of the epiglottis (1) is seen by barium of its superior aspect. Back of tongue (2).

Normal findings

Several indentations can be seen on the swallow that may be normal variants:

- The postcricoid venous plexus or impression has a variable appearance with swallowing, and is not clinically significant. It must be differentiated from pathological narrowings:
  - the impression may disappear after swallowing (Fig. 4.20)
  - the impression is found at the C4 level
  - the venous plexus gives a lobulated anterior filling defect with lots of small indentations.

- Cricopharyngeus is a smooth long posterior defect approximately 1 cm in length: the indentation is found at C5–6 (Fig. 4.21).
- An osteophyte impression may also be posterior but the osteophyte will be visible as a bony prominence: an oesophageal web is a pathological finding and is associated with Patterson–Kelly–Brown or Plummer–Vinson syndrome. It is a short, smooth, constant anterior defect.

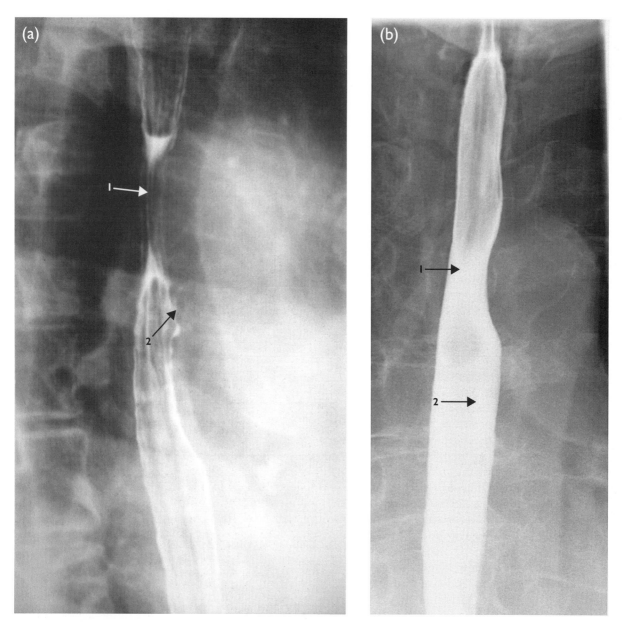

Fig. 4.18 Oblique views of the thoracic oesophagus: (a) mucosal relief view; (b) single contrast view. The two views show the aortic impression (1) on the upper thoracic oesophagus. The left main bronchus (2) can cause an impression below this. The left atrium can cause a third impression below this if enlarged.

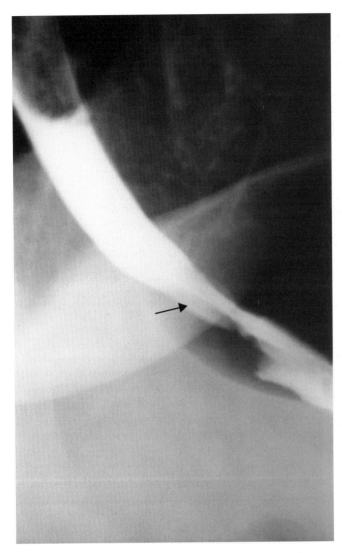

Fig. 4.19 Barium swallow: oblique view of gastro-oesophageal junction (arrow).

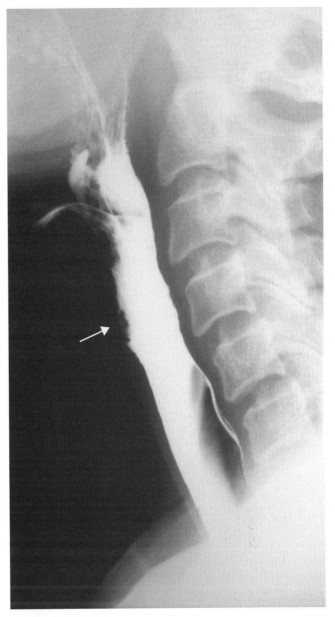

Fig. 4.20 Barium swallow: lateral view neck. The postcricoid venous plexus (arrow) is seen as an anterior filling defect, which disappears on swallowing.

- The thoracic aorta can cause an impression anteriorly on the oesophagus at T4, especially in elderly people.
- The left main bronchus causes an anterior indentation below the aortic arch (Fig. 4.22).
- The left atrium may cause an anterior indentation just above the diaphragm if enlarged.
- An anomalous right subclavian artery may cause a posterior defect which is unusual. When posterior defects are noted in the thoracic oesophagus, there may be an associated vascular ring.

CT of the oesophagus

Indication
CT is used to stage oesophageal malignancy or in mediastinitis.

Technique
Oral and intravenous contrast is used in oesophageal staging. Contrast may be given orally immediately before scanning to enable the oesophageal wall to be seen.

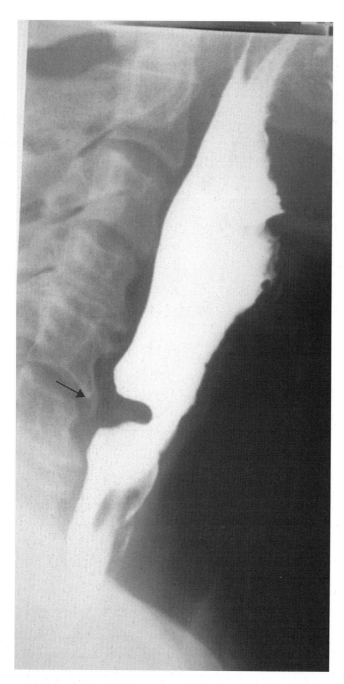

Fig. 4.21 Barium swallow: lateral view of neck shows an impression on the posterior cervical oesophagus due to the cricopharyngeus impression (arrow).

Findings

The wall of the oesophagus should not measure more than 3 mm and more than 5 mm width is abnormal (Fig. 4.23).

- The wall of the oesophagus can be difficult to separate from the left atrium and the trachea.
- Below the diaphragm the oesophagus is attached to the gastrohepatic ligament.

- The regional nodes are divided into thirds according to the blood supply of the oesophagus, which is divided into thirds.
- The upper third drains the cervical and supraclavicular nodes, which are classified as N1 if involved.
- The middle third drains to the perigastric and infradiaphragmatic nodes but not the coeliac nodes.
- The lower third drains to the coeliac nodes.

The stomach and duodenum

Barium meal

Indications

Endoscopy has mainly superseded the use of the barium meal, unless contraindicated. Indications are to assess the lower oesophagus, stomach and duodenum.

Technique

- Denser, 250% w/v contrast is used in a meal, together with sodium bicarbonate granules to give a double-contrast view. The procedure is normally started in the supine position involving controlled rotation of the patient to the prone position to coat the stomach and slowly fill the duodenum. The meal is completed in the erect position to assess the distal oesophagus and GOJ. This technique controls the flow of the barium, enabling the stomach mucosa and distension to be assessed before the barium passes through the pylorus into the duodenum.
- 20 mg hyoscine butylbromide (Buscopan) or 0.2 mg glucagon is given intravenously to produce hypotonia of the duodenum and relax peristalsis, unless contraindicated, enabling good views of the distended duodenum.

Contraindications

- To barium are aspiration, perforation or leak from an anastomotic site. If these are suspected, water-soluble contrast is used.
- Tumours at the cardia or GOJ can be well seen in the left lateral position.

Findings

- The shape and position of the stomach are extremely variable.
- Gastric rugae are linear folds of mucosa that should not measure more than 5 mm in thickness (Fig. 4.24).
- Tiny nodular elevations of mucosa normally seen in the stomach are called areae gastricae. These are 2–3 mm in size.
- The gastro-oesophageal opening is called the cardiac orifice. The fundus lies above this opening.
- Angular incisura is a notch or indentation seen on the lesser curve of the stomach. The antrum lies distal to this and opens into the pyloric canal.

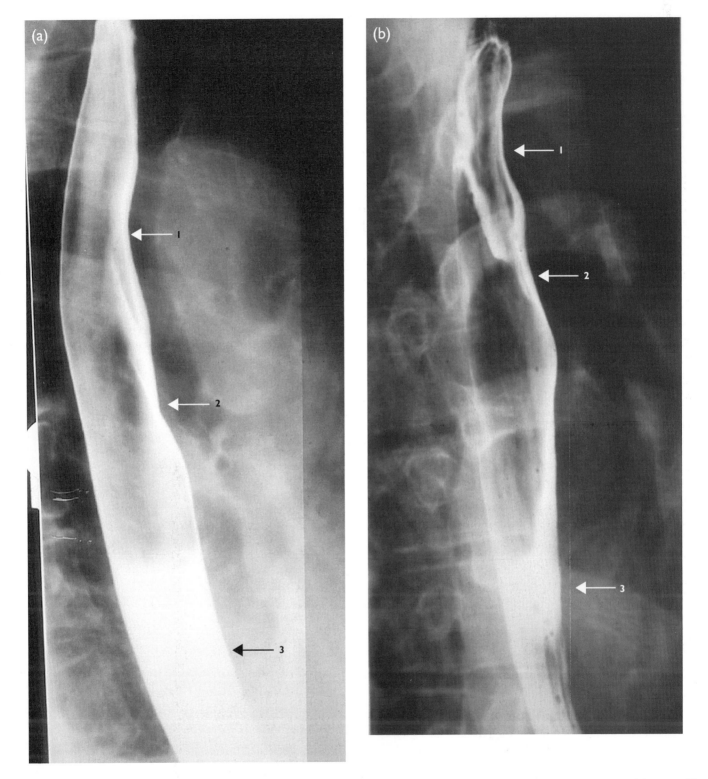

Fig. 4.22 Oblique views of the thoracic oesophagus on barium swallow: (a, b) two different cases showing the normal impression of the aorta (1). Left main bronchus (2), and left atrium (3).

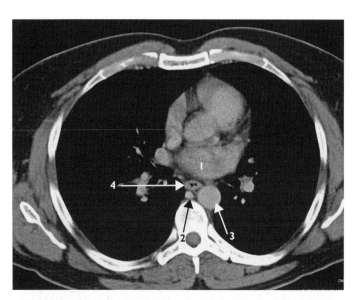

Fig. 4.23 CT of the left atrium (LA) (1): the LA can cause a third indentation and compress the oesophagus if enlarged inferior. Azygos (2), aorta (3), oesophagus (4).

- Prolapsed oesophageal mucosa at the GOJ and prolapsed gastric mucosa at the duodenal cap/pylorus may simulate a mass (Fig. 4.25).
- The spleen or liver may compress the stomach externally, simulating a mass.
- The duodenal cap normally has no visible folds on a barium study following an intravenous relaxant. Filling defects within the duodenal cap may represent an ulcer or a normal variant (Fig. 4.26):
  - ectopic gastric mucosa or gastric heterotopia, filling defects 1–6 mm in size extending from the pylorus into the cap (Fig. 4.27)
  - Brunner's glands.
  - pancreatic rests; islands of ectopic pancreatic mucosa
  - air bubbles.
- In the second part of the duodenum the ampulla may cause a filling defect.
- Duodenal diverticula can occur on the inner curve of the duodenum in the second and third parts.
- All routine barium studies should include one erect view of the whole duodenum to the ligament of Treitz to look for malrotation.

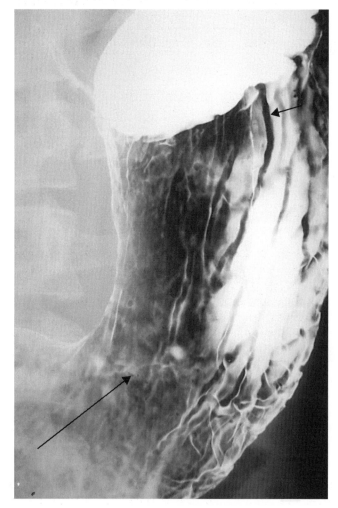

Fig. 4.24 Barium meal: the gastric rugae are the linear folds, which should not measure more than 5 mm in thickness. The area gastricae are seen inferiorly as small nodules measuring less than 3 mm (arrow).

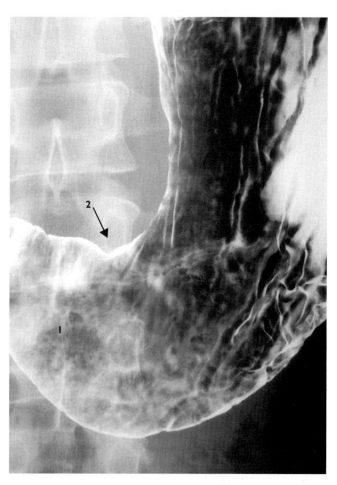

Fig. 4.25 Image of a barium meal showing the antrum (1) and angula incisura (2).

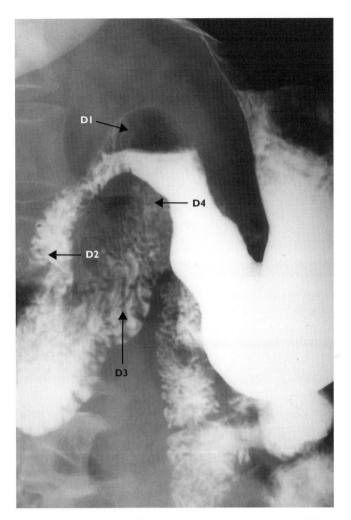

Fig. 4.26 Barium meal erect view showing the duodenal cap (D1), the second part of the duodenum (D2), the third part (D3) and the fourth part (D4) that ascends to the same level as the first part.

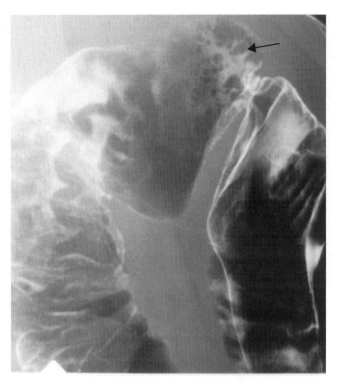

Fig. 4.27 Barium meal: duodenal cap view. Filling defects within the cap of the duodenum are ectopic gastric mucosa (arrow).

CT of the stomach and duodenum

Indications
Staging gastric malignancy, abdominal pain with no abnormality seen on other investigations.

Technique
- The patient should be fasted for a good examination of the stomach.
- Water is given as oral contrast in gastric malignancy and the stomach should be well distended.
- Intravenous contrast is administered and scanning undertaken in the portal venous phase.
- The liver, spleen, adrenals, kidneys and the pelvis are included for staging.

Findings
- The normal gastric wall should be less than 4 mm thick when well distended. However, when collapsed the wall can measure up to 10 mm thick.

- The stomach is in close proximity to the transverse colon, the pancreas and the liver, which are often involved in direct spread of tumour in gastric malignancy.
- Regional spread is to the gastric wall nodes N1, then to the gastrohepatic and gastrosplenic nodes – N2
- Nodal size is taken as 8 mm short axis in the gastrosplenic, gastrohepatic and left gastric regions (Fig. 4.28).

Imaging the whole bowel

Abdominal radiograph

Indications
In the acute abdomen an abdominal radiograph is indicated to assess for bowel dilatation and free intraperitoneal air. Its role has diminished with the increasing use of other imaging modalities such as ultrasound and CT. The bowel gas pattern, soft-tissue calcification and skeletal abnormalities are visible on an abdominal radiograph.

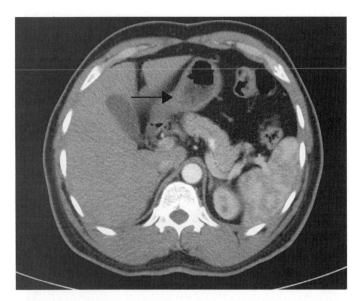

Fig. 4.28 CT of the stomach: the stomach wall (arrow) may appear thickened but if it is normal above the air/fluid levels this is an artefact. Water contrast is used to show the stomach wall.

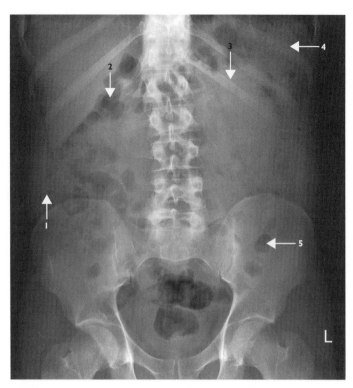

Fig. 4.29 Abdominal radiograph showing the normal bowel gas pattern. Ascending colon (1), hepatic flexure (2), transverse colon (3), splenic flexure (4) and descending colon (5).

Technique

The abdominal radiograph is taken with the patient in the supine position:

- In the acute abdomen, an erect chest radiograph is also performed to look for free intraperitoneal air, which will be seen under the diaphragm.
- If this is not possible, a left lateral decubitus, with the right side raised, may be performed. The patient must stay in that position for at least 10 min before acquisition of the image to allow free air to rise to the highest point.

Findings

- The abdominal cavity includes the pelvis.
- The diaphragm forms the superior border of the abdomen.
- The hernial orifices and symphysis pubis must be included on the inferior aspect of the abdominal radiograph to assess for hernias or bladder exstrophy (Fig. 4.29).
- The bowel gas pattern and calibre can be assessed on an abdominal radiograph (Fig. 4.30).
- Small bowel predominantly lies centrally and large bowel peripherally; however, this is unreliable. (The only reliable difference on a plain abdominal radiograph is the presence of faeces in the large bowel – Fig. 4.31.)
- Large bowel may be interposed between the liver and the diaphragm which may mimic free air and is called chiladitis.
- An infant crying can lead to massive gaseous distension of the stomach mimicking gastric outflow obstruction.

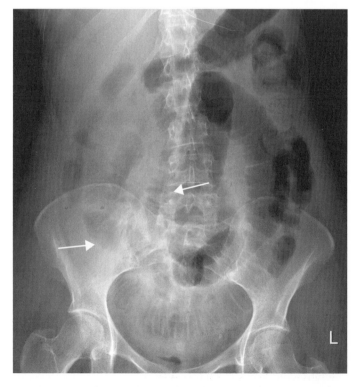

Fig. 4.30 Abdominal radiograph showing dilated small bowel (arrows).

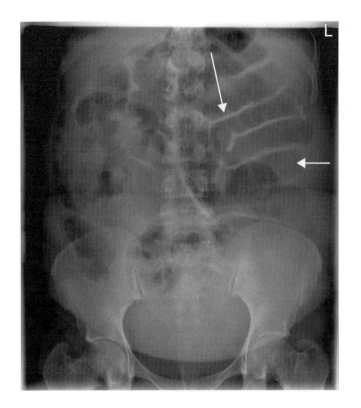

Fig. 4.31 Abdominal radiograph showing dilated small bowel (arrows).

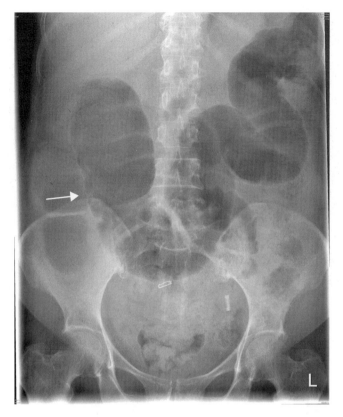

Fig. 4.32 Abdominal radiograph showing a dilated loop of bowel centrally (arrow).

- Short air–fluid levels may normally be seen in small bowel, but more than two fluid-filled dilated loops >2.5 cm in diameter is abnormal on an erect film.
- In the transverse colon a diameter >5.5 cm is abnormal.
- The caecum is very distensible but is at risk of perforation when >9 cm (Fig. 4.32).
- There may be soft-tissue calcification or masses that are relevant.
- The psoas shadows are visualized due to adjacent fat, and loss of clarity may indicate a retroperitoneal mass or collection. It is a normal variant for the right psoas shadow to be absent. In 20% of adults and 50% of children the right psoas shadow is absent.
- The organs are visualized as a result of surrounding fat. The perirenal and perivesical fat, i.e. fat surrounding the bladder and kidneys, enables assessment of their size. The posterior aspects of the liver and spleen are demarcated by fat. In 42% of normal individuals the spleen cannot be identified.
- The liver occupies a larger proportion of the abdomen in a child compared with an adult.
- The retroperitoneal fat line is a lucent line of fat lying between the parietal peritoneum and the transversalis muscle. This is absent in 18% of normal individuals.
- Skin folds or starched bed sheets may cause linear densities across the abdominal radiograph that mimic pathology.
- The skeleton/spine may show signs of spina bifida, collapsed vertebra or an absent sacrum.

When reporting an abdominal radiograph assess:
- The bowel for dilatation: up to five fluid levels are within normal limits in non-dilated small bowel.
- The presence of free air.
- The presence of ascites which displaces loops centrally.
- The hernial orifices for bowel gas, indicating a hernia.
- The size of the kidneys, liver and spleen.
- The spine and bones for abnormality.

Faecal transit time
The radiograph in Fig. 4.33 is taken when a faecal transit study is being performed. Radio-opaque markers are ingested and serial abdominal radiographs taken to assess the transit.

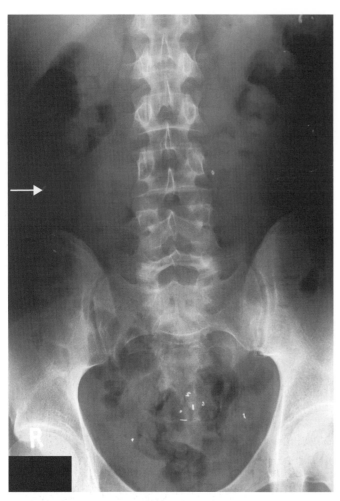

Fig. 4.33 Abdominal radiograph: faecal transit time. Small radio-opaque particles (arrow) are given and their progress through the colon is monitored with serial radiographs.

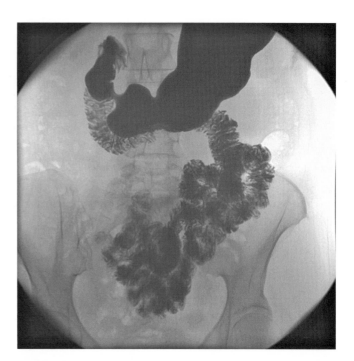

Fig. 4.34 Film from a series of a barium follow-through using high kilo-voltage.

Small bowel

Small bowel meal/follow-through

Indications

The meal or follow-through is performed to assess the mucosal relief of the small bowel. The small bowel enema is reserved for rare instances to gain a superior view of the mucosal relief of the small bowel, but is a time-consuming study for the radiologist who has to be present throughout the whole procedure, which may take over an hour. These are now usually performed only in specialist institutes and have largely been superseded by CT and MRI enteroclysis.

Technique

In a follow-though or small bowel meal, the patient drinks 500 ml of 50% barium. A radiograph is taken at 20 min in the supine position and then repeated at 20- to 30-min intervals with the patient prone, or longer if the passage of barium is slow.

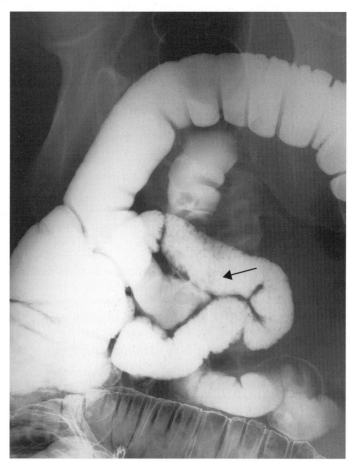

Fig. 4.35 Plain views of the terminal ileum are taken in the barium follow-through series. In this case the terminal ileum shows prominent but normal Peyer's patches, which are small filling defects (arrow).

- Metoclopramide, Gastrografin or other pharmacological agents can be given to speed transit time. Methylcellulose is used in small bowel enteroclysis.
- If the flow is slow, the time is doubled before repeating the radiograph to limit the radiation dose. When barium approaches the terminal ileum the radiologist screens the patient fluoroscopically using a remote cone to identify the terminal ileum and take dedicated spot pictures (Fig. 4.34).
- High kilovoltage is needed to penetrate the dense barium.
- The study is complete when barium flows into the caecum and ideally the appendix is visualized (Fig. 4.35).

Small bowel enema

Technique
- A special catheter is used which should be placed distal to the duodenojejunal flexure. This is to ensure the barium does not reflux backwards, leading to aspiration pneumonitis. The catheter is inserted through the nostril down into the stomach.
- 17–19% w/v barium is used, which is equivalent to one can of 100% barium diluted with four cans of water.
- The barium is poured as a continuous column from a height in a bag on a drip stand. The rapid flow rate causes good distension of the bowel.
- The end point is when the barium reaches the caecum (Fig. 4.36).

Findings
- The mucosal folds should be less than 2 mm thick.
- The calibre of the jejunum and ileum should be less than 4 cm and 3 cm respectively.
- The separation of the bowel loops reflects the thickness of the bowel wall. Increased separation of the loops may be due to a mass within the mesentery or abnormal thickening of the bowel wall.
- The jejunum should lie on the left and the ileum on the right.

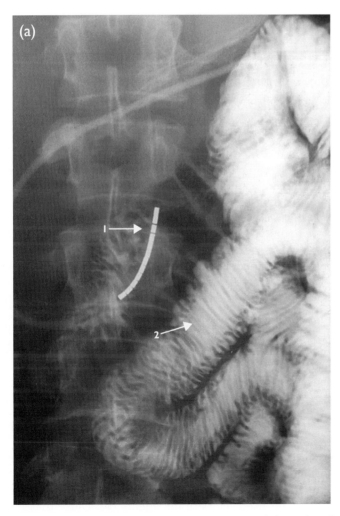 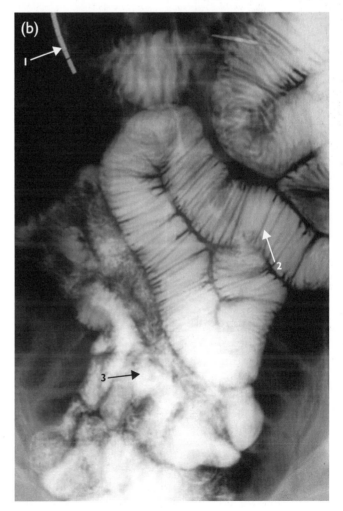

Fig. 4.36 Two views from a small bowel enema series showing the tube used. The tube should lie at the duodenojejunal flexure. (a) The tube (1) lies in the fourth part of the duodenum; (b) the tube (1) has been pulled back and the patient is at risk from aspiration. The jejunum (2) has more valvulae conniventes and a greater calibre. The terminal ileum (3) has more Peyer's patches and a smaller calibre.

- Nodules within the bowel may be present as a pathological finding unless lymphoid follicles.
- The folds may be smoothly or irregularly thickened (Fig. 4.37).

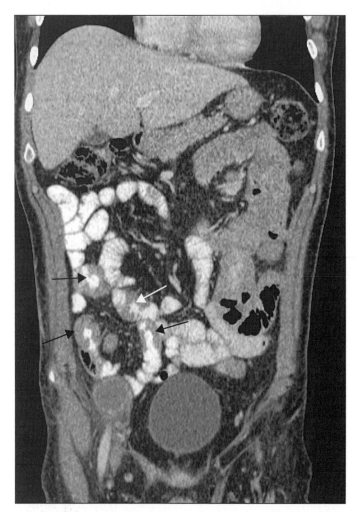

Fig. 4.37 Coronal CT of the abdomen showing multiple loops of thickened small bowel (arrows).

CT of the small bowel

Indication

Currently conventional enteroclysis is the method of choice for diagnosing inflammatory small bowel disease. CT is the investigation of choice for diagnosing extraluminal and extraintestinal complications such as fistulae and abscesses.

The applied radiation dose is high.

Technique

CT can be used for a dedicated small bowel study.

- The use of multidetector CT, neutral oral contrast agents and multiplanar thin section evaluation of the small bowel is known as CT enterography. Neutral contrast

agents are those with a CT number similar to water (10–30 HU), which allows full visualization of the bowel wall. Water in methylcellulose can be used and is better than water alone because there is improved small bowel distension as the water is absorbed less quickly.

- Intravenous contrast is used to enhance the small bowel.
- A nasojejunal tube can be used to distend the small bowel but is more invasive and known as CT enterography rather than CT enteroclysis.

Findings

- When the small bowel is distended with positive contrast, the wall thickness must be no more than 2 mm.
- Underdistension can give a false-positive diagnosis.
- An abnormal small bowel loop is present when the wall thickness is ≥3 mm.
- The mural enhancement pattern and lengths of involvement are important considerations.

MRI enterocyclis

See below for this.

Large bowel

Barium enema

Indications

Strictures, polyps, obstructing lesions.

Technique

- Bowel preparation is given to clear the colon, usually involving a combination of dietary restriction, excessive water drinking and laxatives or osmotic purgatives such as Picolax.
- A double-contrast barium enema can be performed (or colonoscopy or CT colonography).
- A barium enema involves three stages: filling the colon with barium, gas insufflation of the colon and radiography. A standard enema tip is safer than a balloon catheter.
- An intravenous smooth muscle relaxant is given to relax the colon – either 20 mg hyoscine butylbromide (Buscopan) or 0.2 mg glucagon.
- The gas used is air or CO_2 which is better absorbed.
- An instant enema is performed in suspected colitis with no bowel preparation, the rationale being that there is no faecal residue in an inflamed bowel with colitis. CT has largely superseded this.
- In cases of suspected bowel perforation barium is contraindicated due to the risk of severe adhesion formation. Water-soluble hypertonic or isotonic contrast agents can then be used. Hypertonic agents can cause diarrhoea, affect the circulating blood volume and may lead to perforation if they pass proximal to an obstruction because they will absorb water.

Findings
- The large bowel has haustra (Fig. 4.38).
- Normal lymphoid hyperplasia can occur in the terminal ileum, mimicking terminal ileitis.
- The caecum usually lies in the right iliac fossa, although it may lie in the right upper quadrant if undescended.
- The descending colon may normally be devoid of haustra (Fig. 4.39) and on a double-contrast barium enema there is often no haustra distal to the mid-transverse colon. Absence of haustra in the proximal colon is always abnormal.
- The ileocaecal valve can mimic a mass in the caecum on a barium enema, but the presence of fat identifiable on CT helps identify it.

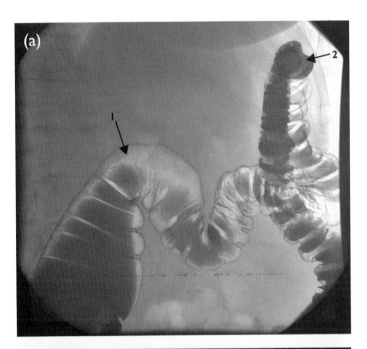

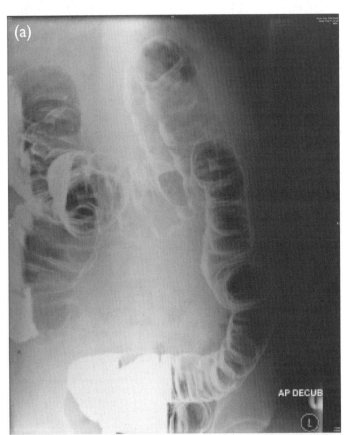

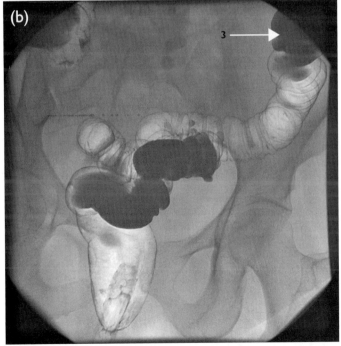

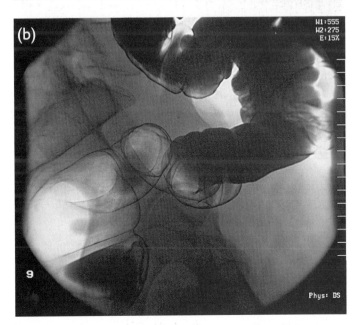

Fig. 4.38 (a, b) Two films from a barium enema series showing: hepatic flexure (1), splenic flexure (2) and descending colon (3).

Fig. 4.39 Large bowel enema showing (a) decubitus view and (b) zoomed view rectosigmoid colon.

- Pelvic lipomatosis, which is an excess of pelvic fat, can elongate and narrow the sigmoid.
- On a lateral radiograph the presacral space measures a maximum of 1–2 cm at the S4 level.

CT of the bowel

Indications
CT has gained increasing use in evaluation of acute appendicitis, inflammatory and small bowel disease, and colonography.
- In the acute abdomen CT can diagnose collections, diverticulitis and colitis.
- CT can evaluate the bowel wall and lumen, and the surrounding structures.
- CT can be used for staging GI, genitourinary and hepatobiliary tumours, assessing for distant spread.
- MR has become routine for local staging of rectal tumours.

Technique
- Oral contrast to opacify the bowel in CT is very dilute, i.e. 4% Gastrografin or similar. Contrast is used to change the density of the bowel and make it easier to identify masses and bowel wall thickening (Fig. 4.40).
- The oral contrast indicated depends on the protocol. For gastric assessment the patient should fast for 6 hours before the test. Water contrast is used for the stomach and a litre is drunk shortly before scanning and 200 CL immediately prior to the scan.
- For optimal visualization of the small bowel, oral contrast with barium or dilute Gastrografin is given: 1000–2000 ml should be given starting at least 90 min before, with cups every 15 min.
- For the large bowel oral contrast at least 90 min before the study is recommended.
- Rectal contrast may be required for distal or rectal lesions.
- Intravenous contrast is administered with image acquisition in the portal phase.
- CT of the abdomen and pelvis is suboptimal for a few days after a barium enema due to image degradation from the high-density barium which causes streak artefacts.

Findings
- The small bowel on a supine CT has intraluminal gas in the anterior lumen.
- The ileum lies predominantly in the right lower quadrant and the terminal ileum can be seen on CT clearly joining the caecum.
- The ileocaecal valve may be very prominent and appear as a soft-tissue mass which can be identified sometimes by the presence of fat (Fig. 4.41).
- In the large bowel, small bubbles of gas are seen in the non-distended colon (Fig. 4.42).
- The bowel should be assessed for:
  - wall thickness
  - dilatation
  - stranding around the bowel
  - masses related to the bowel
  - lymph nodes in the pericolonic or mesenteric fat.

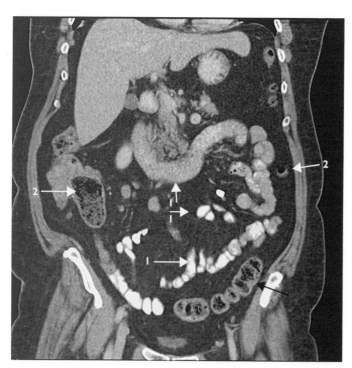

Fig. 4.40 Coronal CT scan of the bowel. The CT shows the small bowel lying centrally (1) and containing all the contrast. The large bowel (2) lies towards the periphery of the abdomen. Coronal imaging is very useful for assessing the bowel. Iliacus muscle (black arrow).

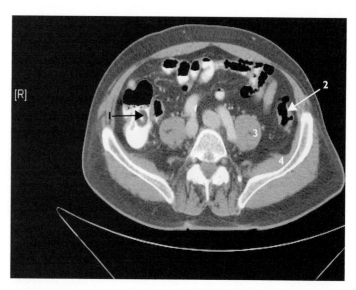

Fig. 4.41 CT of the abdomen showing the ileocaecal valve which is characteristically fatty (1). Descending colon (2), psoas muscle (3) and iliacus muscle (4).

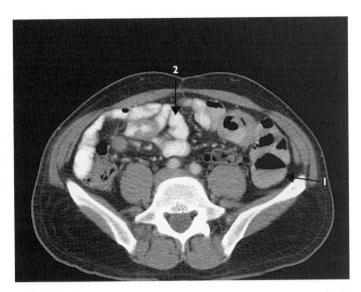

Fig. 4.42 CT of the abdomen showing the large bowel peripherally (1) and the small bowel centrally (2).

- If oral water contrast is used the mucosa will enhance normally following intravenous contrast.
- The large bowel has a wall thickness less than 2 mm and again, after oral water contrast and intravenous contrast, the enhancing normal mucosa can be seen.
- On CT the normal appendix is a thin tubular structure, of variable position, arising from the caecum. If the appendix is air filled on CT, this virtually excludes an inflammatory process. The normal appendix is less than 6 mm transversely. The surrounding fat is 'clean'. An appendicolith, i.e. calcification in the appendix, may be an incidental finding.

Pathology
- Stranding in the fat surrounding the bowel is one of the most important abnormal signs that can be seen in acute appendicitis, diverticulitis or tumour invasion of the surrounding fat. Fat stranding becomes more apparent when comparing the fat in the normal asymptomatic side with the fat density in the symptomatic area. A subtle small increase in fat density could be overlooked (Fig. 4.43).
- The abdomen is lined by peritoneum which is a common site for tumour seedlings from colonic and ovarian cancer.
- The peritoneum and omenta are not usually visible on CT by their fat density, unless involved with tumour or infection, where they become thickened and denser. Peritoneal stranding, omental caking and omental deposits are all quite difficult to visualize. It is best to look in the areas of fat that are normally relatively isolated, i.e. in the left upper outer quadrant near the spleen, towards the heart, underneath the diaphragm and in front of the transverse colon. Omental deposits cause an extra layer of soft tissue anterior to the colon called an omental cake.

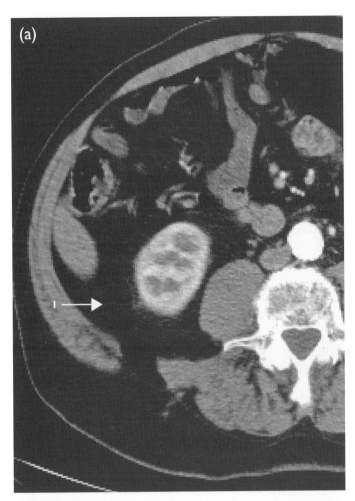

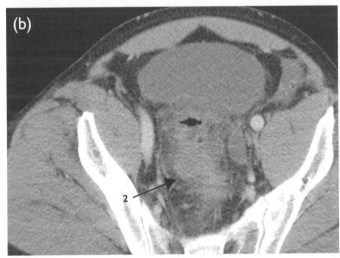

Fig. 4.43 (a) CT of the abdomen showing perirenal stranding (1). (b) CT of the pelvis showing stranding around the sigmoid colon in sigmoid diverticulitis (2).

- CT can just detect the thin mesorectum which confines the rectum (Fig. 4.44).
- CT may detect the transition point between dilated and normal bowel in bowel obstruction.

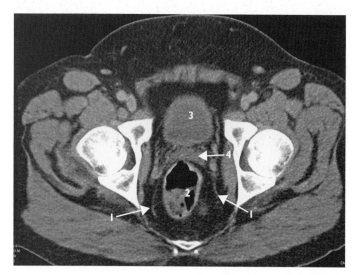

Fig. 4.44 CT of the pelvis showing the mesorectum (1) around the rectum (2). Bladder (3) and seminal vesicles (4).

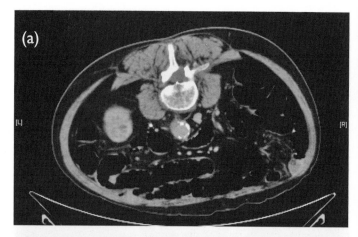

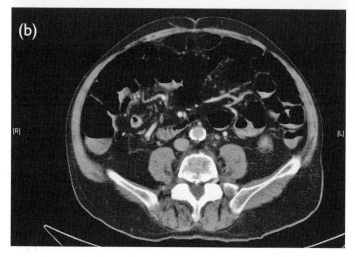

Fig. 4.45 CT enema with (a) prone and (b) supine images.

CT colonography

This can be performed to detect colonic cancer after a failed barium enema or colonoscopy, or as part of a screening programme. In some institutions it is used as a first-line investigation to assess the large bowel, being a focused examination of the colon.

Technique
- A suggested preparation is dietary restriction with clear fluids for 2 days before the procedure and then two sachets of Picolax given 3 h apart the day before.
- In CT colonography faecal tagging can be used, whereby the patient drinks dilute barium and liquid Gastrografin the day before the procedure to tag any solid or liquid faecal residue, which is then removed by the CT colonography software.
- Rectal insufflation with air or CO_2 is used.
- Prone and supine scanning positions are adopted.
- Hyoscine butyl bromide or glucagon may relieve abdominal pain and achieve better distension.
- Software enables virtual colonography (Fig. 4.45).
- Intravenous contrast is not routinely used.

CT of the acute abdomen

Indication
CT is increasingly used in acute abdominal pain.

Technique
- Oral contrast use varies according to the suspected pathology. It may obscure causes of GI bleeding and gastric pathology. It should not be given in high small bowel obstruction due to the risk of aspiration, and is also unnecessary in small bowel obstruction as the dilated fluid filled bowel has its own contrast.
- Water contrast, i.e. negative contrast is used with the stomach in suspected malignancy and upper small bowel disease, and in pancreatitis if the patient can tolerate it.
- Oral positive contrast can be given if the patient can tolerate it to help in inflammation, abscess, diverticulitis, etc.
- In acute appendicitis oral contrast is not given. The abnormal appendix is surrounded by stranding or fluid. There may be reactive surrounding lymphadenopathy and thickening of surrounding caecum or small bowel (Fig. 4.46).

Findings
- Abnormal fat stranding suggests inflammation.

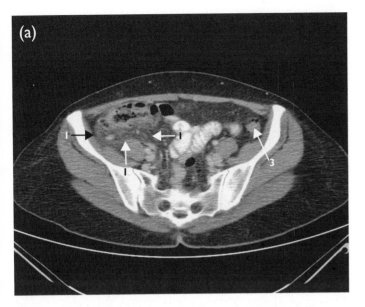

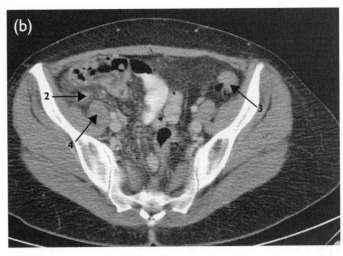

Fig. 4.46 (a) CT of the abdomen showing stranding (1) around the caecal pole. (b) CT of the abdomen showing a dilated appendix with stranding around it (2). Descending colon (3) and iliopsoas muscle (4).

- Free fluid may be found in the paracolic gutters, subdiaphragmatic spaces, Morrison's pouch, i.e. the hepatorenal fossa, and the pelvis. Retroperitoneal fluid is found around the psoas muscles.
- Free gas is easily seen by looking for extraluminal gas through a lung window setting.

MR enteroclysis of the small bowel

Indication
MRI has emerged as an alternative small bowel imaging technique that can be performed without ionizing radiation.

Technique
- Oral contrast agents such as mannitol can be used to image the small bowel. Inflamed small bowel and extraluminal complications in inflammatory bowel disease, particularly Crohn's disease, can be identified without using ionizing radiation.
- MR enterocyclis can distinguish between active and inactive strictures. The images can be used for virtual small bowel endoscopy.

- Dedicated high-resolution T1-weighted three-dimensional FLASH (**f**ast **l**ow **a**ngle **sh**ot MRI) sequences with fat suppression are performed after a suitable oral contrast agent.
- The high filling volume used for the small bowel leads to a secondary paralysis of the small bowel and avoids motion artefacts (Fig. 4.47).

MR of the rectum

Indications
Staging rectal carcinoma, fistula tracts, pelvic floor.

Technique
Angled MR images are taken through the rectum with and without gadolinium.

Findings
The mesocolon, which is the fascia confining the rectum and hence tumour spread, is well visualized with MRI. Fistulae are well seen with STIR images in three planes (Fig. 4.48).

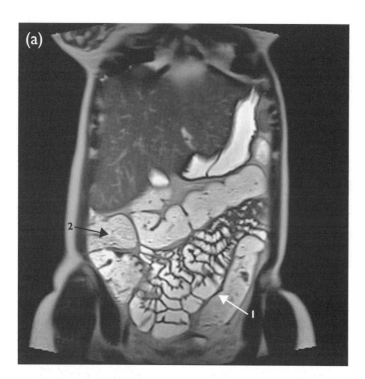

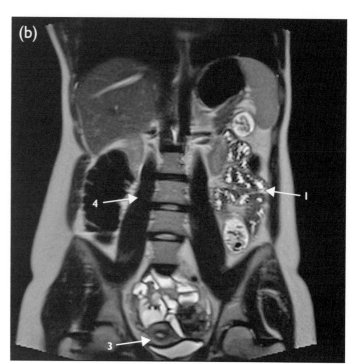

Fig. 4.47 (a) MR enteroclysis coronal MR showing small bowel centrally (1) and large bowel peripherally (2); (b) coronal MR enteroclysis showing small bowel (1), uterus (3) and psoas muscle (4).

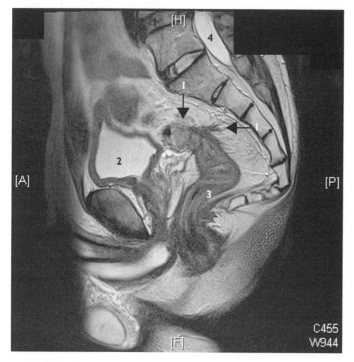

Fig. 4.48 MR of the rectum, sagittal plane, showing a rectosigmoid tumour with stranding in the surrounding fat (1). Bladder (2), rectum (3) and theca (4).

CASES

Case 4.1

Patient presents with dysphagia and iron deficiency anaemia. The initial investigation is a barium swallow (Fig. 4.49).

- There is an anterior constant defect seen in the cervical oesophagus on a lateral barium swallow. The constant nature of the defect differentiates this from a postcricoid venous plexus.
- The defect is found at C5.
- Is a short, sharp thin anterior defect.

An oesophageal web can be associated with Plummer–Vinson syndrome.

The idealized report reads: On the barium swallow in the hypopharynx there is a short anterior filling defect consistent with an oesophageal web, the remaining oesophagus appears normal with no GO reflux seen.

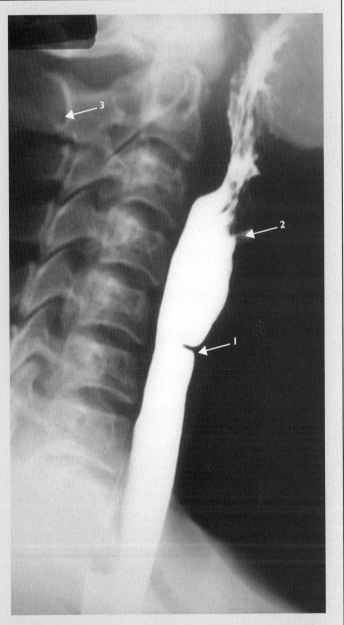

Fig. 4.49 Lateral barium swallow of the neck showing an anterior defect in the anterior oesophagus, which is sharp and constant. It is an oesophageal web (1), epiglottis (2), spinolaminar line (3).

Case 4.2

Patient presents with weight loss and dysphagia for solid food. Investigation: barium swallow (Fig 4.50).

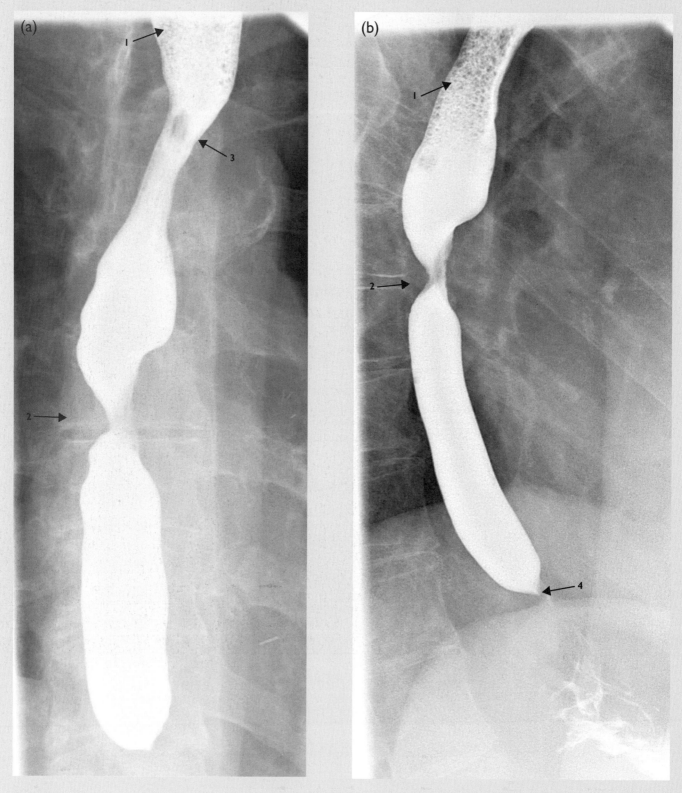

Fig. 4.50 (a, b) Two views of a barium swallow showing food debris (1) above an oesophageal shouldered stricture (2), arch of aorta (3) and GOJ (4).

The whole oesophagus must be examined. The cervical oesophagus appeared normal.

- On the thoracic views of the oesophagus there is a shouldered irregular stricture in the mid-oesophagus. This cannot be distended even on double-contrast views. It is an anterior and a posterior apple-core deformity
- Food debris is seen above the stricture.
- The diagnosis is suggestive of a malignant stricture, but a histological biopsy is required for confirmation.
- Not all strictures are malignant. Evidence of severe reflux with ulceration helps widen the differential to include reflux oesophagitis. Benign strictures can occur after caustic ingestion and occur at the natural hold-up points such as the aortic arch. They are longer and smoother than malignant ones.

The idealized report would read: There is an irregular short stricture in the distal oesophagus just above the GOJ. The differential for the stricture includes malignancy. Biopsy recommended.

Case 4.3

The patient presents with rectal bleeding and weight loss.

A barium enema is performed (Fig. 4.51). Barium has to fill the whole colon and the caecum be visualized. This is recognized by filling of the appendix or reflux into the terminal ileum. A study is incomplete if the caecum is not definitely visualized.

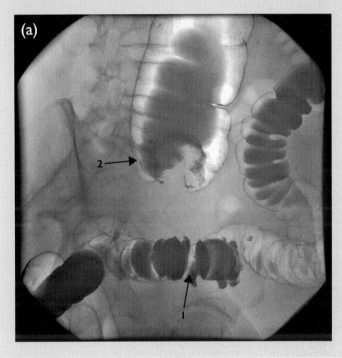
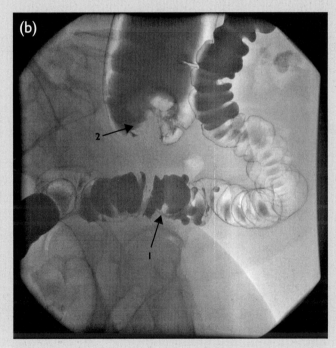

Findings

Initially diverticular disease is seen in the sigmoid colon. The enema also shows an irregular filling defect in the ascending colon. This has the appearance of a carcinoma.

If one abnormality is diagnosed, a second lesion may be present as metachronous bowel tumours. A CT of the abdomen with oral and intravenous contrast is performed for staging. Using a standard system this is reviewed:

- Lung bases: clear
- Liver, spleen, pancreas, adrenals and kidneys normal
- No para-aortic lymphadenopathy
- There is a mass in the caecum
- Then assess for the presence of free fluid, bony lesions, a second bowel lesion and locoregional nodal involvement, and most importantly peritoneal disease.

The idealized report reads: The lung bases are clear. The liver, spleen, pancreas, gallbladder, adrenals and kidneys appear normal. There is a large mass in the ascending colon with multiple enlarged locoregional nodes. Some small peritoneal nodules are present. No free fluid. The diagnosis on CT is of a colonic cancer with locoregional lymphadenopathy and peritoneal nodules.

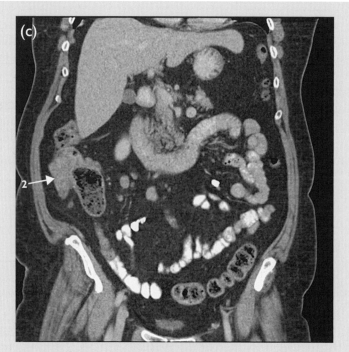

Fig. 4.51 (a, b) Two views from a barium enema and (c) coronal CT abdomen. Sigmoid diverticular disease (1) and a polypoid tumour in the caecum (2).

Case 4.4

A patient presents with left iliac fossa pain and pyrexia.

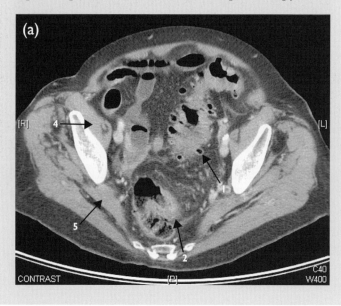

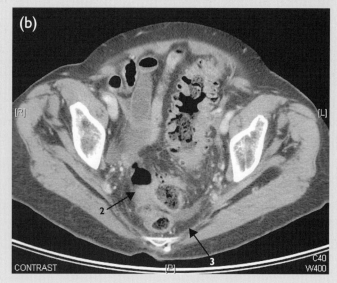

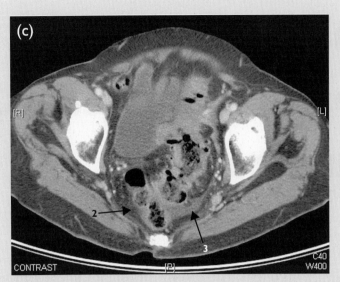
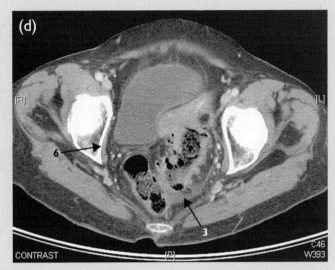

Fig. 4.52 (a–d) Four views from CT of the pelvis showing sigmoid diverticular disease (1) and stranding around the colon (2). (b) A trace of free fluid around the sigmoid colon is shown which may be very small and hard to detect (3). Right iliopsoas muscle with central fatty tendon (4), piriformis muscle (5) and obturator internus muscle (6).

- The history usually indicates the possibility of acute diverticulitis, i.e. there is left iliac fossa pain, acute onset, pyrexia. Ultrasound was and still is commonly unhelpful.
- A CT abdomen is the primary imaging mode which should have adequate bowel preparation with oral contrast at least 90 min before the test and intravenous contrast in the portal phase.
- Follow the system of reviewing the lung bases, liver, spleen, pancreas, gallbladder and adrenal glands.
- The bowel must be carefully assessed from the rectum through to the caecum, but particularly concentrating on the left iliac fossa images due to the symptoms and signs. Colonic diverticula may be present without being symptomatic.
- Wall thickening helps differentiate inflamed diverticula from simple diverticula. By closely analysing for 'dirty' stranded fat around the symptomatic area the pathology and inflammation becomes visible (Fig. 4.52).
- Free fluid may be very subtle around the area of concern. Collections are overlooked if the lumen of the bowel is not carefully traced. Tracks of free air extending from the colon become more apparent on close analysis. If air is present in an uncatheterized bladder suspect a colovesical fistula.
- In this case the findings were in the left iliac fossa with free fluid, stranding and thickened inflamed diverticula. No abscess was present. There was no free air present (checked by reviewing for extraluminal gas on a lung window).

The idealized report should read: Within the pelvis in the left iliac fossa there is acute diverticulitis with thickening of the sigmoid wall, diverticula and stranded, inflamed surrounding fat. A small amount of free fluid is seen around the segment of bowel but no abscess. No other significant abnormality is seen.

5 Gastrointestinal imaging 2: liver, spleen, pancreas, adrenals, biliary tract and aorta

RADIOLOGICAL ANATOMY

The liver

- The liver is divided into right and left lobes according to the arterial supply to the liver and not according to the fissure for the falciform ligament. The fissure subdivides the left lobe of the liver into medial and lateral lobes.
- The liver is then subdivided into eight segments according to the Couinand or bismuth classification, which reflects the vascular supply of the segments. The segments function independently and are numbered according to their relationship with the three hepatic veins and the portal vein. The right lobe comprises segments V, VI, VII and VIII, and the left segments I, II, III and IV.
- The portal vein divides the liver into superior and inferior levels. The level of the portal vein is called the principal plane (Fig. 5.1).

- Segment I, the caudate lobe, lies posterior to the inferior vena cava and the ligamentum venosum (the obliterated ductus venosus) and is part of the left lobe (Fig. 5.2).
- Segment IV, the quadrate lobe, is a large segment divided into IVa cranially and IVb caudally due to the vascular supply. It is part of the left lobe of the liver and lies between the gallbladder fossa and the ligamentum teres (the obliterated umbilical vein).
- The upper segments are segments IVA, II, VII and VIII (Fig. 5.3).
- The lower segments are segments are segments VI, V, IVb and III.
- When reporting CT it is important to accurately ascribe lesions to the correct segment.
- The falciform ligament lies within the fissure and ligamentum teres, which is the obliterated umbilical vein. In cirrhosis with portal hypertension, the umbilical vein may recanalize and flow may be seen in it to the umbilicus.

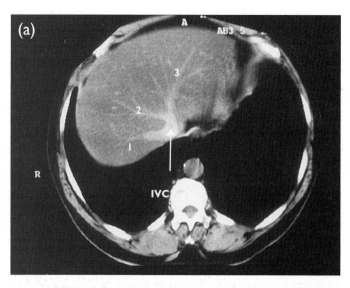
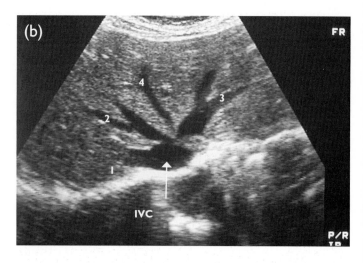

Fig. 5.1 (a) Axial CT of the liver enhanced showing the three hepatic veins dividing the liver into segments. (b) Subcostal ultrasound of the liver showing the hepatic veins joining into the inferior vena cava causing a crows' feet appearance. Right hepatic vein (1), middle hepatic vein (2) and left hepatic vein (3), accessory (4).

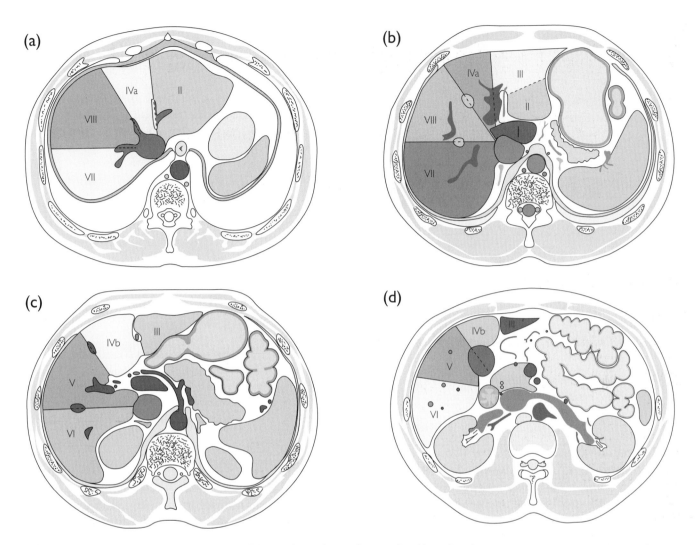

Fig. 5.2 Diagram showing segments of the liver and their relationship to the portal and hepatic veins.

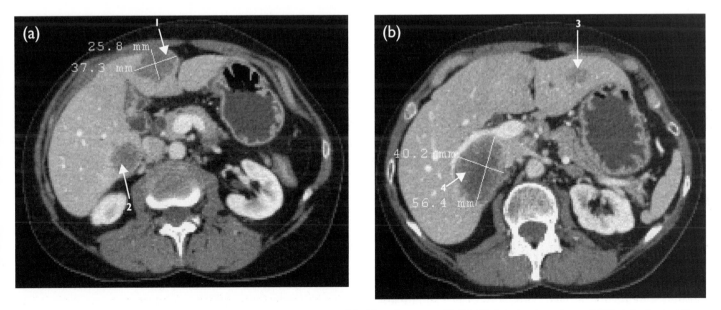

Fig. 5.3 (a) Axial post-contrast CT showing liver lesions in segment IVb (1) and segment VI (2). (b) A lesion in segment III (3) and a further large lesion in segment VI (4).

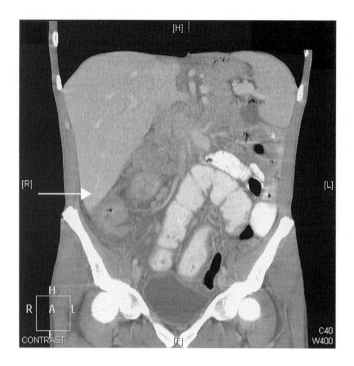

Fig. 5.4 Coronal post-contrast CT shows a normal variant of large Reidel's lobe (arrow) extending into the right iliac fossa.

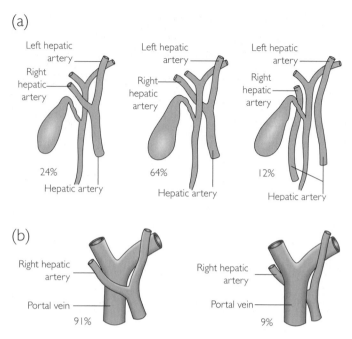

Fig. 5.5 (a) Diagram showing the variations in relationship of the hepatic artery and common bile duct. (b) Diagram shows the usual configuration of anatomy at the porta in 91% with the portal vein posteriorly; the right hepatic artery then normally lies anteriorly in between the portal vein and the common hepatic duct. The other variations are shown.

- Segments II and III lie to the left of the fissure.
- Common anatomical variants are a large left lobe that fills the left dome of the diaphragm and may wrap over the spleen, or a hypoplastic segment IVb.
- The right lobe is normally bigger than the left lobe by a ratio of 3:2. Reidel's lobe is a variant when the right lobe extends inferiorly into the right iliac fossa, seen in up to 10% of women (Fig. 5.4).

Vascular supply to the liver

- The liver has a dual vascular supply with 25% originating from the hepatic artery and 75% from the portal vein.
- The common hepatic artery normally arises from the coeliac axis and becomes the hepatic artery proper after giving rise to the gastroduodenal artery. In the porta, the hepatic artery normally lies posterior to the common hepatic duct and anteromedial to the portal vein. However, a variant is a hepatic artery arising from the superior mesenteric artery (SMA) which may run posterior to the portal vein (Fig. 5.5).
- The portal vein is formed from the confluence of the SMA and the splenic vein at L1–2 behind the neck of the pancreas.
- There are usually three hepatic veins that separate the liver in the vertical plane into segments. There may be accessory hepatic veins. The caudate lobe drains separately into the inferior vena cava (IVC). The caudate lobe may hypertrophy when there is thrombosis or occlusion of the other hepatic veins, draining segments 2–8 in

Budd–Chiari disease, due to its separate venous drainage (Fig. 5.6).
- Hepatic veins have no valves so pulsed Doppler ultrasound reflects a waveform similar to the heart.
- There are many variations in the arterial supply to the liver occurring in 45% of individuals. Vessels can be replaced or accessory. The hepatic arteries right or left

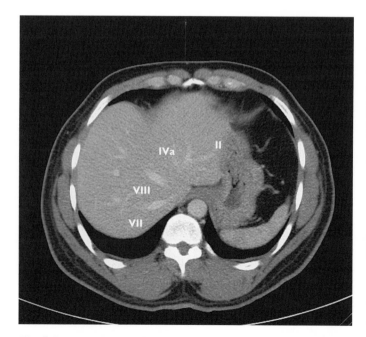

Fig. 5.6 Axial enhanced CT showing the hepatic veins dividing the liver into segments VII, VIII, IVa and II.

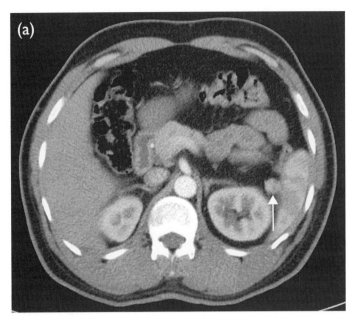
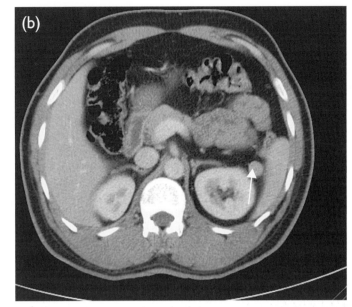

Fig. 5.7 Axial enhanced CT of a splenunculus (arrow) in portal phases.

can arise directly off the aorta, or from the coeliac directly or the SMA.

The spleen

- The craniocaudal length of the spleen has a range of 10–15 cm normally, although in most people the spleen is <12 cm long.
- Small foci of splenic tissue called splenunculi may be visible on CT in up to 10% of adults (Fig. 5.7).
- The spleen lies within the peritoneum.

Vascular supply to the spleen

- The spleen is supplied by the splenic artery, a branch of the coeliac axis. The artery is often tortuous and may calcify, giving rise to the appearance of a 'curly pig tail'.
- The splenic vein joins the superior mesenteric vein (SMV) to form the portal vein. The splenic vein runs posterior to the pancreas forming its posterior border.
- The inferior mesenteric vein drains into the splenic vein (Fig. 5.8).

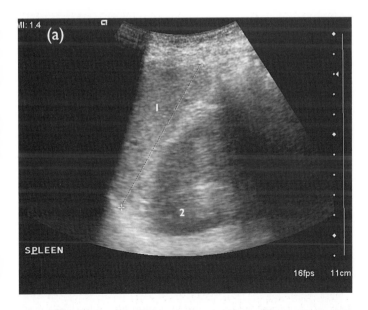
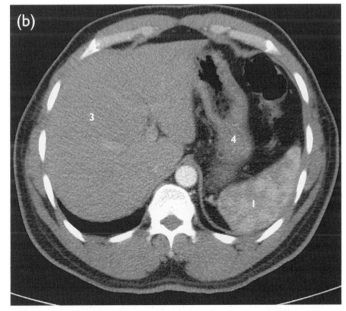

Fig. 5.8 (a) Ultrasound of the spleen (1), which should normally have a convex and a concave border. Left kidney (2). (a) Axial arterial phase-enhanced CT showing the normal heterogeneous filling of the spleen (1) on arterial phase. Liver (3) and stomach (4).

Pancreas

- The pancreas lies at L1 and has a head, neck, body and tail. The head lies more inferiorly than the tail (Fig. 5.9). The tail usually ends intraperitoneally in the splenic hilum.
- The pancreas lies in the anterior aspect of the retroperitoneal space. It is bound posteriorly by Gerota's fascia and anteriorly by the parietal peritoneum.
- The lesser sac lies anterior to the pancreas between the stomach and the pancreas.
- The pancreatic size and shape are extremely variable, but normally the pancreas should gently taper towards the tail. Fatty replacement of the pancreas is common with age.
- The pancreatic head lies within the C-shaped curve of the duodenum.
- The SMA and SMV lie anterior to the uncinate process of the pancreas; identifying the superior mesenteric vessels is a landmark for the position of the uncinate process.
- The SMA is normally completely surrounded by fat with a fat plane seen between itself and the pancreas.
- The main pancreatic duct joins the bile duct to from the common bulbous portion known as the ampulla which drains into the second part of the duodenum at the papilla. The accessory pancreatic duct drains into the duodenum 2 cm proximal to the main duct. There is usually a communication between the two ducts.
- In utero the pancreas is formed from a dorsal and ventral bud. At 6 weeks in utero, the ventral bud rotates and fuses with the dorsal bud.
- The dorsal bud forms the body, head and accessory duct of Santorini.
- The uncinate process of the pancreas is formed from the ventral bud (Fig. 5.10). The ventral bud arises in common with the common bile duct to form the main duct of Wirsung.
- In 9% the two pancreatic ducts, i.e. the ducts of Santorini and Wirsung, are separate giving rise to pancreas divisum (Fig. 5.10b).
- In some the ventral bud fails to atrophy, leaving a ring of pancreas surrounding the duodenum called an annular pancreas.
- Accessory pancreatic tissue called 'rests' can be found in the stomach or duodenum

Vascular supply to the pancreas

- The pancreas is supplied by branches of the coeliac artery and SMA. Having arisen from the common hepatic artery, the gastroduodenal artery gives off the superior pancreaticoduodenal artery, which forms an important anastomosis with the inferior pancreaticoduodenal, a branch of the SMA. The anastomosis is between the coeliac artery and the SMAs.
- The splenic artery gives rise to the dorsal pancreatic artery and pancreatica magna artery.

- The pancreatic head drains to the SMV, but the remaining pancreas drains to the splenic vein (Fig. 5.11).
- The splenic artery runs along the superior surface of the pancreas and the splenic vein forms the posterior border.

Gallbladder and biliary tract

- In the liver, the right and left intrahepatic bile ducts drain the right and left lobes. The bile ducts have a segmental anatomy similar to that of the hepatic arteries. The right and left bile ducts join at the porta to form the common hepatic duct.
- The gallbladder drains via the cystic duct into the common hepatic duct to form the common bile duct.
- The course and length of the cystic duct are variable, being up to 3–4 cm in length.
- The common bile duct (CBD) lies anterior to the porta vein in the porta (Fig. 5.12).
- The CBD runs on the posterior aspect of the pancreatic head and then opens with the pancreatic duct into the second part of the duodenum at the papilla. There is a circular muscle layer called the sphincter of Oddi at the ampulla. A variant is the pancreatic duct and CBD opening separately into the duodenum
- The gallbladder lies in the gallbladder fossa on the under surface of the right lobe of the liver, but its position and size are extremely variable. It usually measures up to 10 cm in length. It may lie surrounded by liver or down in the right iliac fossa on a long mesentery. It is covered by mesentery (Fig. 5.13).
- The gallbladder has a thin smooth wall up to 2 mm thick and the distal portion, which is dilated, is called

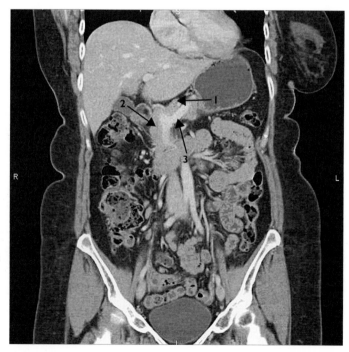

Fig. 5.9 Coronal CT of the pancreas showing how the tail (1) lies higher than the head (2) and the close relationship to the splenic vein (3).

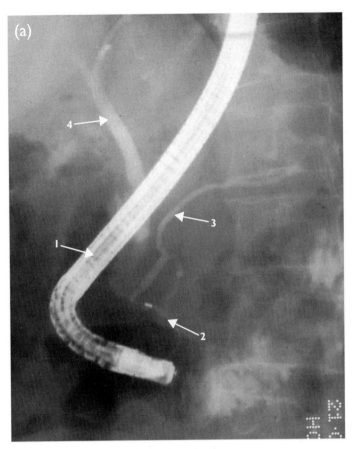

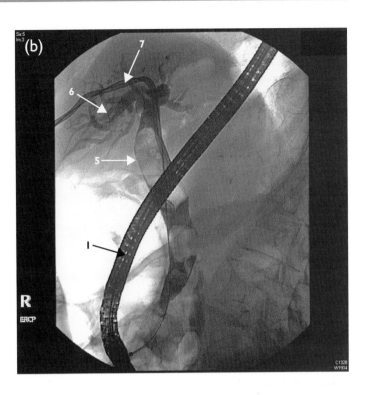

Fig. 5.10 Images from an ERCP: conventional (a) and digital (b) images show the endoscope (1) lying in the second part of the duodenum. The catheter (2) lies in the ampulla. (a) Opacification of the pancreatic duct (3) with the accessory and main duct visualized and the common duct (4). (b) Taken during interventional procedure for a dilated common bile duct (CBD). It shows the CBD full of stones seen as filling defects (5), dilated intrahepatic bile ducts (6) and a percutaneous catheter (7).

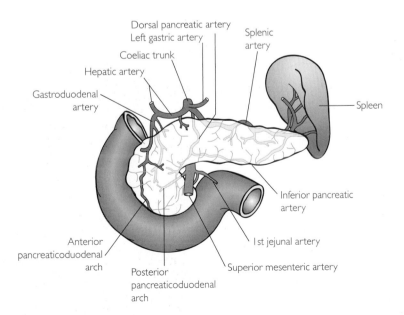

Fig. 5.11 Diagram showing the vascular supply to the pancreas from branches of the hepatic and splenic arteries.

the fundus. The fundus of the gallbladder may be folded over, known as a phrygian cap, making it difficult to assess the lumen.

- A small expansion of the gallbladder neck is called Hartmann's pouch.
- Spiral folds in the neck are called valves of Heister.
- The vascular supply to the gallbladder is the cystic artery, a branch of the hepatic artery.

Openings of the diaphragm

- T8: an opening in the central right tendon of the diaphragm through which the IVC and right phrenic nerve pass.
- T10: to the left of the midline, but the right crus surrounds it, and passes the oesophagus, vagus nerves and gastric vessels.
- T12: behind the median arcuate ligament, anterior to T12 between the crura, passes the aorta, thoracic duct and azygos vein.
- Behind the crura, retrocrural nodes may be seen which can normally measure up to 6 mm in short axis diameter (Fig. 5.14).
- The right crus arises from L1–3 and the left crus from L1–2.

Abdominal aorta

The aorta becomes abdominal at T12 when it passes between the crura with the azygos vein and thoracic duct. The aorta lies to the left and the IVC to the right. There are three main branches arising anteriorly from the abdominal aorta (Fig. 5.15).

- The coeliac axis arises at T12–L1 supplying the liver, spleen, stomach and pancreas.
- Its branches are: common hepatic, splenic, left gastric artery.
- The splenic artery has the appearance of a curly pig tail.
- The left gastric runs vertically upwards and is seen only above the origin of the coeliac axis. It is an important site to assess for left gastric lymphadenopathy in oesophageal stomach and upper gastrointestinal (GI) malignancy (Figs 5.16 and 5.17).
- There is an important anastomosis between the coeliac artery and the SMA through the inferior and superior pancreaticoduodenal branches. This can save the bowel if there is a thrombus at the origin of the SMA.
- The SMA arises from the aorta at L1–2 and descends vertically, parallel to the descending abdominal aorta.
- The SMA supplies the small and large bowel from the second part of the duodenum up to the mid-transverse colon/splenic flexure.

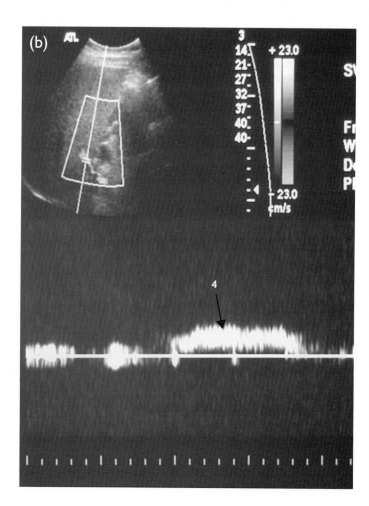

Fig. 5.12 (a) Ultrasound of the porta, showing the portal vein posteriorly (1), the right hepatic artery (2) and the common duct anteriorly (3); (b) a normal Doppler trace of the portal vein with anterograde flow that gently oscillates (4).

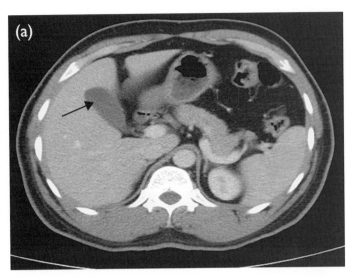

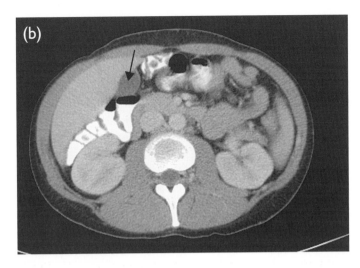

Fig. 5.13 (a,b) CT scan of the gallbladder showing two cases with variable position of the gallbladder.

- The branches include jejunal, ileal, inferior pancreaticoduodenal, middle colic, ileocolic and sometimes a right colic.
- The SMA should be surrounded by fat. Loss of this fat in pancreatic carcinoma implies vascular invasion (Fig. 5.18).
- The relationship of the SMA and SMV is important; the SMA should always lie to the left of the SMV. If the ratio is reversed and the SMA lies to the right of the SMV, there may be an associated malrotation of the small bowel which is at risk of volvulus.

- The inferior mesenteric artery (IMA) arises at L3 from the aorta. This is a very small vessel relative to the SMA (Fig. 5.19).
- The branches of the IMA include the superior rectal, left colic and sigmoid arteries. The wandering artery of Drummond or marginal artery arises from the left colic, which anastomoses with the SMA branches.
- The superior rectal artery forms an important anastomosis with the inferior rectal artery, a branch of the internal iliac vein. This is a portosystemic anastomosis.

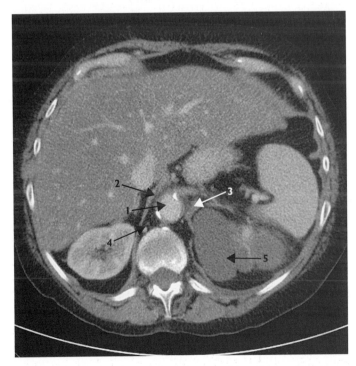

Fig. 5.14 Axial CT of an aortic hiatus: aorta (1), right crus (2), left crus (3), azygos vein (4) and cysts in left kidney (5).

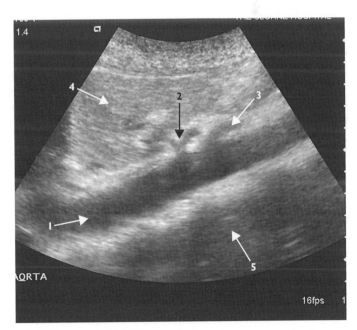

Fig. 5.15 Longitudinal ultrasound of the epigastrium showing the aorta (1) with the left lobe of liver anteriorly (4), the vertebrae posteriorly (5) and the origin of the coeliac artery (2) and the SMA (3).

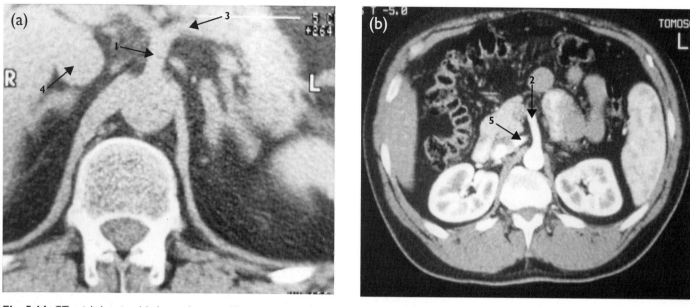

Fig. 5.16 CT axial showing (a) the coeliac axis (1) arising at T12 with a seagull shape and (b) the SMA (2) at L1: splenic artery (3), IVC (4) and left renal vein (5).

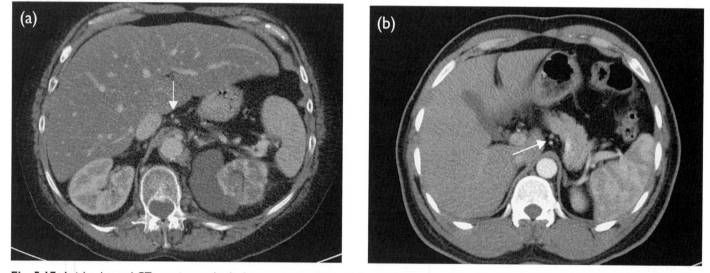

Fig. 5.17 Axial-enhanced CT: two images both showing the position of left gastric artery and lymph nodes (arrow) above the coeliac axis.

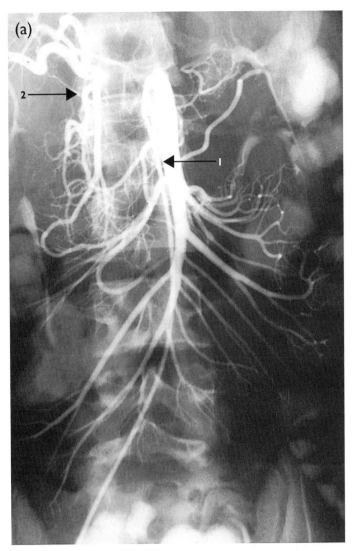

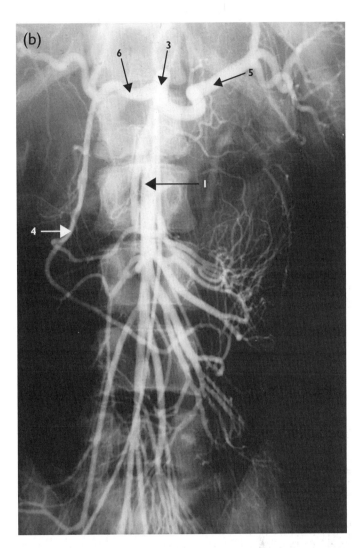

Fig. 5.18 SMA angiogram: (a) direct SMA (1) angiogram showing the anastomosis between the superior and inferior pancreaticoduodenal arteries (2) in the right upper quadrant. (b) Simultaneous coeliac (3) and SMA (1) angiograms done selectively. This also shows the anastomosis between the two vessels via the pancreaticoduodenal branches (4). Splenic artery (5) and common hepatic artery (6).

There are three main pairs arising laterally from the abdominal aorta:

- The adrenal arteries arising at L1
- The renal arteries arising at L1–2
- The gonadal arteries arising at L3.

The aorta also gives rise to the inferior phrenic and lumbar vessels before it bifurcates into the common iliac arteries and median sacral artery.

Inferior vena cava

- The IVC forms at L5 from the common iliac veins.
- The IVC pierces the diaphragm at T8 to enter the heart.
- The IVC has no valves except the one at the atrium.
- Anatomical variants of the IVC include a persistent left IVC below the level of the renal veins (Fig. 5.20).

The retroperitoneum (Fig. 5.21)

The following structures lie in the retroperitoneum:

- The abdominal aorta lies to the left of the midline, directly in front of the lumbar vertebrae. The calibre of the aorta is age dependent, but is about 2–3 cm wide normally.
- The branches of the abdominal aorta are retroperitoneal.
- The IVC varies in size and shape according to respiration. It receives the three main hepatic veins below the diaphragm.
- The kidneys.
- The adrenals.
- The pancreas.
- The second, third and fourth parts of the duodenum.
- Part of the descending colon.
- Part of the ascending colon.

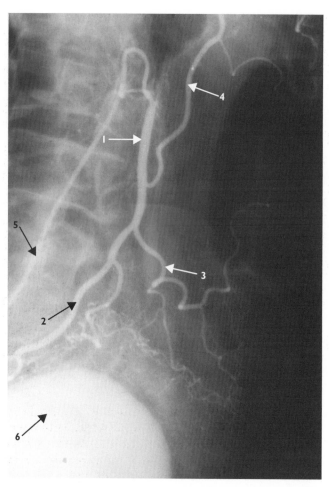

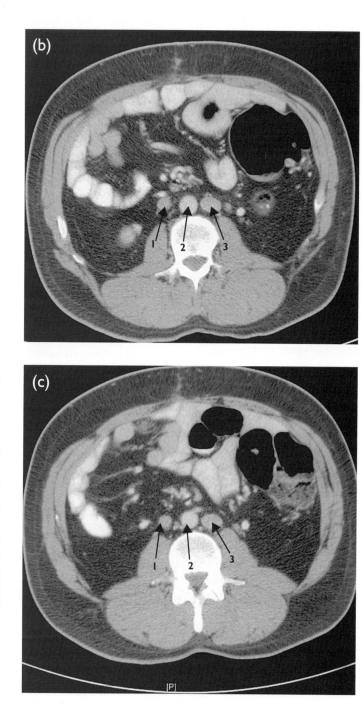

Fig. 5.19 CT of the selective catheterization of the inferior mesenteric artery (1) showing the superior rectal (2), sigmoid (3), left colic (4) and the catheter (5). The bladder (6) is full.

Fig. 5.20 Axial enhanced CT: three images at level (a) of left renal vein (4), (b) of L3, and (c) just above the aortic bifurcation, showing a left inferior vena cava (3) draining into the left renal vein (4). Aorta (2) and right inferior vena cava (1). This case is a double IUC, but right IUC may be absent.

(a)

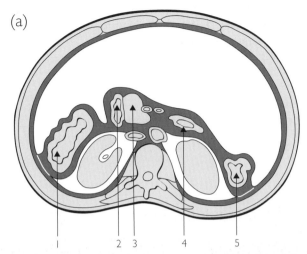

(b)

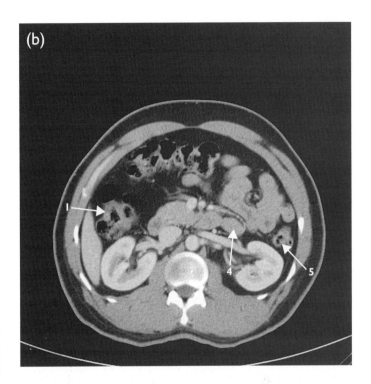

(c)

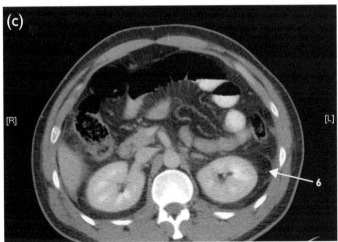

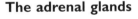

Fig. 5.21 (a) Diagram of the retroperitoneum showing ascending colon (1), second part of duodenum (2), head of pancreas (3), duodenojejunal (DJ) flexure (4) and descending colon (5); (b) axial CT of the abdomen showing ascending colon (1), DJ flexure (4) and descending colon (5). (c) Axial CT of the abdomen showing Gerota's fascia (6).

The adrenal glands

- The adrenal glands are retroperitoneal and each has a body and two limbs. The limbs should not be thicker than the diaphragmatic crus.
- The adrenal shape is extremely variable being linear, V shaped, deltoid or triangular.
- The left adrenal gland is found at the level of the upper pole of the left kidney. It lies anteromedial to the kidney. The left adrenal is usually Y-shaped.
- The right gland is suprarenal and is found above the right kidney behind the IVC. The right adrenal has two limbs which lie in between the liver and the right crus of the diaphragm, i.e. a medial and a lateral limb. The medial limb is fatter. The right adrenal gland is usually V-shaped (Fig. 5.22).
- The adrenal glands are relatively much larger in neonates, being up to one-third the size of the kidney.
- The adrenal thickness varies between 5 and 8 mm and >10 mm is abnormal. The thickness of the medial limb of the right adrenal should be <4 mm or the thickness of the right crus.
- The vascular supply is interesting for multi-choice questions (MCQs) as three arteries supply the glands. The superior adrenal artery arises from the inferior phrenic,

the middle adrenal artery from the aorta and the inferior artery from the renal artery directly.
- The right adrenal vein drains into the IVC and the left adrenal vein into the left renal vein.

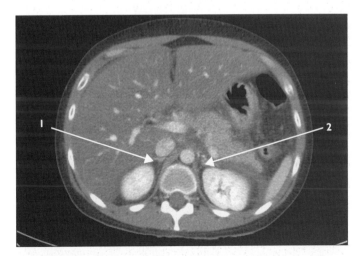

Fig. 5.22 CT scan, portal phase, showing the normal position of the right adrenal gland (1) lying behind the inferior vena cava and the left adrenal (2) anterior to the left kidney.

IMAGING

Liver and spleen

Abdominal ultrasound

Indications

Ultrasound is a non-invasive, easily accessible, fast way of evaluating the abdominal organs without using ionizing radiation. It is the first-line investigation in children and in adults for liver, gallbladder, renal and aortic abnormalities. In pancreatic disease and splenic trauma CT is now the first-line investigation. Doppler ultrasound can assess flow in the hepatic artery, hepatic veins and portal veins.

Technique

- A curvilinear 5-MHz probe is used or a 7-MHz one in children.
- The best views of the liver are obtained intercostally and in the epigastric region. The gallbladder may be best assessed in the left lateral decubitus position.
- Fasting is required to assess the gallbladder and pancreas because this distends the gallbladder and enables emptying of the stomach contents, which can obscure the pancreas.
- A technique of scanning the organs in an organized orderly sequence helps consistency and avoids omission of an organ in error. An example would be to assess initially in this order:
  - the liver for homogeneity, focal lesions, outline, biliary tract dilatation, vasculature
  - the gallbladder for stones and wall thickness
  - the right kidney for length, scarring, pelvicalyceal dilatation, stones, corticomedullary differentiation, the renal brightness relative to the liver; the right kidney is normally less reflective than the liver; the kidneys can be scanned in the supine position using an intercostal or subcostal approach or in the decubitus position; a true length must be obtained
  - the pancreas for size and reflectivity

  - the aorta for aneurysmal dilatation
  - the spleen for size in the left upper quadrant using an intercostal approach
  - the left kidney
  - the paracolic gutters, under the diaphragm, hepatorenal fossa and pelvis, for free fluid.
- Ultrasound can be used to assess paediatric adrenal glands and may detect large adrenal tumours in adults. The adrenals are found at the top of the kidneys on ultrasound.

Findings

- The liver should have a smooth outline and homogeneous reflectivity. A fatty liver will have increased reflectivity. The portal vein walls, which are normally echogenic, cannot be visualized in a bright liver. A fatty liver is more reflective or brighter than the right kidney (Fig. 5.23).
- The hepatic veins draining into the IVC make a 'crows' feet' appearance in the transverse oblique plane (Fig. 5.23).
- At the porta, the portal vein always lies posteriorly, with the CBD anteriorly and the right hepatic artery in between the portal vein and the common duct. Doppler ultrasound of the portal vein shows anterograde flow up towards the right upper quadrant (RUQ) normally.
- Portal vessels have white walls on ultrasound whereas hepatic veins have dark walls, unless they lie parallel to the probe, i.e. perpendicular to the beam (Figs 5.24 and 5.25).
- The diameter of the common duct is usually 6 mm, although it could be 8 mm in older people. After cholecystectomy it may reach 10 mm.

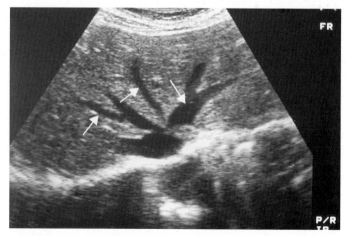

Fig. 5.23 Ultrasound of the liver showing the smooth outline of the normal liver and the hepatic veins (arrows).

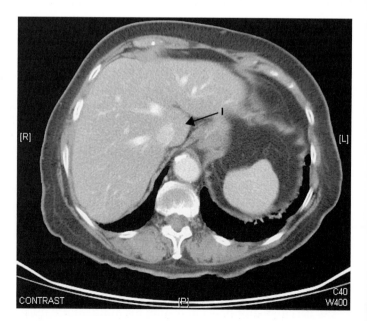

Fig. 5.24 Abdominal CT showing the position of the hepatic veins and the caudate lobe (1) of the liver.

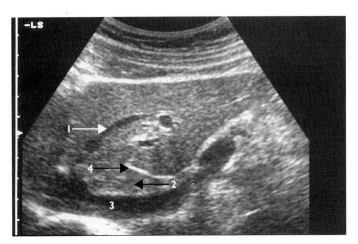

Fig. 5.25 Longitudinal ultrasound showing the left hepatic vein (1) and the caudate lobe (2). Inferior vena cava (3) and ligamentum venosum (4).

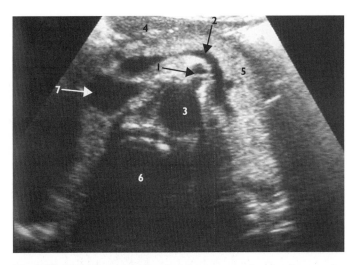

Fig. 5.26 Transverse ultrasound of the pancreas showing the superior mesenteric artery (1) in cross-section surrounded by echogenic fat. The splenic vein lies anteriorly (2). Aorta (3), left liver lobe (4), pancreas (5), vertebral body (6) and inferior vena cava (7).

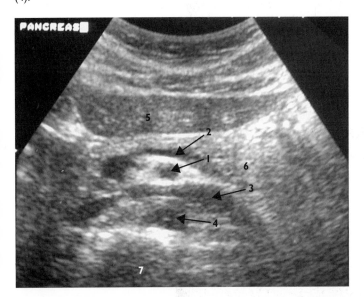

Fig. 5.27 Another transverse ultrasound of the pancreas in a different series showing the superior mesenteric artery (1) in cross-section surrounded by echogenic fat. The splenic vein lies anteriorly (2) and the left renal vein (3) posteriorly. Aorta (4), left liver lobe (5), pancreas (6) and vertebral body (7).

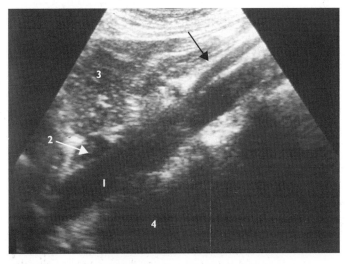

Fig. 5.28 Longitudinal ultrasound of the aorta showing the superior mesenteric artery (black arrow) running parallel to this. Aorta (1), gastro-oesophageal (2) junction, left liver lobe (3) and vertebrae (4).

- The gallbladder wall should be <2 mm thick. It may be folded giving an impression of septa. Stones may become apparent only in the left lateral decubitus position.
- The pancreas is seen in the transverse plane at about L1, but it may be obscured by bowel gas (Fig. 5.26). The relationship of the pancreas with the SMA and splenic vein aids its detection; the splenic vein forms the posterior border of the pancreas. The pancreas becomes increasingly fatty with age, making it more reflective or hyperechoic (Fig. 5.27).
- The spleen normally has one concave and one convex border and measures, in most people, up to 12 cm in length (although a spectrum of people will have a normal spleen at 14–15 cm).

- In the longitudinal position the aorta and IVC run caudally. The SMA runs anterior and parallel to the aorta (Fig. 5.28).
- The coeliac artery is seen as similar to a 'seagull' in the transverse plane (Fig. 5.29).
- The gastro-oesophageal junction can be visualized in the longitudinal plane (see Fig. 5.28).

CT of the abdomen

Indications

Adrenal masses, staging malignancy, suspected inflammation or collections, the acute abdomen, for small bowel or large bowel studies, aortic and vascular assessment.

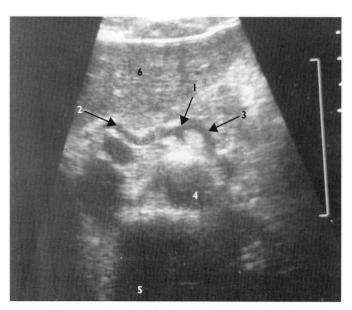

Fig. 5.29 Transverse ultrasound of the coeliac axis (1) dividing into the common hepatic (2) and splenic arteries (3). The left gastric is not seen as it ascends at its origin. Aorta (4), vertebrae (5) and left liver lobe (6).

Technique
- The standard window setting for an abdomen is 40/400. Liver windows are 100/200.
- Ideally, as many structures are enhanced as possible to exploit contrast and density differences between organs. Unenhanced scans will show calcification in chronic pancreatitis, renal stone disease, choledochal stones, calcifying liver lesions, etc. (Fig. 5.30).

- Oral contrast is given, which may be water or very dilute 4% (w/v) contrast depending on the indication. Any stronger oral contrast will cause extensive artefact. If the pancreas and stomach are being assessed, water contrast may be used to provide greater contrast for the bowel, stomach wall and pancreas. The timing of drinking depends on the indication: for oesophageal lesions a drink is given immediately before imaging and, for distal small bowel, ingestion of oral contrast may commence 45 min–1 h before imaging (Fig. 5.31).
- Intravenous contrast is administered with the timing of intravenous contrast planned according to the indication: hepatocellular carcinoma, some liver metastases and pancreatic cancer are best seen in the arterial phase because they derive their blood supply from the hepatic artery.
- The liver has a dual supply. The portal vein supplies 75–80% and is best visualized at a 45- to 60-s delay. The hepatic artery supplies 20–25% of the liver blood supply and the arterial phase is seen with a 25-s delay.
- The liver may be scanned in an unenhanced arterial, portal or delayed phase. Most inflammatory and other malignant abnormalities are best seen in the portal phase.
- The IVC is best seen on a delayed phase. This depends on the volume and the rate of injection. Delayed scanning assesses haemangiomas for nodular mural filling in. Post-intravenous contrast scans should be taken in both the arterial and the portal phases in suspected pancreatic malignancy:
  - arterial phase 25 s
  - portal phase 45–60 s
  - delayed phase 90 s.

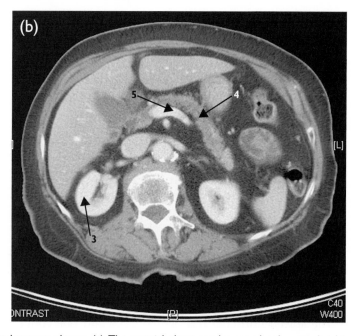

Fig. 5.30 CT scan of the pancreas showing both (a) arterial and (b) portal venous phases. (a) The arterial phase can be seen by the very bright contrast in the aorta, the heterogeneous spleen (1) and the kidneys with prominent cortical medullary differentiation (2) on the arterial phase. (b) On the portal phase the renal cortex and medulla are homogeneous (3). Pancreas (4) and splenic vein (5).

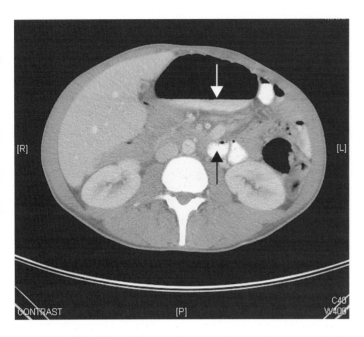

Fig. 5.31 CT of the abdomen showing dense oral contrast in the bowel (arrows).

• Establishing which phase has been performed in the absence of information about the timing can be made by looking at the density of the aorta. If the aorta is denser than the portal vein, the phase is arterial. The spleen usually looks very heterogeneous in an arterial phase scan (Fig. 5.32).

Hepatic angiography and angioportography

Indications
MRI has superseded some indications for these.

Technique
• Hepatic arteriography is performed with a catheter in the coeliac axis or the hepatic artery itself. It may be performed for embolization of a bleeding tumour or after trauma.
• A hepatic venogram can be performed via the internal jugular vein in the neck. A catheter is passed through the internal jugular vein, through the right heart and into the IVC in order to cannulate the hepatic veins. This approach may be used for TIPSS (**t**ransjugular **i**ntrahepatic **p**ortosystemic **s**tent **s**hunt procedure to treat portal hypertension when a shunt is placed between the IVC and the portal vein.

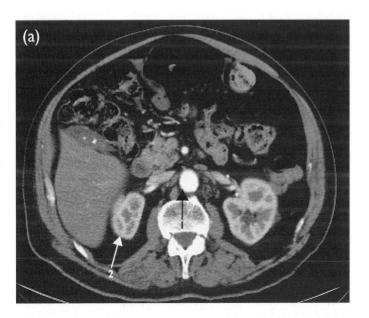

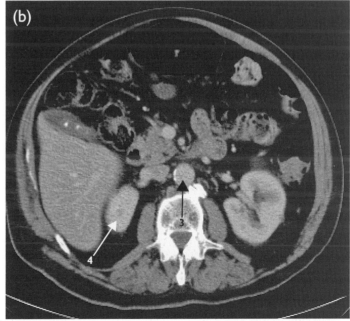

Fig. 5.32 (a) Arterial phase CT showing the dense aorta (1) and corticomedullary differentiation (2); (b) the late phase with less dense aorta (3) and homogeneous cortex and medulla (4).

Findings

When performing CT assess each organ individually and develop a consistent system. Standard sections show the anatomy (Figs 5.33–5.37).

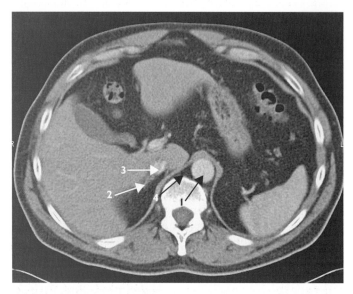

Fig. 5.33 CT of the aortic hiatus at T12. Retrocrural nodes occur here in the retrocrural region (4) and are part of the mediastinum. Their upper limit is 6 mm in short axis. Aorta (1), right adrenal gland (2) and inferior vena cava (3).

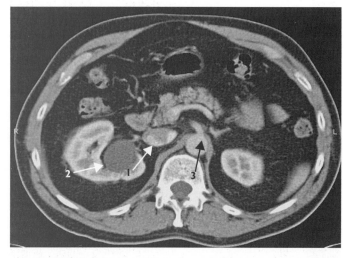

Fig. 5.34 CT of the abdomen showing flow artefact in the inferior vena cava (1) due to unopacified blood from the legs mixing with opacified blood from the kidneys. There is an incidental simple cyst in the right kidney (2). Aorta (3).

The liver

• The bare area of the liver lies posterosuperiorly. Here the liver adheres to the peritoneum preventing free fluid collecting at this site.

• The liver contours should normally be smooth in outline. Slips of the diaphragm may invaginate the liver superfi-

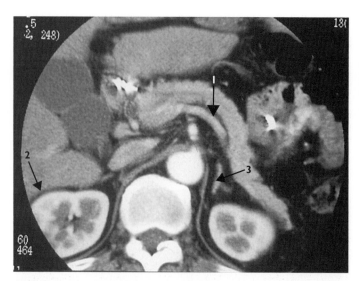

Fig. 5.35 Arterial phase of a CT of the pancreas showing the splenic veins posterior to the pancreas. The fat plane between the pancreas and the splenic vein can mimic the pancreatic duct (1). Hepatorenal fossa or Morrison's pouch (2) and left adrenal gland (3).

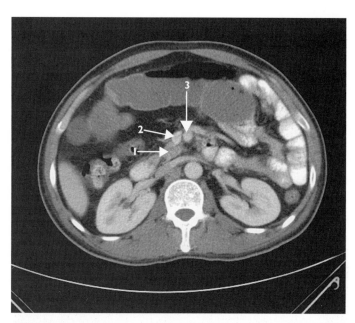

Fig. 5.36 Axial CT of the uncinate process of the pancreas (1); superior mesenteric vein (2) and superior mesenteric artery (3).

cially and mimic subcapsular deposits on CT (Fig. 3.38). An irregular liver suggests cirrhosis or deposits.

• The normal attenuation value of the unenhanced liver is 40–70 HU and the unenhanced liver is usually denser than the spleen by about 8 HU. After intravenous contrast this ratio is reversed.

• The Hounsfield unit of fat is −40 and therefore a fatty liver is of lower density than normal. Focal fatty change is common around the fissure and gallbladder fossa and in the caudate lobe. A hyperdense liver is seen with amiodarone and haemochromatosis (Fig. 5.39).

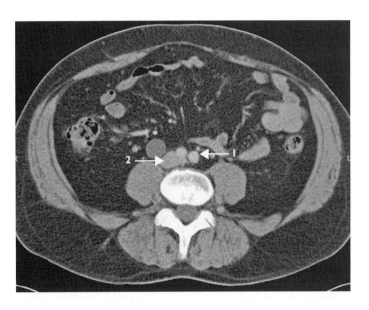

Fig. 5.37 Axial enhanced CT of aortic bifurcation (1) at L4. The IVC (2) has already formed at L5.

- Unopacified hepatic veins may cause pseudolesions, i.e. mimic tumours. Later phase post-intravenous contrast images show normal opacification of the hepatic veins (Fig. 5.40).
- The presence of air within liver lesions or calcification or fat may alter the diagnosis, e.g. calcification may be seen in hydatid disease or certain metastases. Air within a liver lesion may imply a gas-forming abscess or previous intervention. The clinical details help the interpretation of findings.
- Dilated intrahepatic bile ducts appear as fluid-density intrahepatic lesions, which may or may not appear linear (see Fig. 5.40).

- In a fatty liver some areas may be spared from the fatty infiltration and remain of normal density, which causes the areas to mimic focal lesions (Fig. 5.39b).
- Focal liver lesions should be described according to which segment they lie in and the number of lesions; the presence of calcification, enhancement and a subcapsular position should be reported.

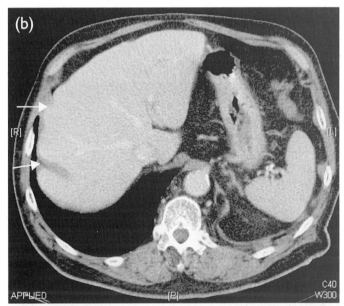

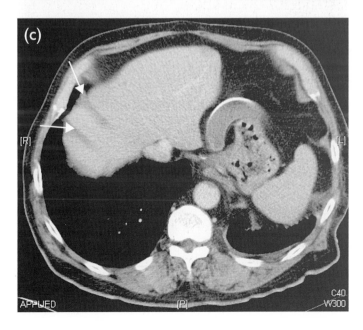

Fig. 5.38 (a, b, c) CT scans of the abdomen showing how slips of the diaphragm (arrows) can mimic subcapsular liver deposits where they insert.

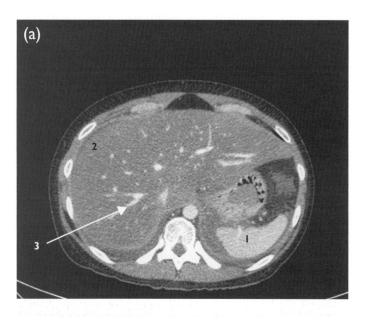

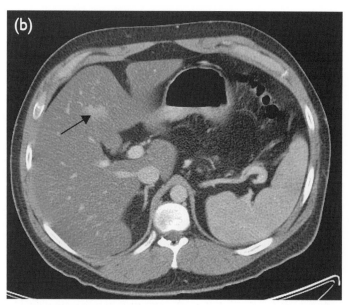

Fig. 5.39 (a) CT axial post-contrast portal phase: a fatty liver (2), showing how the hepatic veins (3) stand out against the liver background. There are multiple cysts in the left kidney. The spleen (1) is usually denser than the liver post-contrast but this is much denser. (b) CT axial post-contrast portal phase showing a fatty liver with focal fatty sparing (black arrow).

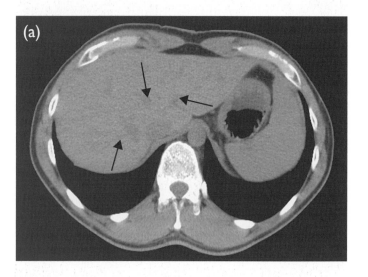

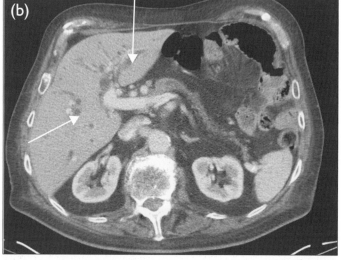

Fig. 5.40 CT of unopacified hepatic veins mimicking bile ducts. (a) Unopacified hepatic veins (arrows). (b) Dilated bile ducts (arrows) on unopacified CT.

The pancreas

- When reviewing the pancreas on CT, assess three things: the calibre of the pancreatic duct, the contour of the pancreas and the enhancement of the pancreas.
- The splenic vein forms the posterior border of the pancreas and the fat plane between the splenic vein and the pancreas may mimic the pancreatic duct. On unenhanced scans this makes the pancreas appear fatter on axial imaging. Enhanced scans reveal the true anatomy.
- The uncinate process of the pancreas lies behind the SMA and SMV.
- The tail of the pancreas lies higher than the body and is seen on more superior axial cuts. This can be appreciated on coronal imaging. If there has been a left nephrectomy,

the tail of the pancreas may lie even higher and lie under the left hemidiaphragm in the left renal bed. This may cause confusion with a recurrent left renal mass.

- The pancreatic duct is normally visible on CT and can measure up to 2 mm in diameter with a consistent calibre throughout its length. Sudden changes in calibre or an abrupt dilatation of the pancreatic duct may imply a tumour at the transition point. Variation in pancreatic duct calibre can be seen, however, in chronic pancreatitis where a beaded appearance may be present (Fig. 5.41).
- The pancreas should have a slightly smooth, lobulated contour. If there is a sudden bulge in the contour, this may indicate a tumour even if there is no obvious difference in contrast enhancement. The uncinate process

should normally have one convex and one concave border, like a beak. If it is convex on both sides it may imply a tumour (Fig. 5.42).
- After intravenous contrast, areas of hypo- or hyperperfusion may represent tumours or necrosis depending on the clinical context. Both arterial and portal venous phases should be performed to maximize tumour detection. In acute pancreatitis, only the portal venous phase can be used to assess for pancreatic necrosis.
- In acute pancreatitis the fat surrounding the pancreas may be stranded or 'dirty' due to inflammation, which causes an increase in density in the fat. Tumour invasion of the fat may also cause this appearance.

- Lymph nodes in the left gastric, gastrohepatic and gastrosplenic region may be involved by a pancreatic malignancy. The normal short axis of these nodes is usually 8 mm.

The adrenal glands
- On CT the right limb of the adrenal gland should be <4 mm thick or less than the thickness of the right crus of the diaphragm (Fig. 5.43).
- The adrenal glands are arrow, V- or Y-shaped.
- The right adrenal lies behind the IVC. The medial limb may only be seen behind the IVC. The left adrenal gland lies anterior to the upper pole of the left kidney.

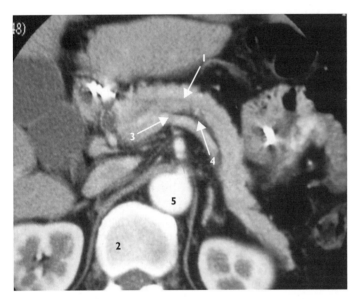

Fig. 5.41 CT of the pancreatic duct (1), which is normally visible, being 2 mm. The duct should be smooth in calibre with no abrupt transitions of calibre. Aorta (5), vertebral body (2), splenic vein (3) and fat in between the pancreas and the splenic vein (4).

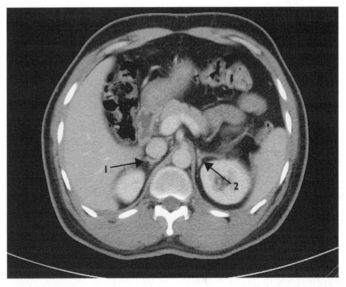

Fig. 5.43 CT scan of the adrenal glands post-intravenous contrast showing the relationship of the right adrenal (1) to the inferior vena cava and the relationship of left adrenal (2) to the top of the left kidney.

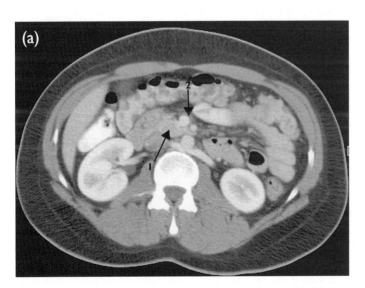

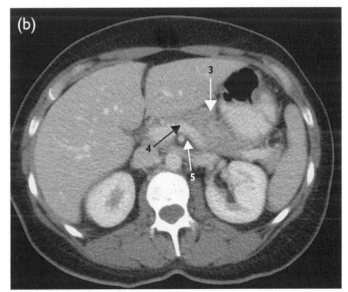

Fig. 5.42 Axial CT of the pancreas: two images showing (a) the uncinate process (1) tucked behind the superior mesenteric vessels (2); (b) the body of the pancreas (3) anterior to the splenic vein (4) and superior mesenteric artery (5) surrounded by fat.

- Incidental adenomas are commonly seen on CT scans of the abdomen in the adrenal glands. There are several ways of further evaluating these: on CT adenomas are usually <4 cm in size and of fatty density on an unenhanced phase, i.e. the CT number is <10 HU.
- A delayed CT contrast scan may be helpful to see if there is washout of enhancement.

The spleen

- In the arterial phase of scanning, i.e. early scanning, the spleen invariably looks heterogeneous and pathology can be overdiagnosed. The spleen should always be assessed in the portal phase of scanning (Fig. 5.44).
- Splenunculi are seen commonly on CT.
- CT is the modality of choice in splenic trauma.

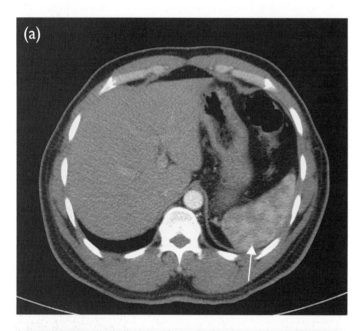

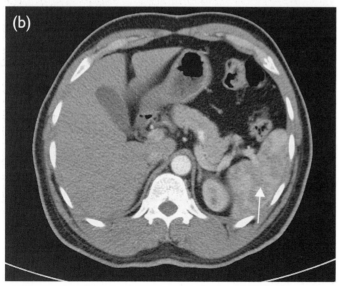

Fig. 5.44 Two cases of axial CT of the arterial abdomen showing the spleen (arrows) with heterogeneous filling on arterial phase.

The kidneys
See Chapter 6.

Other areas of review in the abdomen and pelvis
After review of the liver, spleen, kidneys, adrenal glands and bowel on CT, assess in a systematic order:
- For free fluid that may collect in the hepatorenal fossa, subphrenic spaces, paracolic gutters and pelvis. In patients who are recumbent fluid settles initially in the pelvis (Fig. 5.45).
- The peritoneum and omentum for thickening or nodules.
- The presence of free intra-abdominal gas in the context of the acute abdomen. This can be done using a lung window looking for extraluminal air.
- The aortic calibre for aneurysmal change.
- The SMA position: the SMA should lie to the left side of the SMV. The artery may lie in front of the vein but should never lie to its right.
- The SMA should be surrounded by fat. Loss of fat definition around the SMA is abnormal. Fat around the SMA is seen on CT as a grey ring and on ultrasound as an echogenic ring around the vessel.
- The vertebra and ribs on bony windows for alignment, metastases or trauma.
- There may be a breach in the anterior abdominal wall and groin in the case of possible hernias.
- The IVC forms at L5. Flow artefact is commonly seen in the IVC at the level of the left renal vein, as a result of unopacified blood from the legs mixing with contrast opacified blood from the renal veins (Fig. 5.34).
- The left renal vein runs posterior to the superior mesenteric artery to join the IVC. An anatomical variant is the retroaortic left renal vein, which runs behind the aorta (Fig. 5.46).
- The third part of the duodenum runs posterior to the SMA. The SMA can cause a 'nutcracker' effect with compression of the duodenum.

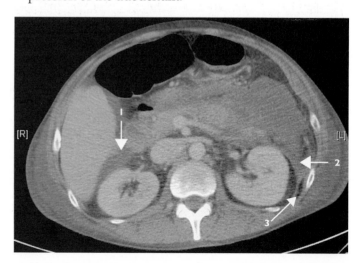

Fig. 5.45 Enhanced axial CT of the abdomen showing free fluid in the hepatorenal fossa (1) and left paracolic gutter (2). Gerota's fascia (3) surrounds and protects the kidneys.

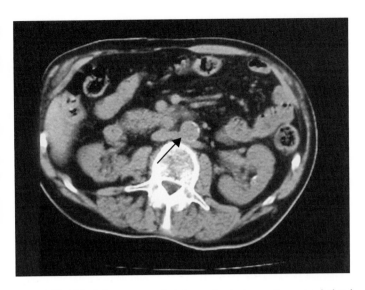

Fig. 5.46 CT of the retroaortic left renal vein (arrow) running behind the aorta.

- The right crus of the diaphragm runs from L1 to L3 compared with the left (L1–2). A lumpy crus may mimic lymphadenopathy (see Fig. 5.47).

Size of abdominal nodes
- Abdominal nodes are measured for size in their short axis.
- Retrocrural nodes should normally measure <0.6 cm in short axis.
- Para-aortic, coeliac axis and superior mesenteric nodes should measure <1 cm.
- Gastrohepatic, left gastric and gastrosplenic nodes should measure <0.8 cm in short axis.
- Numerous nodes in the mesentery itself or around organs may be pathological even if not enlarged.

MRI of the abdomen and pelvis

- The anatomy is the same whatever the technique, whether it is CT or MRI. By remembering this principle, MRI interpretation becomes easier. If struggling with interpretation of MRI, imagine it is a CT scan and things often become more apparent. On MRI the bony landmarks are less apparent, which often throws the individual.
- Comparing the CT scan of the abdomen with an MR scan (see Fig. 5.47b), the same liver segments apply and the gallbladder is in the same position. The vascular structures appear on an unenhanced MR scan as signal voids. Knowledge of the anatomy enables you to identify these more easily.

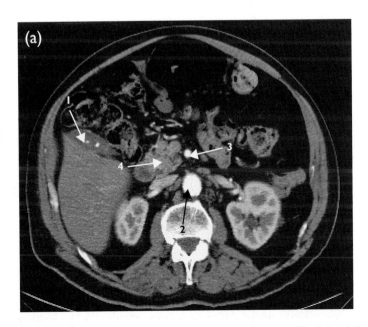

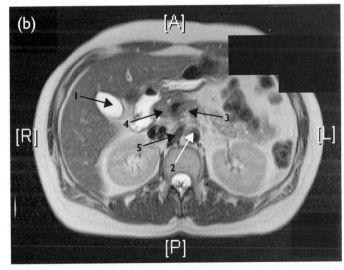

Fig. 5.47 (a) Post contrast CT abdomen. (b) T2 axial MRI of the abdomen. Gallbladder (1), aorta (2), superior mesenteric artery (3), uncinate process of the pancreas (4) and lumpty right crus (5).

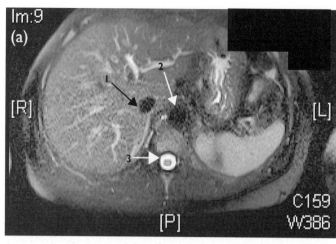

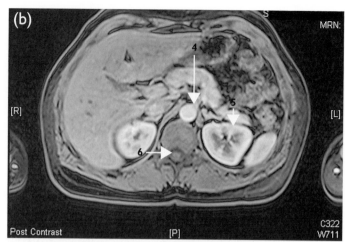

Fig. 5.48 MRI of the abdomen: (a) axial T2-weighted showing flow void in the inferior vena cava and (1) aorta (2). The cerebrospinal fluid (CSF) in the spinal canal is bright (3). (b) Axial post-contrast T1-weighted MRI of the abdomen showing the aorta (4) and corticomedullary differentiation in the kidneys (5). Note CSF around the spinal canal is low signal (6).

- The cerebrospinal fluid (CSF) in the spinal canal helps ascertain whether it is a T1-weighted or T2-weighted series: T2-weighted images have bright CSF; T1-weighted images have dark CSF (Fig. 5.48).
- Due to the bowel and aortic motion, fast imaging is required within the abdomen and pelvis. Gradient echo imaging is therefore widely used which is much faster than spin echo series.

MRI of the liver

Indication
MRI of the liver helps in lesion characterization, i.e. differentiating simple cysts and haemangiomas from metastases, and in lesion detection. It is used in problem-solving cases when CT is indeterminate or if surgical resection of liver metastases or tumours is planned when the presence of other lesions may prohibit surgery. It is also indicated in patients with iodine allergy who cannot undergo contrast-enhanced CT.

Technique
- A standard imaging protocol for the liver is axial gradient, echo, T2-weighted imaging, short inversion time, inversion recovery (STIR) imaging and T1-weighted imaging with dynamic enhancement. Enhanced images are performed with T1-weighted scanning.
- Contrast enhancement on MRI may use iron oxide. This is taken up by the reticuloendothelial system and lowers the signal of the normal liver. Liver tumours do not take up the iron oxide contrast and appear as hyperintense foci in a low signal background.

- Manganese dipyridoxyl diphosphate is a T1-shortening agent that is taken up by the liver hepatocytes and eliminated in bile. It can aid detection of metastases that do not take up the contrast and aid detection of primary hepatocellular carcinoma, which takes up the contrast but cannot excrete it.
- Using moderately and heavily T2-weighted imaging and also dynamic T1-weighted enhanced images, metastases can be differentiated from benign lesions such as cysts and haemangiomas (Fig. 5.49).

Findings
- Haemangiomas and simple cysts are heavily T2 weighted, unlike metastases which do not show up as brightly on heavily T2-weighted imaging.
- Areas of fatty replacement within the liver can cause confusion with liver deposits. STIR imaging or in- and out-of-phase imaging can help differentiate fatty change from pathology. In- and out-of-phase imaging exploits the difference between fat and water chemical shift artefact. Fatty lesions lose signal on out-of-phase imaging.
- Usually on T1-weighted imaging the liver is higher signal than the spleen.
- To help work out if contrast has been administered look at the aorta. On T1-weighted imaging the aorta will enhance with gadolinium (Fig. 5.50).
- STIR sequence images show fat as low signal areas and fluid or CSF as high signal.
- On MRI ghost artefacts can mimic liver lesions (Fig. 5.51).

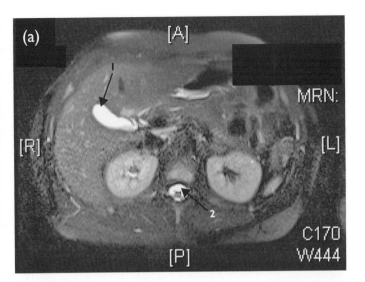

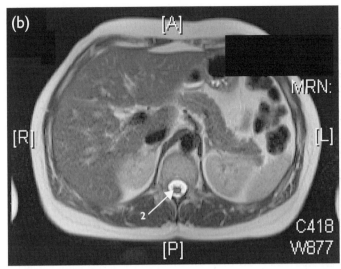

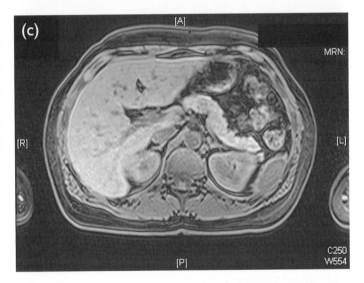

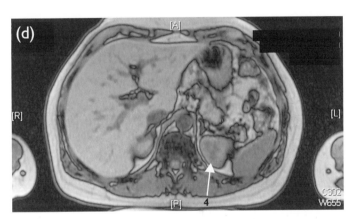

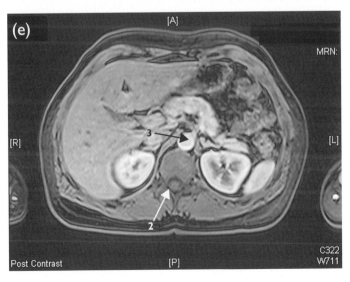

Fig. 5.49 MRI of the liver: (a) STIR image which makes fluid in the gallbladder very bright (1) and in the theca (2). (b) Axial T2 with moderate T2 weighting with bright fluid in the theca (2). (c) In-phase and (d) out-of-phase axial images showing the 'black line' (4) around the organs on out-of-phase imaging. (e) Post-contrast T1-weighted MRI of the liver showing high signal in the aorta (3) from contrast and low-signal cerebrospinal fluid in the spinal canal (2).

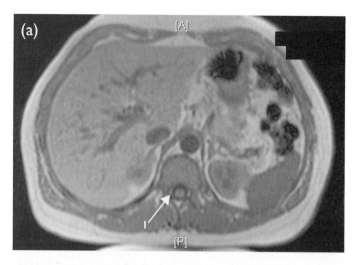

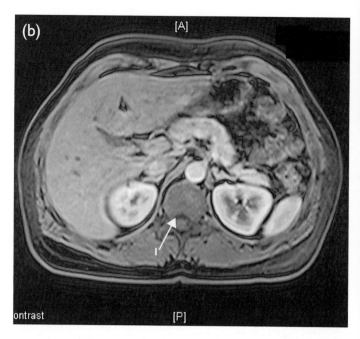

Fig. 5.50 MRI of the abdomen dynamic T1-weighted: (a) pre- and (b) post-contrast. Use the cerebrospinal fluid (1) to establish the series being T1-weighted as the fluid is low signal on T1-weighted.

The biliary tract and pancreatic ducts

Endoscopic retrograde cholangiopancreatography

Indications

ERCP (endoscopic retrograde cholangiopancreatography) is performed to assess the pancreatic and bile ducts. Due to its invasive nature, ultrasound and then magnetic retrograde cholangiopancreatography (MRCP) are used initially or to assess the ducts. ERCP is indicated only for therapeutic or interventional procedures such as dilatation of the sphincter of Oddi, for stone extraction and stent insertion, unless MRI is contraindicated when MRCP cannot be performed.

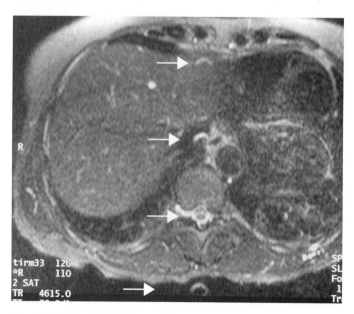

Fig. 5.51 MRI axial STIR image showing ghost artefact (arrows) of the cerebrospinal fluid propagated at regular intervals across the image.

Technique

- ERCP involves performing endoscopy under sedation. The duodenal papilla in the second part of the duodenum is canulated at the sphincter of Oddi. Contrast is injected carefully into the ducts in small aliquots. It is an invasive procedure with a significant complication rate, one of which is acute pancreatitis. Overdistension of the ducts increases the incidence of acute pancreatitis.
- To see the left intrahepatic ducts the patient may need to be turned prone.

Findings

- The pancreatic duct is 16 cm long with a maximum width of 4 mm in the pancreatic head (Fig. 5.52)
- The accessory pancreatic duct may fill if connected to the main duct.
- Complications are increased pancreas divisum, as the main and accessory pancreatic ducts do not communicate and overdistension of one is more likely.

Magnetic resonance cholangiopancreatography

Indications

MRCP is now used as the first-line investigation of the intra- and extrahepatic bile ducts and pancreatic duct. MRCP is a non-invasive technique using MRI to assess the bile duct.

Technique

A fluid-sensitive sequence such as a heavily T2-weighted fat-suppressed image is used. The static fluid in the ducts is hyperintense. Maximum intensity projection (MIP) image is used

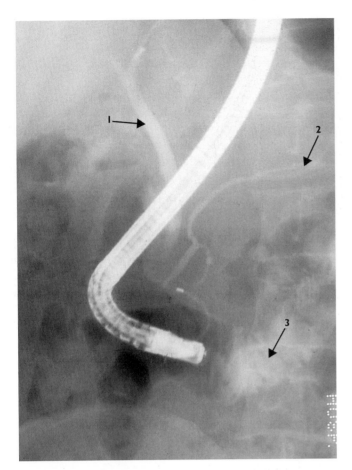

Fig. 5.52 Endoscopic retrograde cholangiopancreatography showing the common bile duct (1) and pancreatic duct (2). The accessory duct drains into the duodenum 2 cm proximal to the main duct. Contrast is seen in the duodenum (3).

Findings

The ureter, the CSF and the bowel are all visible and may overlap the image (Fig. 5.53a).

Percutaneous transhepatic cholangiogram

Indications

To visualize the biliary tract when ERCP cannot be performed, mainly for interventional procedures and stent insertion or TIPSS.

Technique

A fine Chiba needle is used to cannulate the intrahepatic ducts when dilated percutaneously. Contrast can be injected via the Chiba needle. A complication is a pneumothorax (Fig. 5.53b).

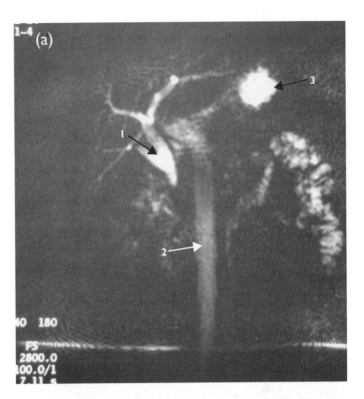

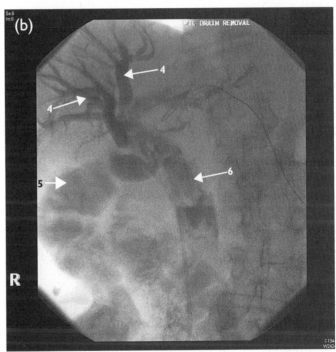

Fig. 5.53 (a) Magnetic retrograde cholangiopancreatography showing the common duct (1) and superimposed cerebrospinal fluid in the spinal canal (2) and contrast in the duodenum (3). (b) Percutaneous transhepatic cholangiogram contrast is injected percutaneously into the bile ducts (4) by puncturing the liver. Duodenum (5) and common bile duct full of stones (6).

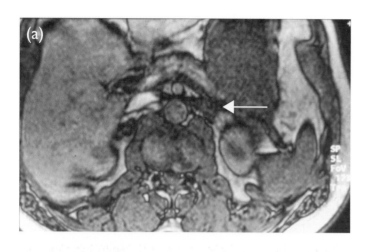

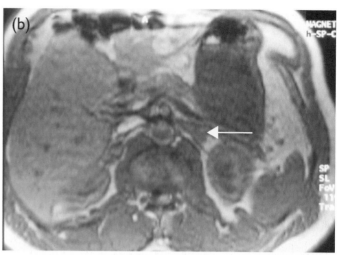

Fig. 5.54 Adrenal glands: (b) in- and (a) out-of-phase imaging. Out-of-phase imaging has a black line around the organs due to chemical shift. Fat-containing lesions drop signal relative to the spleen on out-of-phase series. The left adrenal mass loses signal relative to the spleen on out-of-phase images confirming the presence of fat (arrow).

MR of the adrenal glands

Indication
MRI of the adrenal glands aids in the investigation of incidental adenomas.

Technique
In- and out-of-phase imaging can evaluate the adrenal glands. This exploits the difference between fat and water using chemical shift artefact.

Findings
If the adrenal gland mass drops signal relative to the spleen this would confirm fat within the gland and the mass being an incidental adenoma (Fig. 5.54).

Angiography

Indications
Embolization of tumours, bleeding from trauma to the liver.

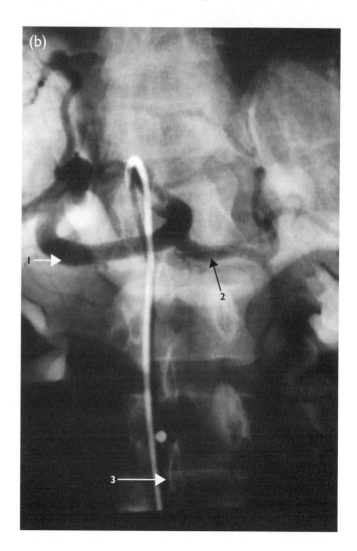

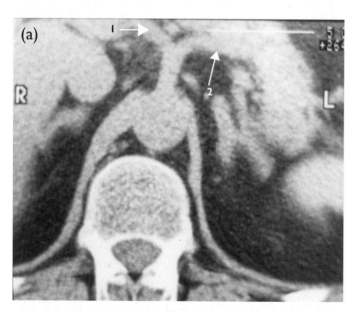

Fig. 5.55 (a) Coeliac axis CT and (b) coeliac angiogram of common hepatic (1) and splenic arteries (2). The catheter (3).

Technique
- The femoral artery at the groin is punctured and a pigtail catheter over a guidewire is inserted to perform a flush aortogram. The aortogram enables the anatomy of the origins of the mesenteric vessels to be visualized.
- Using a sheath, the catheter is then exchanged for a selective catheter. A selective catheter has one end-hole to enable even contrast injection and various catheters are available, including a sidewinder or shepherd's hook.
- Contrast is injected using a pump to simulate physiological flow at between 5 and 10 ml/s depending on the vessel.

- The timing of the images depends on whether the arterial or the portal phase is being investigated. Late-phase imaging is called indirect portography. The portal vein is visualized 60 s after contrast injection into the splenic or coeliac artery.

Findings
Flow artefact can be seen in the portal vein at indirect portography via mixing from the splenic vein and SMV unless catheters are put into both arteries and injections are performed simultaneously (Fig. 5.55).

The portal vein
Can be imaged with Doppler ultrasound (Fig. 5.56), CT with contrast, MRI or indirect angiography.

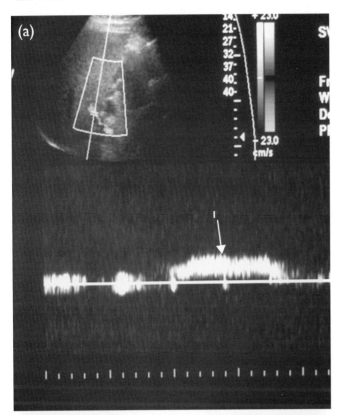

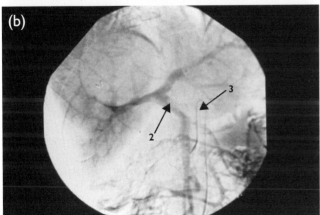

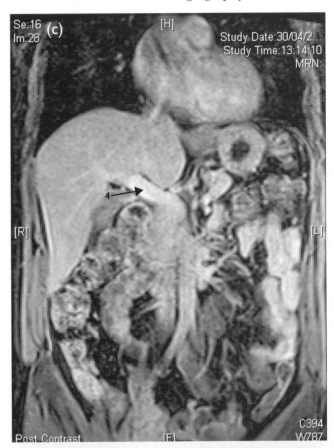

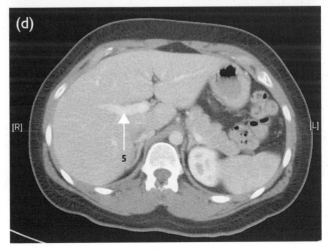

Fig. 5.56 (a) Portal vein Doppler ultrasound showing normal waveform (1); (b) indirect portal venography with a catheter (2) in the superior mesenteric artery in late phase angiography (3). (c) Coronal post-contrast CT showing the portal vein (4). (d) Axial CT showing the portal vein post contrast (5).

The IVC

Can be imaged by CT, MRI sometimes ultrasound but not usually well seen by venography.

Venography is mainly used for intervention such as filter insertion for pulmonary embolism (Fig. 5.57).

Box 5.1 Reporting a CT of the abdomen

- Have a system
- Start with the liver, spleen, pancreas, adrenal glands and gallbladder; Review organ by organ
- Look for free fluid and ascites
- Check the para-aortic region for lymphadenopathy and the retrocrural space
- Assess the lung bases on lung windows
- Assess the peritoneum and mesentery for tumour spread, particularly anterior to the colon in the greater omentum, and in the gastrosplenic and gastrohepatic regions

---

CASES

When assessing for inflammation, i.e. cholecystitis, diverticulitis, inflammatory bowel disease or pancreatitis, the same principles apply:

- Concentrate on looking for dirty stranded fat around the symptomatic site.
- Look for free fluid in the abdomen, hepatorenal fossa, paracolic gutters and pelvis.
- Look at thickness of the wall, i.e. the gallbladder, bowel and sigmoid colon.

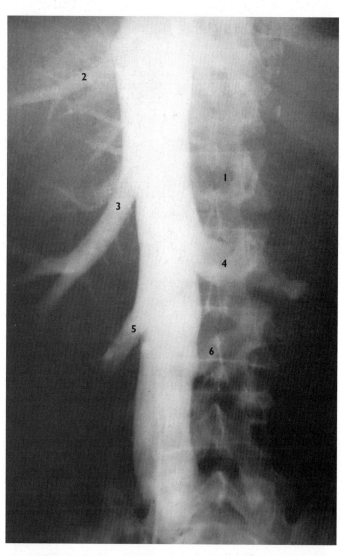

Fig. 5.57 Inferior venocavogram: first lumbar vertebra (1), hepatic veins (2), right renal vein (3), left renal vein (4) and lumbar veins (5, 6).

Case 5.1

A patient presents with acute abdominal pain radiating through to the back. The serum amylase is raised. A CT abdomen is performed

The CT protocol must be planned. An unenhanced scan is indicated to look for pancreatic calcification, gallstones and choledochal stones which may be missed if only post-contrast scans are taken. A portal phase CT is also indicated to look for necrosis of the pancreas and vascular complications (Fig. 5.58).

- On the unenhanced scan look for calcification in the pancreas indicating chronic pancreatitis. Is the pancreas swollen? Remember that, on an unopacified scan, the unenhanced splenic vein may make the pancreas look fatter. Look for stones in the common bile duct, i.e. choledochal stones. These may be visible only in the duct within the head of the pancreas and should be very closely looked for.
- There is no calcification of the pancreas in this case.
- On the post-contrast images look for biliary tract dilatation and pancreatic duct dilatation. Look at the gallbladder for gallstones and the biliary tree, remembering that ultrasound is more sensitive for gallstones and they may not be seen. Look for free fluid around the pancreas and in the remaining abdomen and pelvis. In this case there is free fluid around the pancreas and liver.
- Look for stranding around the pancreas within the fat suggesting inflammation (Fig. 5.58b).
- On enhancement of arterial and portal veins look for homogeneous enhancement of the pancreas. Areas of non-enhancement suggest necrosis which is a poor prognostic sign (Fig. 5.58a). The case shows focal areas of non-enhancement in the body and tail of the pancreas.
- Look for pseudocysts within the pancreas or remaining abdomen, which may warrant drainage. These are walled-off fluid collections.
- Remember that areas or collections, i.e. phlegmons, and areas of necrosis indicate a poor prognosis and warrant follow-up with CT.
- Assess the vessels, in particular the SMA, SMV and splenic vein for thrombosis and vascular complications of acute pancreatitis. In this case the splenic vein appears normal and the SMA was normal.

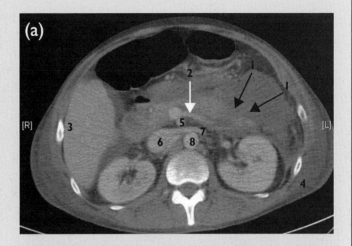

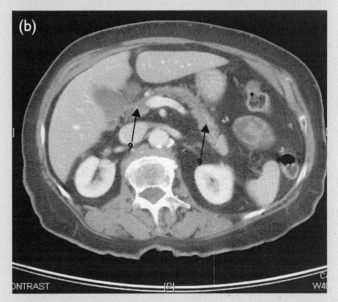

Fig. 5.58 Acute pancreatitis: (a) axial CT of the pancreas in portal phase post-intravenous contrast. There is ascites that spares the renal area, which is protected by Gerota's fascia. The pancreas is blurred and indistinct. The tail and distal body of the pancreas show poor enhancement (1). Splenic vein (2), liver (3), left Gerota's fascia with trace fluid (4), superior mesenteric artery (5), inferior vena cava (6), left renal vein (7) and aorta (8). (b) Normal CT of the pancreas post-contrast portal phase for comparison (9), normal pancreas.

- Anatomy can help you in cases of severe pancreatitis. Sometimes it is not possible initially to see what the main problem is. By careful review of each organ the lack of definition and oedema of the pancreas become more apparent.
- In conclusion, in this example there is free intra-abdominal fluid. The pancreas is swollen with loss of definition and there are focal areas of hypoperfusion in the body and tail, representing necrosis. There are no vascular complications. The findings are consistent with severe acute pancreatitis with necrosis seen.

The idealized report reads: The pancreas is ill defined and there are areas of poor enhancement with the body and tail. The findings are consistent with acute pancreatitis with focal areas of necrosis in the body and tail. There is ascites seen throughout the abdomen. No vascular complications are seen and no cause for the pancreatitis is visible.

Case 5.2

A patient presents with haematemesis. A CT of the abdomen is performed. A portal venous phase is performed, but, should there be a history of cirrhosis, then an arterial phase would also be required to look for hepatocellular tumours, which are more prevalent in cirrhosis.

- Work through the CT with a system.
- The lung bases are clear.
- Liver: no focal lesions, small liver with a slightly macronodular outline, normal density, no biliary tract dilatation.
- Portal vein abnormal with multiple vessels seen in the porta.
- The spleen is absent.
- The adrenals and kidneys appear normal.
- The gallbladder is normal.
- The aorta is of normal calibre.
- No abnormality is seen in the para-aortic region.
- There is no free fluid in the abdomen.

Anything else: there are multiple serpiginous enhancing structures consistent with varices in the porta and along the lesser curve of the stomach. These are varices, and become more apparent when looking at the normal portal vein (Fig. 5.59d) and the normal appearance on CT of the stomach (Fig. 5.59e). The long enhancing appearance aids in the diagnosis of a vascular abnormality, i.e. varices.

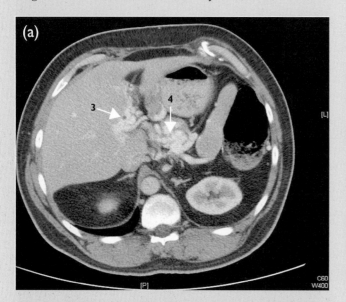

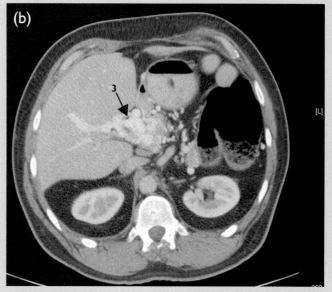

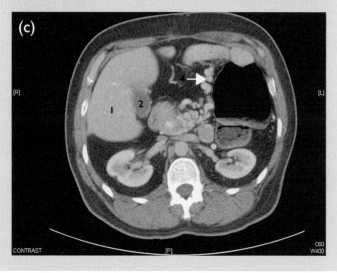

Fig. 5.59 CT of the abdomen: (a–c) varices and cavernous transformation of portal vein. Liver (1), gallbladder (2), cavernous transformaion of portal vein (3) and varices (4). (d) A normal CT of the abdomen with a normal portal vein (5). (e) The normal gastrohepatic region and normal nodes and vessels (6).

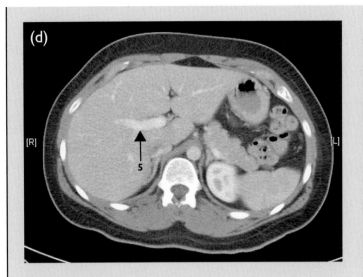

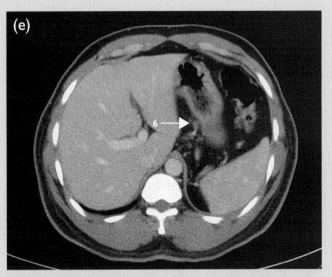

In conclusion there are varices and the portal vein is abnormal with cavernous transformation. The diagnosis is not as important at this stage as the approach to the CT, listing all the correct findings and giving an accurate differential diagnosis.

Case 5.3

A 76-year-old presents with an acute distended abdomen, being very unwell with a raised lactate. A CT of the abdomen was performed. A raised lactate is associated with bowel ischaemia in this context.

Use a systematic review of the images:
- The lung bases are clear.
- There are no focal lesions liver lesions; the liver outline is smooth, with normal liver density. There are multiple gas-filled branching structures in the liver which extend to the periphery. This is gas in the portal veins.
- The spleen is normal.
- The adrenal glands are normal and the kidneys.
- The gallbladder, aorta and para-aortic region are normal.
- Free fluid: there is a very small amount in the left iliac fossa (Fig. 5.60b, block arrow).

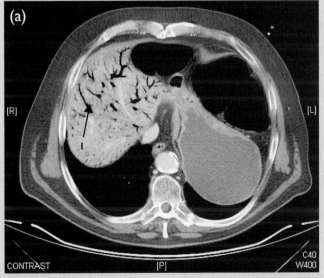

Anything else: the bowel is abnormal. The large bowel is distended with intramural gas. This gas extends circumferentially around the bowel even in a dependent position (Fig. 5.60b–d) as opposed to normal bowel (Fig. 5.60f).

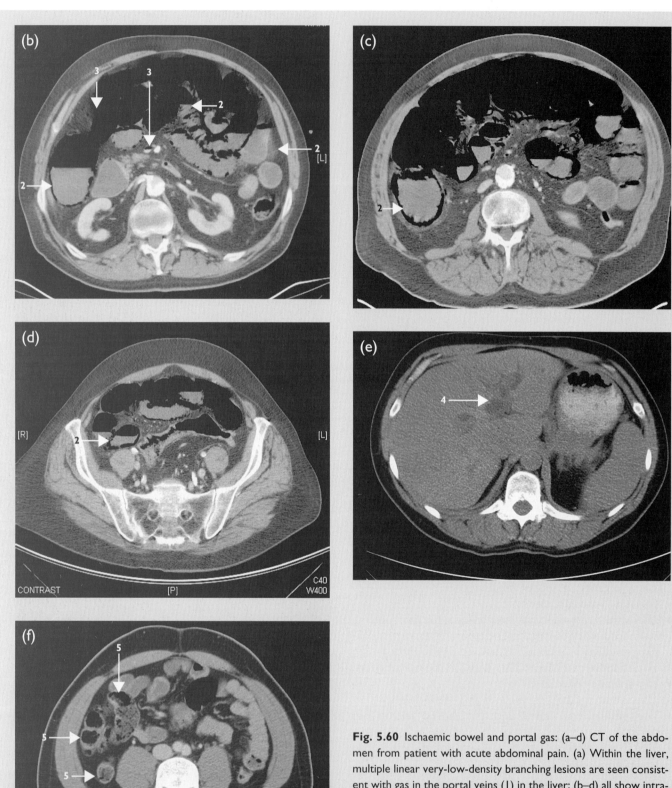

Fig. 5.60 Ischaemic bowel and portal gas: (a–d) CT of the abdomen from patient with acute abdominal pain. (a) Within the liver, multiple linear very-low-density branching lesions are seen consistent with gas in the portal veins (1) in the liver; (b–d) all show intramural gas in the large bowel (2). Gas in the superior mesenteric vein (3). (e) CT of the liver showing dilated intrahepatic bile ducts (4) and how they are fluid density as opposed to (a) when there is gas density in the portal veins. (f) CT of the abdomen showing normal bowel (5).

The findings are of portal gas in the liver and intramural gas consistent with ischaemic colitis.

Case 5.4

A 74-year-old woman presents with a 2-week history of abdominal distension and vomiting. A CT of the abdomen was performed on call. Post-contrast CT of the abdomen was performed.

Review the images systematically:
- The lung bases are clear.
- The liver has no focal lesions; it is smooth in outline, of normal density, with no biliary tract dilatation.
- Portal vein is normal.
- The spleen is normal.
- The kidneys, gallbladder and aorta are normal.
- In the para-aortic region there are some slightly enlarged para-aortic nodes. The normal para-aortic node size is 10 mm in short axis.
- There is extensive free intra-abdominal fluid or ascites.

Anything else: look at the peritoneum and mesentery. There is a soft-tissue mass in the omentum anteriorly (Fig. 5.61a). Look at Fig. 5.61b to see how the large bowel normally has fat anterior to it only between the bowel and the abdominal wall. This is an important review area for soft tissue that can easily be overlooked and mistaken for bowel.

The findings are of an omental cake and ascites, which are commonly seen in ovarian malignancy at presentation or in colonic malignancy. Application of anatomy and use of review areas aid detection of the omental cake.

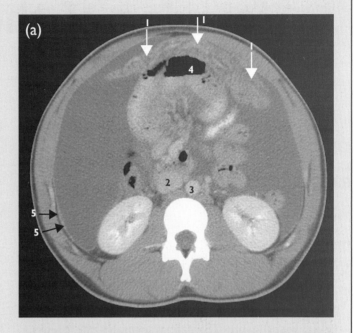

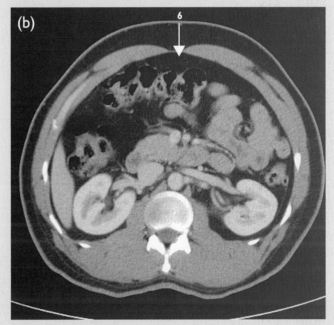

Fig. 5.61 (a) CT of the abdomen post contrast: omental cake (1). Inferior vena cava (2), aorta (3) and transverse colon (4). The arrow (1) shows an extra layer of soft tissue anteriorly outside the bowel, consistent with an omental cake from metastases to the omentum. (5) shows thickening of the peritoneum, consistent with seedlings. (b) A normal CT of the abdomen with normal fatty omentum that is not usually visible (6).

6 Imaging of the genitourinary tract

RADIOLOGICAL ANATOMY

The kidneys

Relations

- The kidneys are retroperitoneal and related to the psoas muscles medially. They are surrounded by perirenal fat and confined by the anterior and posterior perirenal fascia, known as Gerota's fascia and Zuckerkandl's fascia, respectively. The fascia separates the perirenal space from the remaining retroperitoneum, limiting spread of inflammation and infection between the compartments (Fig. 6.1).
- Morrison's pouch or the hepatorenal fossa, a continuation of the peritoneal cavity, lies between the right kidney and the liver.

Size

- The renal size increases from birth up to the age of 20 years.
- At birth the kidney measures approximately 4.5–5 cm. The neonatal premature kidney should measure 1 mm for every week of life, i.e. at 28 weeks the kidney should measure 28 mm in length.
- The kidneys are quoted as measuring 9–12 cm in length which is reflected on ultrasound. Intravenous urograms (IVUs) can cause magnification and there is an apparent increase in length. The range of renal length is actually wider depending on age, individual build and gender, and the normal kidney can measure between 7 cm and 14 cm in length with normal renal function.
- The renal size can be estimated comparing the length of the kidney on plain film to the vertebrae. The renal length should be approximately three and a half vertebral bodies including intervertebral discs.
- The IVU overestimates the renal size due to divergence of the X-ray beams. The range of renal size is therefore 11–16 cm on an IVU.
- Pregnancy causes an increase in renal size.
- The left kidney can be larger than the right kidney by up to 2 cm.
- The left kidney is usually higher than the right kidney (Fig. 6.2).
- Respiratory excursion and the erect position can cause excursion of the kidney by up to 6 cm (Fig. 6.3).

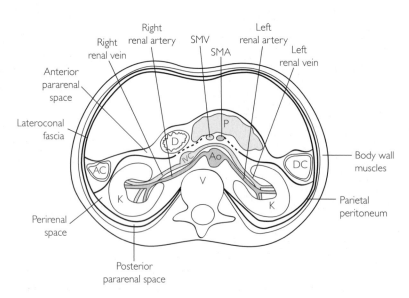

Fig. 6.1 Diagram of the renal anatomy. The kidneys lie surrounded by the perirenal fascia called Gerota's fascia anteriorly and the lateroconal fascia laterally.

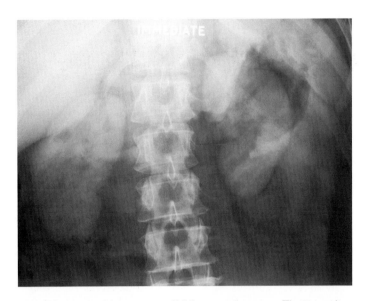

Fig. 6.2 Intravenous urogram (IVU) or nephrogram. The immediate phase of the nephrogram shows how the left kidney normally lies higher than the right kidney by up to 2 cm. The position of the kidneys is also seen with the upper pole lying closer to the midline.

Outline

- There may normally be a bulge in the left renal outline called the dromedary hump or splenic hump. This may simulate an expanding lesion, but the adjacent calyx should be elongated into the bulge and the parenchyma has a uniform thickness. This is a developmental adaptation of the kidney to surrounding organs
- The primitive kidney develops from about 14 lobes in utero which fuse, but traces of fetal lobation can persist in adult life. These are notches that lie in between the renal calyces, which tend to lie centrally and in the lower part of the kidneys, and must be differentiated from renal scars which lie over the calyces (Fig. 6.4).
- The upper pole of the kidney is more medial and posterior than the lower pole of the kidney (Figs 6.5 and 6.6).
- The renal hilum is made up of the renal vein, renal artery and ureter which have a constant relationship at the hilum from anterior to posterior, i.e. VAU – vein, artery, ureter.
- The kidneys have a fibrous capsule. They have a cortex, outer layer and inner layer, the medulla. The cortex and medulla can be separated by imaging with ultrasound and CT/MRI. This is termed 'corticomedullary differentiation'.
- Columns of cortex extend centrally as columns of bertin into the central kidney. These columns separate the medulla into pyramids. The top of the pyramid is pointed and called the papilla (Fig. 6.7). On ultrasound a very thick column of bertin may mimic a renal mass.
- The renal sinus is the central part of the kidney containing the collecting system and vessels, which are all surrounded by fat that is echogenic on ultrasound. The renal pelvis usually lies within the sinus fat, but may lie outside and is known as an extrarenal pelvis.

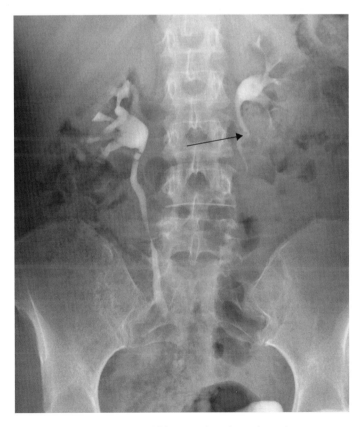

Fig. 6.3 An image from an IVU series that shows how the ureter can move due to respiratory excursion of the kidneys. This causes apparent kinking of the ureter (arrow).

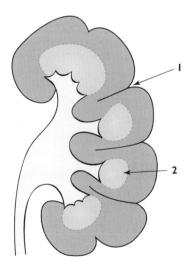

Fig. 6.4 A diagram of fetal lobation. The primitive kidney develops from lobes in the ureter which fuse. The systems of the lobes cause notches that lie in between the renal calyces, which differentiate from scars that lie over the calyces. Notches from fetal lobation (1), the papilla (2).

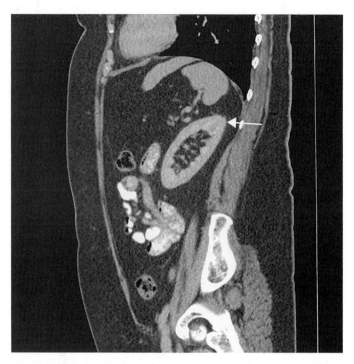

Fig. 6.5 This is a sagittal CT showing the position of the kidney and how the upper pole lies more posteriorly than the lower pole. The arrow marks the upper pole.

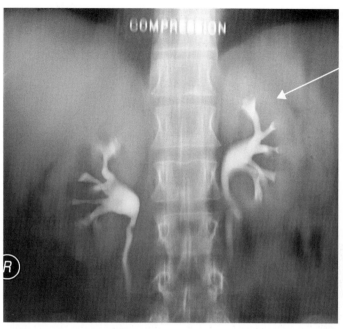

Fig. 6.6 A tomogram image from an IVU series. The upper pole of the left kidney is well seen at 9 cm. The lower pole would be seen at 10 and 11 cm, as it lies more anteriorly.

Vascular supply

- Twenty per cent of individuals have accessory renal arteries supplying the kidneys. This is more common on the left and can be quoted as 40% in some series (Fig. 6.8a,b).
- The right renal artery is longer than the left artery due to its longer course from the aorta, which lies to the left of the midline.

- The renal artery has a large anterior branch which supplies the inferior and anterior poles of the kidney. This is important to remember when performing selective embolization. The posterior branch supplies the superior and posterior aspects of the kidney (Fig. 6.8c,d).

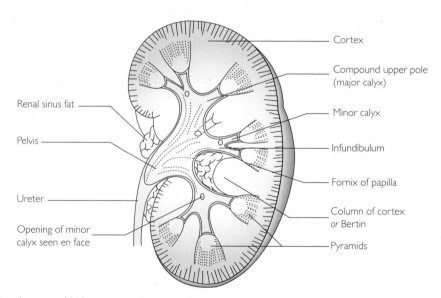

Cortex

Compound upper pole (major calyx)

Minor calyx

Infundibulum

Fornix of papilla

Column of cortex or Bertin

Pyramids

Renal sinus fat

Pelvis

Ureter

Opening of minor calyx seen en face

Fig. 6.7 A diagram showing the normal kidney structure.

- The renal vessel divides into lobar, interlobar, arcuate and interlobular arteries.
- A secondary renal artery may arise from the ipsilateral iliac artery, phrenic artery or directly off the aorta.
- The left renal vein crosses the midline to join the inferior vena cava (IVC) underneath the superior mesenteric artery (SMA). The third part of the duodenum and the left renal vein are found between the SMA and the aorta; a further variant is a retroaortic left renal vein.

Congenital renal anomalies

- Renal agenesis occurs 1 in 1500. This is complete absence of one kidney at birth, more common on the left side.
- Renal ectopy occurs if the kidney in utero fails to progress cranially and the ectopic kidney may lie in the pelvis.
- Rarely cross-fused ectopia occurs, i.e. the ectopic kidney is fused to the opposite kidney. The normally sited kidney has fusion of its lower pole with the upper pole of the ectopic kidney which lies on the same side. This is prone to pelviureteric junction (PUJ) obstruction or reflux.

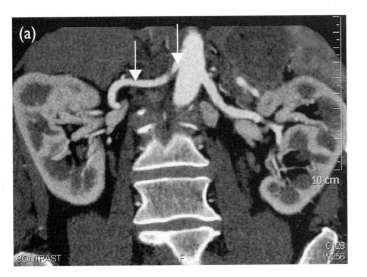

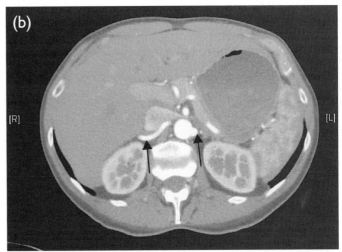

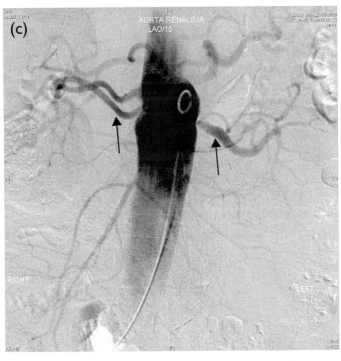

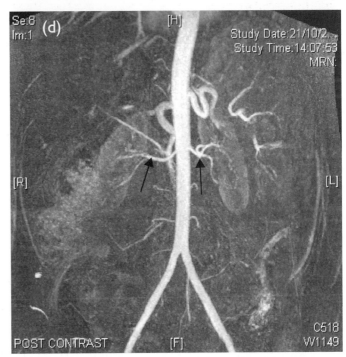

Fig. 6.8 CT renal angiogram showing single renal arteries (arrows) to each kidney on (a) coronal images and (b) axial. The position of the renal arteries coming off laterally from the abdominal aorta at L2 is noted. Twenty per cent of individuals will have multiple renal arteries which can be seen on CT. (c) Conventional renal angiogram and (d) a MRI renal angiogram. The renal arteries are shown by the arrows.

- Rarely, a pancake kidney occurs with two pelvic kidneys fused together in the pelvis.
- A horse-shoe kidney is a congenital variant occurring in 1 in 400. The kidneys are fused by a bridge or isthmus of tissue at their lower poles. This is a fibrous or active connecting band that usually lies at L3 in front of the aorta and IVC and is more prone to trauma. The polarity of the kidney is altered facing anteriorly and the kidneys are more vertical. It is associated with an increased incidence of PUJ obstruction and calculi. The fused kidney is more susceptible to trauma and there is a connection with Wilms' tumours (Fig. 6.9).

- Duplex kidney: 10% of individuals have some form of duplex that ranges from a bifid renal pelvis to a complete duplex in 4%. The upper moiety has a tendency to obstruct and has the lower more distal inserting ureter. The lower ureter inserts ectopically into the bladder and is associated with a dilatation called a ureterocele, which may obstruct. The lower moiety has a tendency to reflux (Fig. 6.10).
- A ureterocele is a dilatation of the distal ureter at its insertion into the bladder, usually associated with an upper pole moiety of a duplex system (Fig. 6.11).

Ureters

- The ureters are 25 cm long.
- They travel along the psoas muscle into the pelvis in the retroperitoneal space.
- The ureters cross the iliac vessels at the pelvic brim/sacral promontory and may show a slight dilatation proximal to this.
- There are three natural hold-up points of the ureter: PUJ, vesicoureteric junction (VUJ) and pelvic brim.
- There is a varied blood supply to the ureters. There are multiple supplies arising from any local vessel, i.e. renal artery, directly off the aorta, gonadal, iliac and superior vesical vessels.
- The intravesical ureter runs obliquely through the bladder wall for 2 cm.

The bladder

- The bladder is pyramid shaped with the base lying posteriorly and the apex lying behind the symphysis pubis.
- The ureters open into the bladder at the superior angles of the trigone.
- The urethra leaves the bladder at the inferior angle of the trigone.
- The urachus, which is the median umbilical ligament, passes up from the anterosuperior surface of the bladder and inserts into the umbilicus.
- The trigone has a smooth mucosa whereas the remaining bladder has a rugose mucosa.
- The superior surface of the bladder is completely covered by peritoneum and related to bowel. The bladder itself is an extraperitoneal structure.
- The bladder wall thickness is 2–3 mm in a distended bladder.
- The bladder may be intra-abdominal in a child.
- The bladder is attached to the umbilicus via the urachus.
- The bladder is related to the rectum posteriorly, in men the prostate inferiorly and seminal vesicles posteriorly, the peritoneum superiorly, and in women the uterus posteriorly and the vesicouterine pouch. The pouch of Douglas or rectouterine pouch is not related to the bladder.

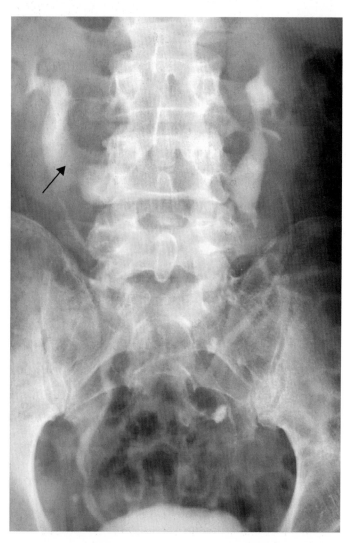

Fig. 6.9 Intravenous urogram of a horse-shoe kidney. See how the polarity of the kidney is abnormal with the kidneys joining or being fused at the L3 position. The ureters come off in an unusual direction. The arrow shows the outward facing polarity of the right kidney.

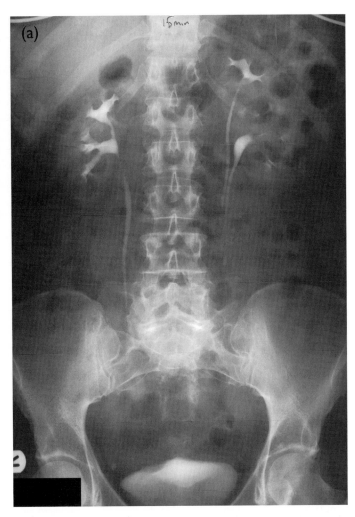

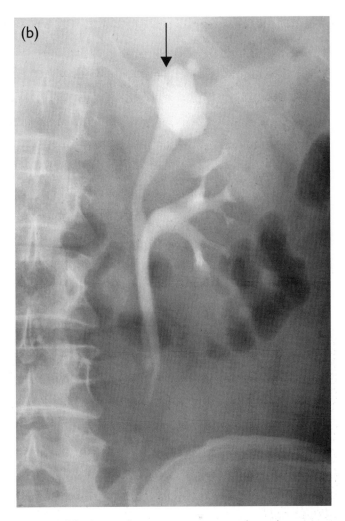

Fig. 6.10 This shows two examples of a duplex kidney. On (a) the right kidney has a bifid pelvis on the intravenous urogram, but only one ureter. The left kidney, however, has two ureters, which were seen to go down to the bladder themselves. (b) A left duplex kidney with a complication of the duplex system, which is of an obstructed upper pole moiety (arrow). This is usually secondary to the ureterocele at the distal ureter.

IMAGING

Kidneys and Ureters

Plain film – KUB

Indications

- Renal colic.
- A plain film or KUB (which stands for kidney, ureter and bladder) is performed to assess for renal tract calcification.

Technique

- The symphysis pubis and renal outline should be included on the image.
- Low kilovoltage of 55 kV is used to detect subtle calcification.
- Oblique views or inspiration/expiration views can be performed to see if calcification is projected over the renal outline or truly lies within the parenchyma.

Intravenous urogram

Indications

Renal stone disease, ureteric obstruction from stones, ureteric pathology.

Contraindications

Allergy to contrast.

Technique

- Using a 19- or 21-gauge intravenous cannula, 50–100 ml non-ionic iodinated contrast medium is injected as quickly as possible to give a bolus. The volume of contrast should be related to the weight of the patient.
- A low kilovoltage is used during the IVU to enhance the renal detail, i.e. 55–65 kV. The contrast in the collecting systems is very dilute so to visualize it low kilovoltage is required.

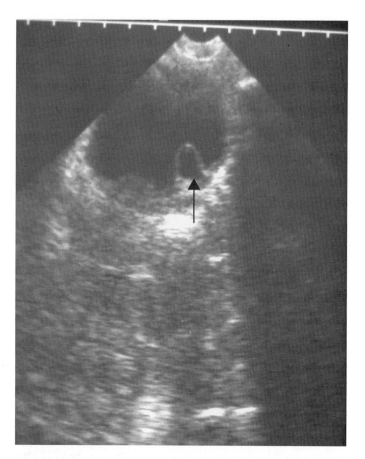

Fig. 6.11 This is an ultrasound showing a ureterocele (arrow) at the distal end of the left ureter. This can lead to obstruction of the upper pole.

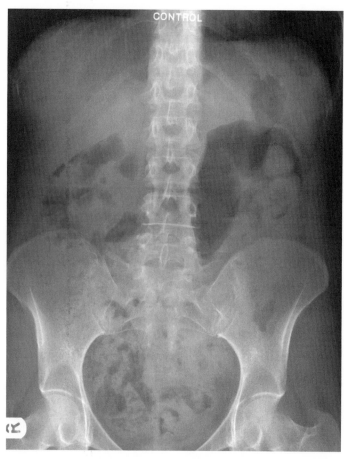

Fig. 6.12 Control film of an IVU series. The symphysis pubis should be included on the film. Any calcification in the line of the renal tract should be identified. If there is any doubt then additional views with inspiration or oblique can be helpful.

- The nephrogram density is affected by the rate of injection, dose of contrast injection and glomerular filtration rate (GFR).
- Dehydration does not affect the nephrogram density. Fluid restriction is no longer used and care should be taken in diabetes, myeloma and impaired renal function to ensure adequate hydration.
- During the nephrogram phase contrast lies in the proximal convoluted tubules.
- The pyelogram/urogram phase is affected by dehydration and sodium salts.
- Hepatobiliary excretion occurs in obstruction or with large doses of contrast injected. It can be normal to visualize contrast in the gallbladder at 24 hours.

Film series

Control film
- Must be taken to visualize any calcific opacities in the renal parenchyma, collecting system or bladder as the iodinated contrast medium will obscure any stones. The control view also ensures that the kidneys are included in the views shown in Fig. 6.12, by seeing the perirenal fat or diaphragms.

Nephrogram immediate
- This is no longer indicated in most cases as ultrasound gives a superior view of the renal outline without using ionizing radiation. The 'nephrogram' view was taken

immediately after intravenous contrast when the contrast was in the proximal convoluted tubules in the cortex to give a cortical nephrogram image

Five-minute views

- The 'urogram' phase – a coned renal area view at 5 min shows the calyces well because contrast is normally excreted into the collecting system at 5 min. If the calyces are poorly distended on the 5-min view and there is no evidence of obstruction, a compression band is applied and a renal area view is repeated 5 min later. The compression belt is normally placed at the top of the iliac crests to compress the ureters as they cross the pelvic brim. In suspected obstruction the first film taken may be a full length 10-min film to show the ureters in their entire length (Figs 6.13 and 6.14). If only one kidney is seen on the immediate 5-min film then a full-length film may show a pelvic kidney.

Contraindications to compression

- Postoperative
- Children
- Abdominal masses
- Renal obstruction
- Renal colic.

Full-length release

- Following removal of the compression band a full-length view is taken when the ureters are well visualized due to the sudden release of contrast from the renal pelvis.
- Postmicturition: finally a full-length view including the bladder area is taken. There should be no hold up of contrast in the ureters (Fig. 6.15).

Additional views

- Tomograms: thick slice tomography is used to blur out overlapping structures obscuring the renal outline such

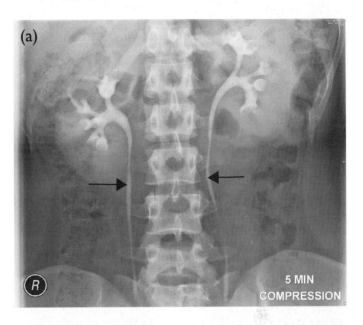

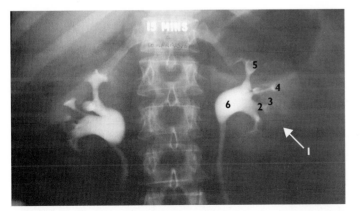

Fig. 6.13 A 15-min series filmed from an intravenous urogram with compression and showing good distension of the upper pole collecting system. The anatomy can be well identified. Fetal lobation (1), infundibulum (2), fornix (3), papilla (4), complex calyx (5) and pelvis (6).

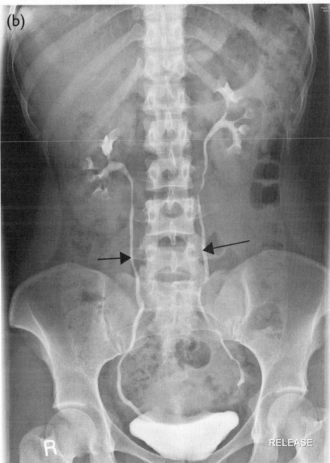

Fig. 6.14 This shows two films from an intravenous urogram series showing: (a) a 5-min compression film; (b) a release film taken when the compression band has been released. Good visualization of the ureters is obtained (arrows).

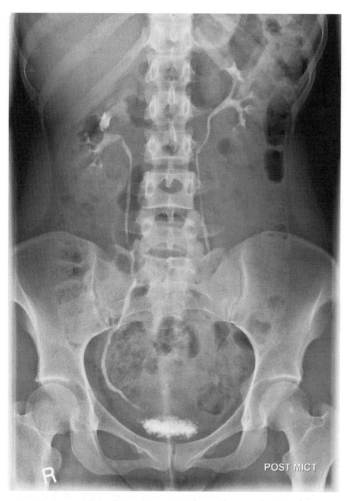

Fig. 6.15 Postmicturition film from an intravenous urogram showing the empty bladder and the drainage from the renal collecting systems. A postmicturition film will show any hold-up of the contrast to the level of a calculus, leading to a 'standing column'.

- The renal pelvis may be intrarenal or lie completely extrarenally. This may mimic obstruction on CT.
- The infundibulum connects the renal pelvis to the minor calyx and terminates in the sharp crescent moon-shaped fornices; every fornix should be sharp and pointed, but if seen en face may be difficult to visualize. The papilla is the pyramid-shaped medulla projecting into the calyx.
- The interpapillary line is an imaginary line that can be drawn between the cortex and the medulla across the papillae connecting all the fornices; the renal cortex should be of even thickness beyond the line. Any defects due to scarring are easier to appreciate using the line. A faint nephrogram may be present at 24 hours after a contrast injection in normal individuals (Fig. 6.16).
- The upper and lower poles of the kidneys have an apparent thickening of the cortex compared with the midpoles due to the obliquity of the lie of the kidneys.
- A complex calyx is seen at the upper pole of the kidney where several minor calyces arise from one infundibulum. More than one papilla drains into the calyx and it is easier to detect the effects of reflux.
- The ureter can kink with respiration. Another variant is a retrocaval ureter where the right ureter runs behind the IVC and is seen to run medially abruptly at L3. The two can cause confusion with retroperitoneal fibrosis where both ureters are displaced medially at L4–5 and narrowed by a focal extrinsic process.
- The papilla is closely related to the minor calyx. Insults to either the papilla as, for example, papillary necrosis, or the calyx, e.g. from obstruction or reflux nephropathy, cause the same appearance as in clubbing, blunting of the calyces (Fig. 6.17).
- The renal vessels can run across the calyces and cause indentations that simulate filling defects.

as bowel, to obtain a sharp view of the renal calyces. It can be used with compression applied to visualize the calyces further. The position of the tomogram reflects the anatomy of the kidney as the upper pole lies more posteriorly, i.e. nearer the tabletop. Tomogram slices are taken as the distance from the tabletop. When planning the tomogram position, if the midpole of the kidney is seen at 9 cm, then the upper pole would be better seen at 8 cm due to its closer proximity to the tabletop and the lower pole better at 10 cm due to it being further from the tabletop.

- Oblique and prone views are used to visualize the ureters as supplementary views if it is important that the whole length is seen as in urothelial tumours. CT IVU is superseding the need for these.

Findings

- There are two to four major calyces and seven to fourteen minor calyces. These drain via their infundibula into the renal pelvis.

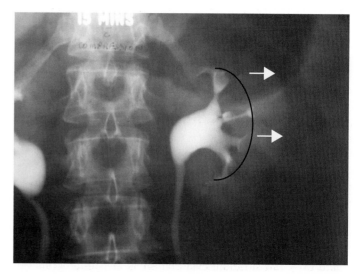

Fig. 6.16 Intravenous urogram: magnified image of the left kidney at 15 min with compression showing the interpapillary line (black line). The cortex should be an even thickness around the renal outline (arrows).

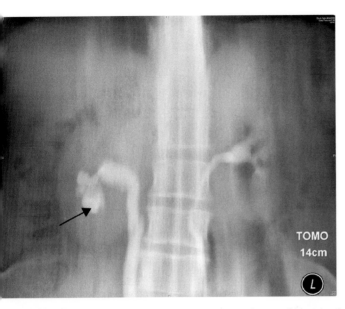

Fig. 6.17 Intravenous urogram: 14 cm tomogram showing blunting of the calyces in the left kidney.

Renal ultrasound

Indication

Ultrasound is a quick, safe, non-invasive investigation of the kidneys not involving ionizing radiation. It is the first-line investigation in children and adults now except in renal colic. It will differentiate solid from cystic masses and can assess bladder volume before and after micturition.

Technique

A 5- or 7-MHz curvilinear probe is used.

Findings

The cortex and medulla can be differentiated on ultrasound due to their different reflectivity; the medullary pyramids are less reflective than the cortex and are seen as echo-poor oval structures. The reflectivity of the kidneys themselves can be referenced to the adjacent liver or spleen. The normal renal cortex is less reflective than the adjacent liver or spleen, assuming that they are normal. If the renal cortex is brighter than the liver it suggests renal parenchymal disease. At the junction between the cortex and medulla, small highly reflective foci are seen in which the arcuate vessels are. The cortex should be an even thickness on ultrasound.

- Children have a different renal appearance on ultrasound to adults. They have increased corticomedullary differentiation, i.e. the renal cortex appears bright normally and does not imply pathology. The cortex is thinner and the pyramids much larger and more echo poor and they can simulate cysts. There is less renal sinus fat (Fig. 6.18).
- The echo-poor areas on ultrasound are the renal papillae or medulla.

- The renal sinus of the kidney or centre is very echogenic due to sinus fat.
- The kidneys sit on the psoas muscle, which can be seen on ultrasound behind the kidneys as a striated structure.
- The hepatorenal fossa or Morrison's pouch lies between the right kidney and the liver, and is a site where abnormal free fluid may be found.
- The renal length can easily be foreshortened on ultrasound. The average length is 10–12 cm.
- In the paediatric bladder using Doppler ultrasound to identify the ureteric jets of contrast enables location of the ureteric orifices.

Renal CT

Indications

- Low-dose unenhanced CT is accurate in renal colic, detecting more ureteric stones than conventional methods.
- CT with contrast for suspected or staging of renal tumours.
- Renal trauma.
- Complications of infection.
- Assessing renal vasculature before renal transplantation or renal surgery.

Technique

Planning the CT depends on what the suspected pathology is. Four phases are possible:

1. To look for calcification non-contrast images are required. Unenhanced scans are also useful in assessing haemorrhage and fat density in cysts and masses. A baseline for cysts should be obtained without contrast to evaluate any enhancement after intravenous contrast. The advantage of a CT KUB compared with an IVU for visualization of renal tract calcification is that intravenous contrast medium is not required. In the cases of asthma and iodine allergy, this is a quick accessible alternative to an IVU and alternative pathologies can be detected at the same time (Fig. 6.19a).

2. The corticomedullary phase is early with a delay of 20–35 s. The cortex opacifies at about 1 min. It may miss renal medullary tumours but is indicated in haemorrhage after trauma and to assess for hypervascular tumours. Arterial phase CT is used to assess renal vasculature pre-nephrectomy and transplantation. There is a high percentage, 20%, of individuals with multiple renal arteries supplying the kidney. This can be seen on CT arising from a range of vessels including the aorta and the phrenic artery.

3. The nephrogram phase or parenchyma phase has a scan delay of 100–180 s. The cortex and medulla are equally attenuating and appear homogeneous while lesions are less dense. This is the ideal phase for evaluation of the kidney. Small cysts in this phase may show partial volume effects and pseudoenhancement. After 120 s the medulla may appear brighter than the cortex. This phase is not part of a routine abdominal CT (Fig. 6.19b).

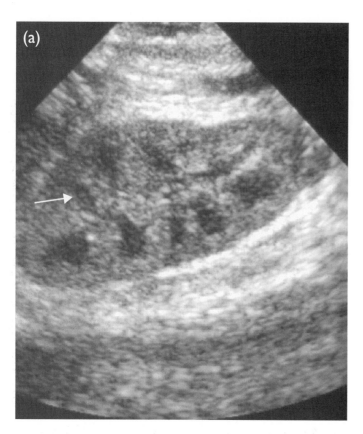

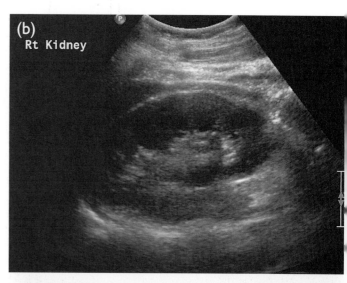

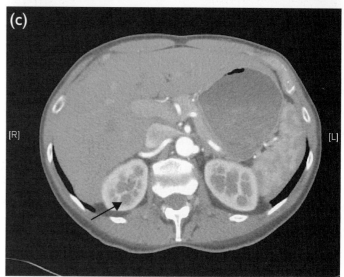

Fig. 6.18 Renal ultrasound images in a child (a) and adult (b). (c) CT of the kidneys, arterial phase. (a) This shows normal cortical medullary differentiation visible on ultrasound, particularly prominent in a child. (b) Shows less marked corticomedullary differentiation in an adult. (c) Axial CT arterial phase showing corticomedullary differentiation. The papillae (arrows) are identified by the echo-poor triangular areas on ultrasound and the low-density triangular areas on CT.

4. Excretory phase/CT urography/CT IVU: indicated to look for urothelial abnormality. The intravenous contrast is given in two phases: a suggested protocol is 40 ml given immediately after the unenhanced CT and then 60 ml given 5 min later as a portal venous phase CT. The earlier bolus will opacify the collecting system and the later bolus the renal parenchyma (Fig. 6.20). In renal failure when the creatinine is >130 μmol/l the risk of renal damage from the contrast must be considered.

Findings

On pre-intravenous contrast scans the kidneys are isodense with muscle, the units being 30–60 HU. There is no corticomedullary differentiation on unenhanced CT, the kidneys appearing of homogeneous density.

Post-intravenous contrast enhancement, during the arterial phase, corticomedullary differentiation is visible within the first 30 s. At 2 min the medulla may appear brighter than the cortex. If assessing for a renal tumour or to evaluate a complex cyst, triple phase scanning is used with unenhanced and dual post-intravenous contrast in the arterial and late portal phase. A delayed scan is required to assess for tumour thrombus in the renal veins and the IVC.

During the venous nephrographic phase the kidneys are homogeneous (Fig. 6.21a). In the delayed excretory phase the contrast is in the collecting systems. An extrarenal pelvis may mimic hydronephrosis but there is no ureteric or calyceal dilatation (Fig. 6.21b/c).

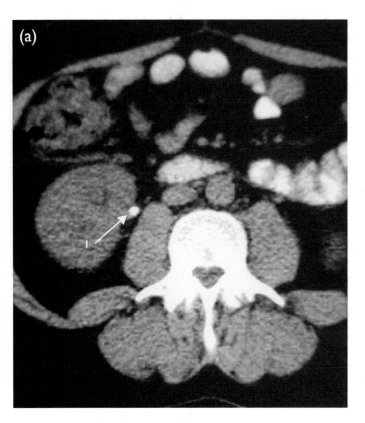

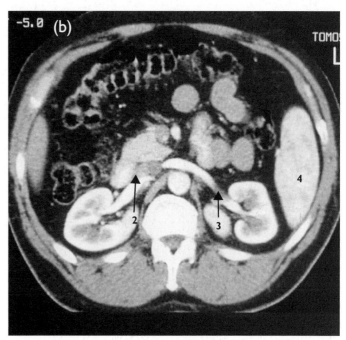

Fig. 6.19 CT kidneys: (a) unenhanced and (b) cortical medullary phase. (a) CT KUB: an unenhanced scan through the renal tract shows a small calcific density in the proximal right ureter (1). No cortical medullary differentiation is seen on unenhanced CT. (b) CT, arterial phase: in the arterial phase corticomedullary differentiation is seen. Flow artefacts can be seen in the inferior vena cava (2) and left renal vein (3). The spleen in this early phase has a heterogeneous appearance (4).

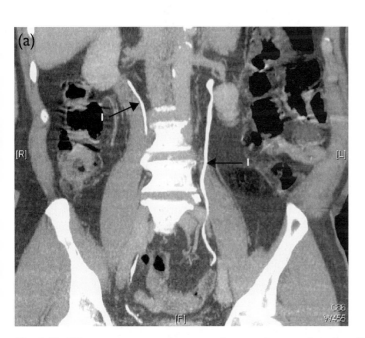

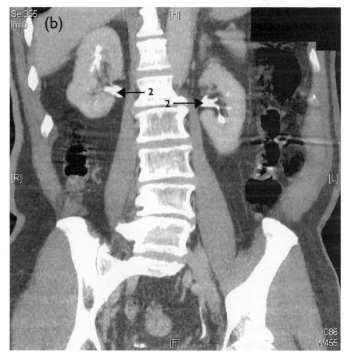

Fig. 6.20 CT intravenous urogram: coronal images. Images taken after 40 ml of intravenous contrast, followed by 60 ml as a 5-minute delay with a portal venous phase. (a) The ureters (1) and (b) the renal pelvis (2).

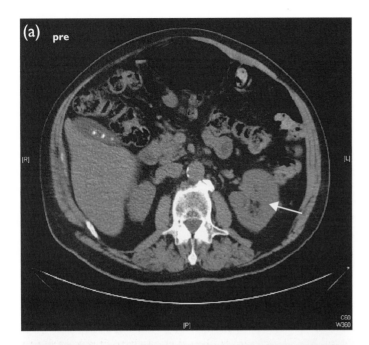

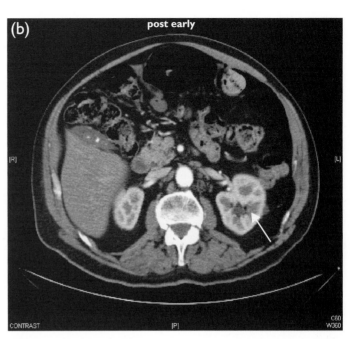

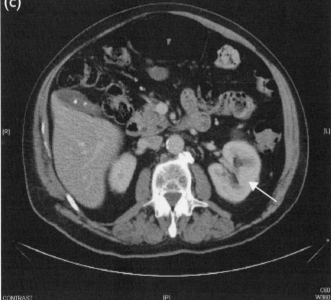

Fig. 6.21 Triple phase CT of the kidneys. (a) Pre-contrast: arrow shows no differentiation of cortex and medulla. (b) Early phase post-contrast showing corticomedullary differentiation (arrow). (c) Late phase showing loss of corticomedullary differentiation.

The polarity of the kidneys is the direction that the hilum faces. On axial CT the renal hilum should face forwards and inwards. In the case of a horse-shoe kidney the polarity is altered and the kidneys may face outwards. If the polarity is abnormal, fusion of the kidneys with a horse-shoe kidney may be present and the fused tissue lies at L3. It is important to detect horse-shoe kidneys due to the increased incidence of obstruction from a stone, PUJ obstruction and an increased incidence of Wilms' tumours

The left renal vein may run behind the aorta and not anterior as is its usual course (Fig. 6.22).

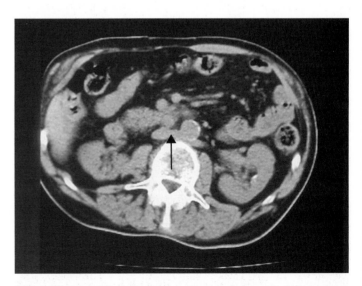

Fig. 6.22 Axial CT of the kidneys shows a retroaortic left renal vein (arrow). Usually the left renal vein runs anterior to the aorta to join the inferior vena cava. A variant is when the left renal vein runs behind the aorta and is retroaortic.

In a CT KUB the signs of acute ureteric obstruction are perirenal stranding, ureteric dilatation and a calcific density within the ureter. In the pelvis the course of the ureter is important to follow as phleboliths may mimic ureteric stones. Perirenal stranding can be seen bilaterally in normal individuals.

When assessing the kidneys for a possible tumour, which is required after an indeterminate ultrasound or incidental finding on ultrasound, a triple phase renal CT is required.

Cysts within the kidney should be simple. There should be no calcification in the wall, which is best seen on the unenhanced scan, there should be no septa and no enhancement within a simple cyst. The CT number before intravenous contrast should be 0–20 HU and the cyst should enhance by less than 10 HU.

Renal MRI

Indications
To assess renal vasculature and for renal artery stenosis, if renal CT is indeterminate.

Findings
On MRI the inherent contrast between the cortex and medulla can be appreciated on both T1- and T2-weighted images (Fig. 6.23). On T1-weighted images the cortex is brighter than the medulla and on T2-weighted images the medulla is brighter, i.e. this ratio is reversed. Intravenous contrast will show the same phases of enhancement as CT. On T1-weighted images the perinephric fat is very bright or intense whereas the urine is of low signal.

MR can be useful to detect fat in lesions with fat-sensitive suppression sequences. MR using flow-sensitive sequences such as time of flight can image the renal vessels or enhanced MR images can show renal vasculature (see Fig. 6.8a).

MR urography using fluid-sensitive sequences and HASTE (**h**alf-Fourier **a**cquisition **s**ingle-shot **t**urbo spin-**e**cho), which are heavily weighted T2-weighted images, can depict the renal collecting system avoiding ionizing radiation.

Retrograde urogram

Indications
To evaluate the urothelial system but has largely been superseded by CT urography. However, the benefit is biopsy and intervention can be performed at the same time.

Technique
- The procedure is performed after cystoscopy and insertion of fine ureteric catheters in theatre.
- Retrograde urogram has a higher infection rate than an anterograde study of 6%.

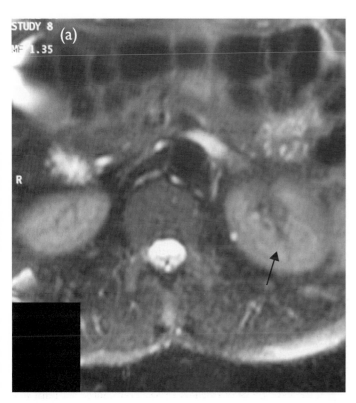 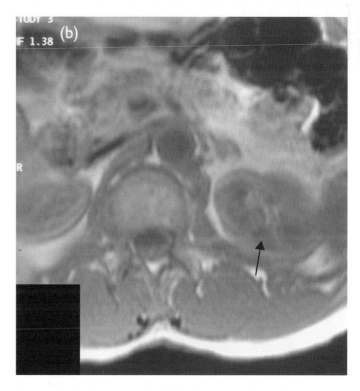

Fig. 6.23 MRI of the kidney. Axial T2- and T1-weighted images. On T2-weighted images (a) the medulla is brighter than the cortex. On T1-weighted images (b) the cortex is brighter than the medulla. To recognize one of the images T1 or T2, look at the cerebrospinal fluid around the theca, which is bright on T2 and dark on T1. A medullary pyramid is marked by the arrow.

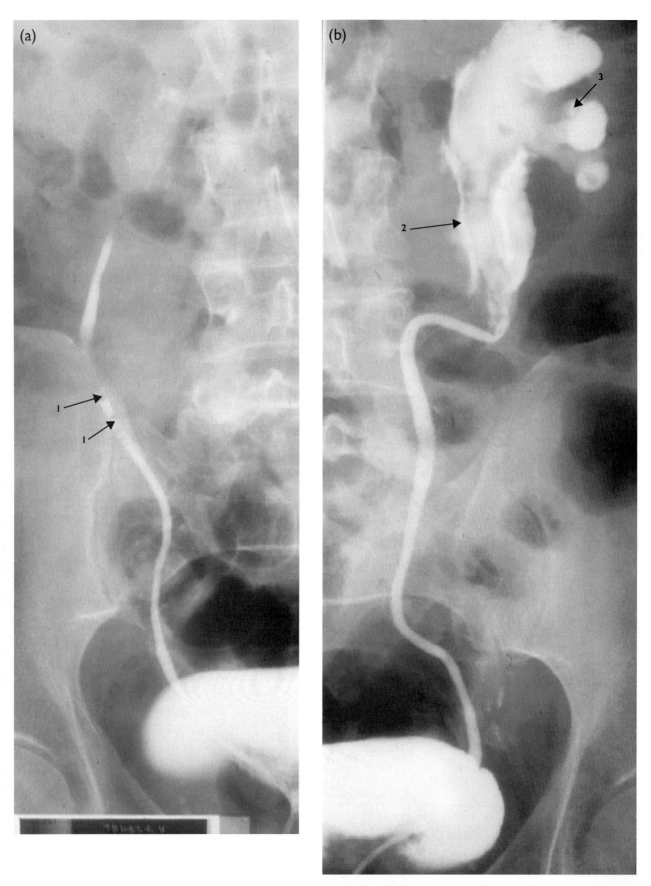

Fig. 6.24 Retrograde urogram: (a) contrast injected from a catheter in the right ureter. Small bubbles of air (1) mimic filling defects within the right ureter; (b) ureteric injection on the left side with a complication of extravasation of contrast into the renal sinus fat and renal tubules, i.e. pyelosinus (2) and pyelotubular reflux (3).

- The renal pelvis has a normal volume of 2–3 ml. Very small aliquots of contrast are injected into the pelvis to avoid extravasation of contrast.
- Back flow of contrast due to overinjection can be into the renal tubules (pyelotubular), into lymphatics (pyelolymphatic), veins (pyelovenous), renal sinus fat (pyelosinus) and renal tissues (pyelointerstitial).
- Prophylactic antibiotics are always used.
- Injected bubbles can mimic filling defects (Fig. 6.24).

Micturating cystogram

Indications

Following a urinary tract infection to assess for vesicoureteric reflux (VUR). It is an uncomfortable examination.

Contraindications

Infection, allergy to contrast.

Technique

- The urethra is catheterized using a feeding tube in a child; the bladder should be filled with the patient supine and the table may be tilted downward. The bladder is filled until the patient voids and oblique views of the ureters are taken to assess for reflux (Fig. 6.25).
- Films should be taken during filling and micturition. Slightly oblique films will show the posterior urethra during micturition for posterior urethral valves.

Findings

There are four grades of ureteric reflux depending on how far up the ureter the urine refluxes and whether there is ureteric or renal pelvic dilatation or intrarenal reflux.

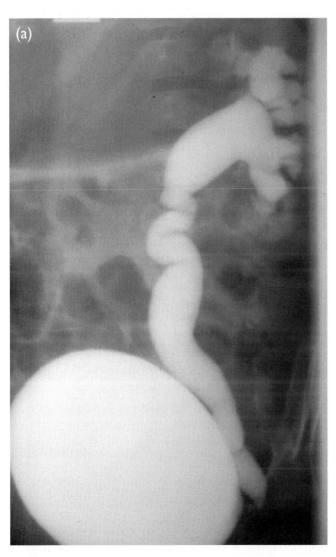 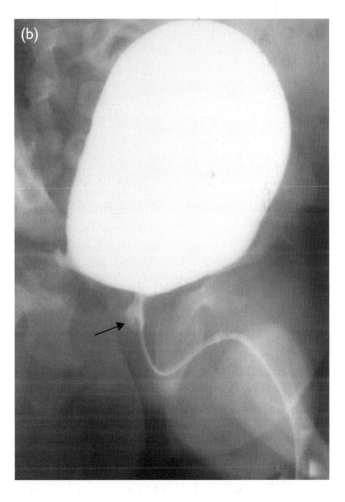

Fig. 6.25 Micturating cystogram in a young child. The bladder has been filled using a feeding tube. (a) There is a grossly dilated left ureter and pelvis secondary to severe vesicoureteric reflux. (b) The micturating phase of a micturating cyst, showing the posterior urethra (arrow).

Anterograde urogram (nephrostomy)

Indications
Percutaneous puncture of the collecting system is performed to relieve an obstructed renal collecting system if infected in renal colic or to chronically drain the system in malignancy if stents have blocked. Stones can be extracted and strictures dilated using this technique (Fig. 6.26).

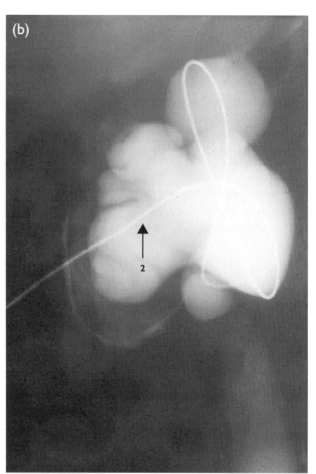

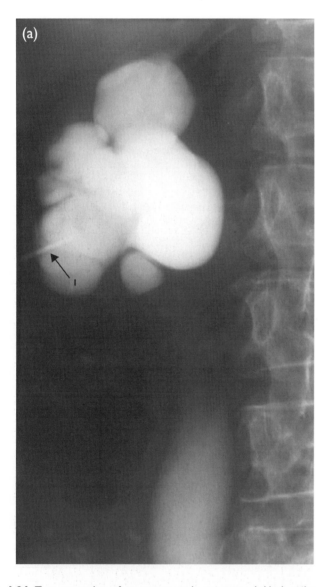

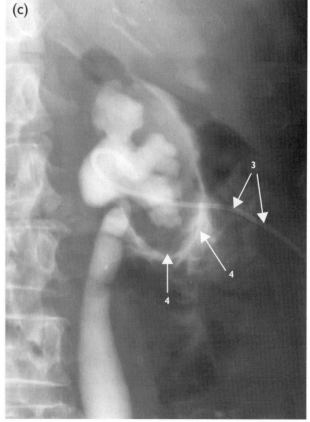

Fig. 6.26 Two examples of an anterograde urogram. (a,b) A right anterograde urogram in a dilated renal collecting system: (a) insertion of a fine Chiba needle under ultrasound guidance into the renal collecting system (1); (b) insertion of the fine guidewire through the needle into the pelvis (2). (c) A left anterograde urogram with a dilated renal collecting system and pigtail drainage catheter in situ (3). Contrast has extravasated around the renal capsule (4).

Technique
- A fine needle is inserted percutaneously under ultrasound or fluoroscopic guidance into the renal collecting system. An example would be a Chiba needle 22G.
- A fine platinum wire is then passed through the needle into the pelvis, i.e. Cope Mandril.
- An exchange system can then be used to exchange the fine or a stiff wire.
- A Lunderquist and Amplatz stiff wire is used.
- The prone position is used.
- This has a lower infection rate than a retrograde urogram.
- A chest radiograph is performed after the procedure to exclude a pneumothorax.

Renal angiography

Indications
Include embolization of renal trauma or tumour. Intervention for renal artery stenosis, renin sampling.

Technique
- In a selective renal angiogram 3–5 ml/s of contrast is injected simulating physiological flow. Digital subtraction angiography enables use of a smaller dose of contrast with smaller catheters. Before performing a selective angiogram a flush aortogram is performed (Fig. 6.27).
- A flush aortogram is performed first to locate the renal arteries and see if multiple vessels are present.
- A catheter exchange system is used to exchange the catheter for a selective renal angiogram catheter with one end hole. Rate of contrast injection is decreased to physiological levels of 8 ml/s.
- A selective catheter such as a cobra, Simmon's or femororenal catheter is used.

Findings
The inferior branch is the anterior division and the superior branch is the posterior division.

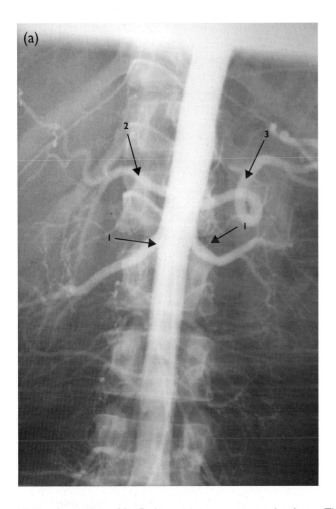 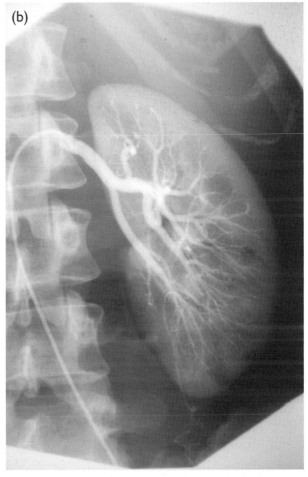

Fig. 6.27 Renal angiogram: (a) a flush aortogram using a pigtail catheter. The renal arteries (1) with their typical posterolateral origin from the aorta. (b) A direct renal angiogram with selective catheterization of the renal artery showing the anterior and posterior branches. The inferior branch is the anterior division and the superior branch of the posterior division. Common hepatic artery (2), splenic artery (3).

Renal nuclear medicine studies

Static scan: ^{99m}Tc-DMSA (dimercaptosuccinic acid)

Indication

A static scan used to look for scarring, pseudotumours. The radioactive substance used in dynamic scanning is taken up by the kidney and fixed within the renal parenchyma with no significant excretion (Fig. 6.28).

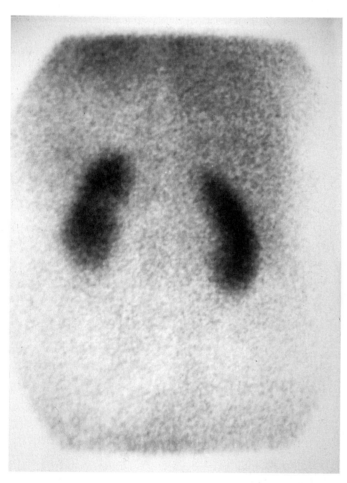

Fig. 6.28 An image from a DMSA scan, which is a static nuclear medicine scan to look for scarring.

Technique

The substance is injected and images are taken at 3 hours.

Dynamic scans: look at divided renal function, total function and differential blood flow to the kidneys. The two main ones are:

- ^{99m}Tc-DTPA (diethylenetriaminepentaacetic acid):
  - used to assess renal function and GFR
  - this is excreted by glomerular filtration.
- MAG-3 (mercapto-acetyl-tri-glycine):
  - used to assess renal function and GFR
  - this is excreted by glomerular filtration and tubular excretion.

Technique

Images are taken at 3 min after injection and then every 5 min for 30 min.

Ascending urethrogram

Indication

Urethral stricture.

Technique

Water-soluble contrast is introduced using Knutson's clamp or a Foley catheter. Films are taken in the oblique position. An ascending and descending phase may be required and then the bladder needs filling and views taken during voiding.

The male pelvis anatomy

The prostate gland

- The prostate gland is no longer considered by lobes, but by zones. The inner gland surrounds the urethra and is called the transitional zone and lies above the verumontanum. The outer gland is made of the peripheral and central zones.
- The prostate gland has a capsule and a normal volume of 25 ml, measuring 4 cm in the lateral plane, 2.5 cm in the AP (anteroposterior) plane and 3.5 cm in the vertical plane (Fig. 6.28).
- The peripheral zone constitutes 70% of prostatic volume and is the site of origin of 70% tumours.
- The central zone constitutes 25% of volume and gives rise to 5–10% of cancers
- The transitional zone is 5% of prostatic volume and gives rise to 10% of cancers.
- A non-glandular fibromuscular stroma: zone lies anteriorly.
- The neurovascular bundle lies at 5 o'clock and 7 o'clock.
- The fascia of Denonvillier lies between the posterior surface of the prostate gland and the anterior wall of the rectum.
- The ejaculatory ducts enter the prostate gland superiorly and insert in the urethra at the verumontanum.
- The obturator internus muscles and levator ani are closely related to the lateral prostate.

Seminal vesicles

- The seminal vesicles are situated behind the bladder and appear like a moustache behind the bladder on CT. They lie above the prostate gland (Fig. 6.29).
- Fat lies in the angle between the bladder and the seminal vesicle (Fig. 6.30).

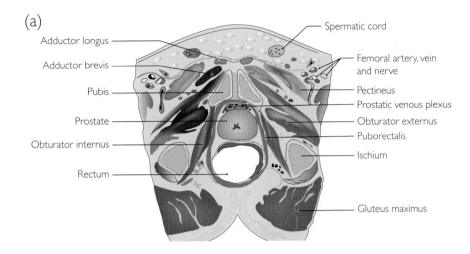

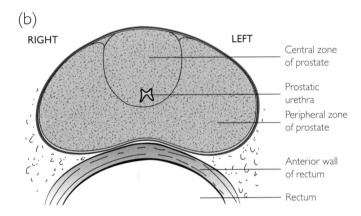

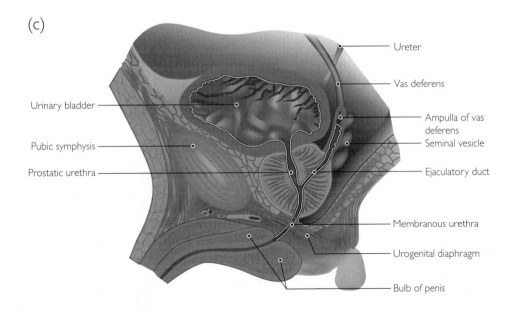

Fig. 6.29 (a) and (b) Diagram of the prostate glands. (a) This shows the peripheral zone posteriorly and the transitional zone centrally. (b) A close relationship with the rectum through the anterior wall of the rectum is noted. (c) Diagram of the relationship of the seminal vesicles, prostate and the posterior aspect of the bladder. The ejaculatory duct arises from the seminal vesicles and runs into the prostate gland to join the prostatic urethra.

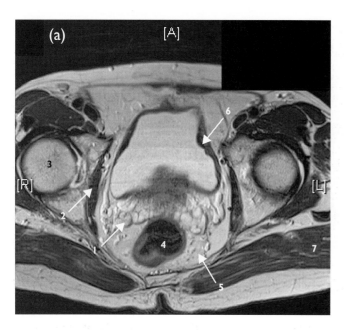

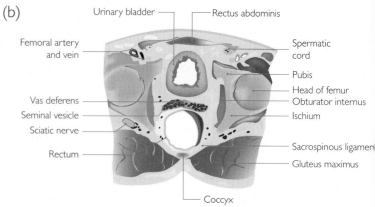

Fig. 6.30 (a) An axial T2-weighted MRI showing the seminal vesicles of high signal intensity behind the bladder (1). The obturator internus muscle (2) is well visualized forming the lateral wall of the pelvis: femoral head (1), rectum (2), mesocolon (3), bladder wall (4) and gluteal muscles (5). (b) Axial diagram of the prostate.

- The seminal vesicles drain into the vas deferens. The vas deferens is a continuation of the epididymis and ascends through the inguinal canal within the spermatic cord, and joins the excretory duct of the seminal vesicle to become the ejaculatory duct.

- The tunica albuginea is a thin membrane that lines each scrotal sac and is closely related to the fibrous capsule of the testis itself (Fig. 6.32).
- The testicular artery, a branch of the abdominal aorta, supplies the testes.

Scrotum, epididymis and urethra

- The testes lie within the scrotum which is divided by a midline septum into two halves.
- The testes are ovoid in shape, measuring on average 5 cm × 3 cm × 3.5 cm.
- Several hundred septa run through the testis and converge on the mediastinum of the testis. The rete testis is adjacent to the mediastinum where seminiferous tubules converge.
- The efferent ductules at the head of the testes empty into the head of the epididymis which can be seen on ultrasound posterior to the testes (Fig. 6.31).
- The vas deferens extends from the epididymis, enters the inguinal canal and then runs through the prostate to join the urethra.
- The ejaculatory ducts from the seminal vesicles enter the urethra within the prostate gland.
- The head of the epididymis lies anterior to the upper pole and the tail lies at the lower pole of the testis.

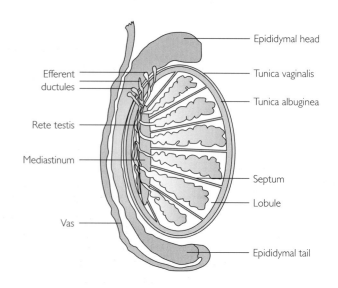

Fig. 6.31 Diagram of the anatomy of the scrotum.

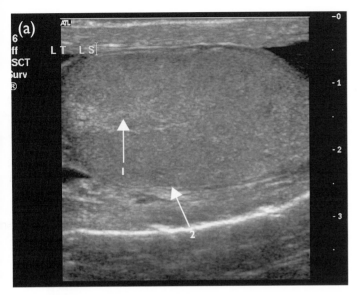 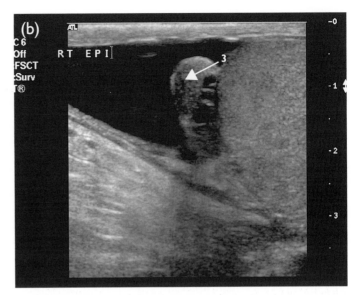

Fig. 6.32 An ultrasound of the testes: (a) the testis itself, with the mediastinum at the testis running through the central aspect with a linear echogenic line (1). The spermatic cord is seen posterior to the testis (2). (b) The head of the epididymis seen at the upper pole of the left testis (3).

- The right testicular vein drains into the IVC and the left testicular vein drains into the left renal vein.
- There is a pampiniform venous plexus that drains the testes.

Imaging of the prostate

MRI of the prostate

Indication
MRI is the modality of choice for staging prostatic malignancy. The prostate is relatively featureless on CT.

Technique
Axial, coronal and sagittal T2-weighted images, supplemented by T1-weighted axial images, are a suggested protocol. Intravenous contrast is helpful for problem-solving, e.g. post-treatment.

Findings
- The zonal anatomy of the prostate is best seen on T2-weighted MRI.
- On T1-weighted images the prostate appears amorphous and the zones cannot be identified. The gland itself appears overall low signal intensity (Fig. 6.33). On a post-gadolinium T1-weighted MR image the central/transitional zone can be differentiated from the peripheral zone which has a less intense enhancement.
- The peripheral zone lies posteriorly and is horse-shoe shaped. This has a high signal normally on T2-weighted imaging which can be differentiated from the lower signal transitional/central zone. Seventy per cent of carcinomas lie within the peripheral zone and are seen there as areas of low signal.
- The transitional zone is taken to be the central part of the whole of the rest of the gland and is a central low-signal zone on T2-weighted images. Benign prostatic hypertrophy occurring within this zone appears as calcification or cysts. Tumours cannot be separated within this normally low-signal zone.
- The periprostatic venous plexus can be seen as a high-signal intensity rim along the rim of the prostatic margins on proton density imaging.
- A breach of the prostatic capsule at 5 and 7 o'clock is more likely to lead to haematogenous spread if the neurovascular bundle is invaded.
- The seminal vesicles appear on T2-weighted imaging as high-signal structures, again as a moustache behind the bladder as seen on CT. A fat plane should be visible between the bladder and the seminal vesicles on CT. The signal intensity of the seminal vesicles is usually high unless there has been radiotherapy change or hormone replacement therapy. In the case of prostatic carcinoma invasion of the seminal vesicles by a tumour will lead to low signal within the seminal vesicle. The seminal vesicles appear as low signal on T1-weighted imaging.
- The bladder wall is seen on MRI as a thin black line. Bladder involvement by tumour will transgress this line (Fig. 6.34).
- Transgression of the prostatic capsule by a tumour shows as 'pointing' or 'beaking', i.e. an acute bulge in the contour of the gland.

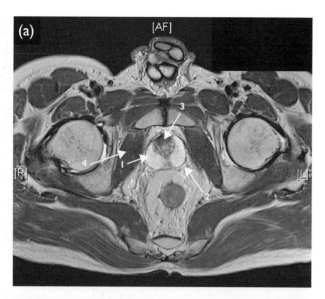

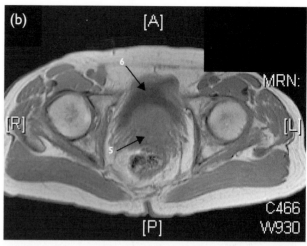

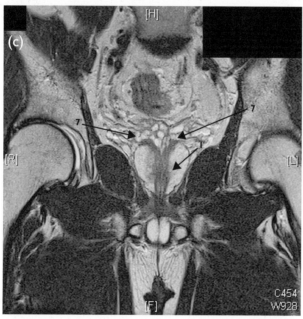

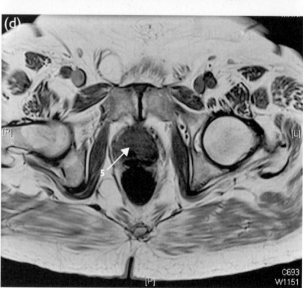

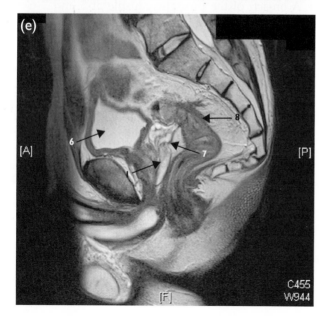

Fig. 6.33 The images of the prostate gland: (a) axial T2-weighted images through the prostate showing the high-signal peripheral zone (1). The prostatic capsule (2) is seen around the edge with the transitional zone centrally in the prostate (3). Obturator internus (4). (b) An axial T1-weighted image of the prostate showing the homogeneous appearance of the prostate (5) with no differentiation of zonal anatomy. The bladder contains low-signal urine (6). (c) Coronal T2-weighted image of the prostate posteriorly showing the peripheral zones posteriorly (1) and the seminal vesicles superiorly (7). (d) A lower image of the prostate T1 weighted at the level of the symphysis pubis (5). (e) A sagittal T2-weighted image through the prostate with the rectum seen posteriorly (8), the bladder superiorly (6), the peripheral zone at the prostate (1) and the seminal vesicles (7).

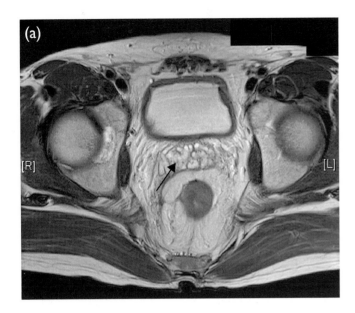
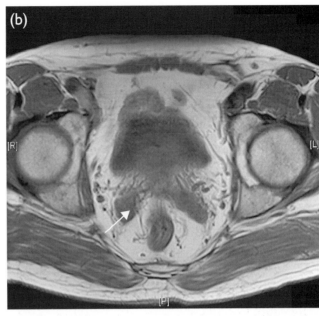

Fig. 6.34 An axial (a) T2- and (b) T1-weighted images through the seminal vesicles (arrows) situated posteriorly to the bladder. The seminal vesicles are usually of high-signal intensity on T2-weighted images, unless the patient has undergone radiotherapy and chemotherapy. Low signal on T2 indicates tumour invasion from a prostate tumour if the patient had not undergone any treatment.

- Lymph node involvement is initially to the obturator nodes, the normal short axis limit is 7 mm, and they lie near the obturator internus muscle.

Ultrasound of the prostate

Indication
Ultrasound is used to screen for prostatic malignancy and in those with an abnormal PSA (prostate-specific antigen) or an abnormal DRE (digital rectal examination).

Technique
- A high-resolution rectal probe is used. A biplanar probe is used to allow for axial and sagittal imaging. The probe is covered by a rubber sheath. Patients are examined in the left lateral decubitus position with the knees flexed.
- Axial and sagittal planes are used.
- Antibiotic prophylaxis is usually given before transrectal ultrasound scan (TRUS) biopsy.

Findings
- The peripheral zone is seen on ultrasound as an echogenic or reflective horse-shoe ring posteriorly.
- Tumours are seen within the peripheral zone as echo-poor lesions. However, TRUS is very operator dependent and not all tumours are detected.

- The central and transitional zones cannot be distinguished on ultrasound and are heterogeneously echo poor.
- Biopsy of the prostate can be performed using ultrasonic guidance.
- The seminal vesicles can be seen behind the prostate gland. They are usually echo poor and measure up to 1 cm in width and are fairly symmetrical.
- Denonvillier's fascia lies between the prostate and the rectum (Fig. 6.35).

Spermatic cord, epididymis and penis

Disease of the spermatic cord, testis, epididymis and penis is primarily evaluated with ultrasound.

Ultrasound of the testes

Indication
Ultrasound is the primary modality for scrotal disease. Tumours, infection, varicocele, hydrocele and ischaemia can all be assessed with ultrasound.

Technique
A high-resolution linear-array probe is used.

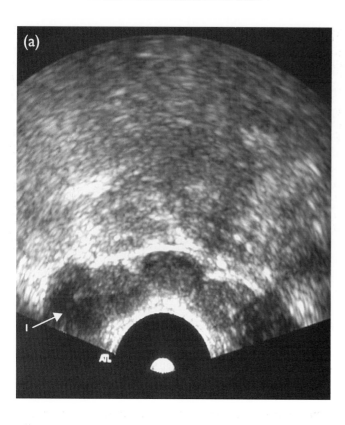

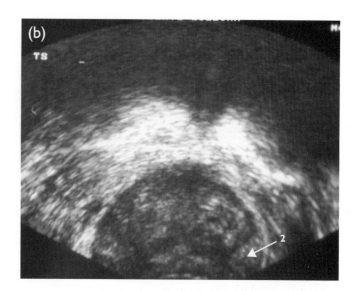

Fig. 6.35 Images of ultrasound of the prostate: (a) the seminal vesicles (1); (b) an axial image of the prostate gland showing the echogenic horse-shoe-shaped peripheral zone (2).

Findings

- The testes should measure a maximum of 5.0 cm in length and be homogeneous in reflectivity.
- A thin echogenic band runs through the long axis of the testis, called the mediastinum of the testes; fine echo-poor strands can be seen radiating into the mediastinum; this is where the blood supply of the testes enters and colour and power Doppler ultrasound show the flow in the vessels in the septa (Fig. 6.36).

- The head of the epididymis is of similar reflectivity to the testis. The head of the epididymis lies at the upper pole of the testes. The spermatic cord is a linear echo-poor structure seen inferior to the testis (Fig. 6.36b).
- Veins at the inferior aspect of the testes, which may represent a varicocele. Use of Doppler ultrasound helps differentiate a varicocele from a spermatocele.

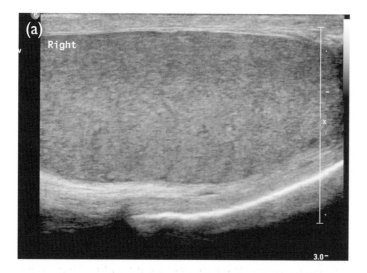

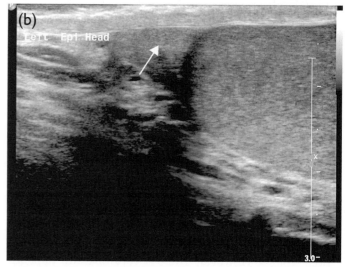

Fig. 6.36 (a) A normal testicular ultrasound and (b) a normal left head of epididymis (arrow). The testis should be homogeneous in reflectivity.

Ultrasound of the seminal vesicles

Indications
Infertility, haematospermia, perineal pain, prostatic malignancy.

Technique
Can be seen at TRUS.

CT of the pelvis

Indications
- For the male pelvis only for lymph node staging or tumour spread, collections or colonic disease. The testes are excluded from the CT imaging volume to protect them from radiation exposure. CT is not used to detect prostatic or testicular malignancy, but it is used for nodal (N) and metastatic (M) staging of tumours.
- The primary modality for imaging the bladder is cystoscopy. CT is inferior to MRI for differentiating layers of the bladder wall. CT is mainly used for staging and postoperative complications (Fig. 6.37).

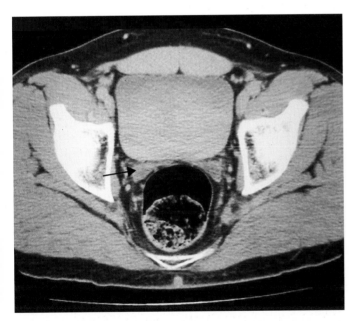

Fig. 6.37 A normal CT axial image of the male seminal vesicles (arrow).

Technique
The bladder should be adequately distended by water drinking and clamping an indwelling catheter 30 min before the procedure (Fig. 6.38).

Findings
- The bladder wall should measure <3 mm, if well distended.
- Ureteric jets may be seen after contrast injection in the bladder (Fig. 6.39).

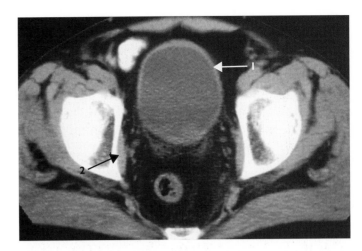

Fig. 6.38 Axial CT of bladder shows the bladder wall (1) and the obturator internus muscle (2).

Anatomy of the female pelvis

Uterus

- The uterus is covered by peritoneum which extends along the posterior wall and the anterior rectal wall to form the pouch of Douglas.
- The peritoneum continues laterally from the uterus as two layers called the broad ligament which extends to the pelvic sidewall. This is a 'mesentery' of the uterus and tube.
- The parametrium is the soft tissue enclosed by the broad ligament laterally, containing the fallopian tubes.
- The parametrial ligaments anchor the cervix to the walls of the pelvis. These are the cardinal, pubocervical and uterosacral ligaments.
- The round ligament can be seen on CT extending from the uterus as a fibromuscular band to the inguinal canal ending in the labium majus.
- The shape, size and position of the uterus are extremely variable.
- The ovary is attached to the broad ligament by a mesentery of its own and to the uterus by the ligament of the ovary (Fig. 6.40).
- The uterus may show failure of embryological development resulting in duplication of the uterus, cervix and even the vagina. This may result in a muscular septum dividing the endometrial cavity into two. A bicornuate uterus can be detected on transverse scanning when two apparent endometrial cavities are noted, side by side (Fig. 6.41).
- The normal uterus has a fundus, a body and a cervix. The cervical canal has an internal and an external os. The tubes open into the uterine cornua.
- Other variants of the uterus include retroversion and retroflexion which make the uterus difficult to assess with ultrasound.

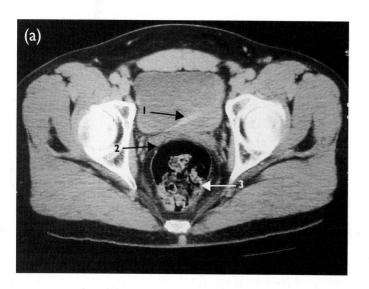

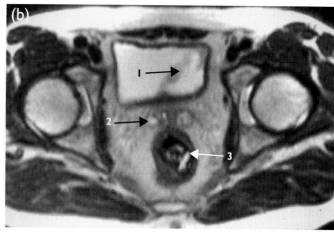

Fig. 6.39 (a) An axial CT and (b) an axial T2-weighted MRI, both showing a ureteric jet contrast (1) into the bladder from the right ureter. The seminal vesicles (2) can be seen behind the bladder with the rectum posteriorly (3).

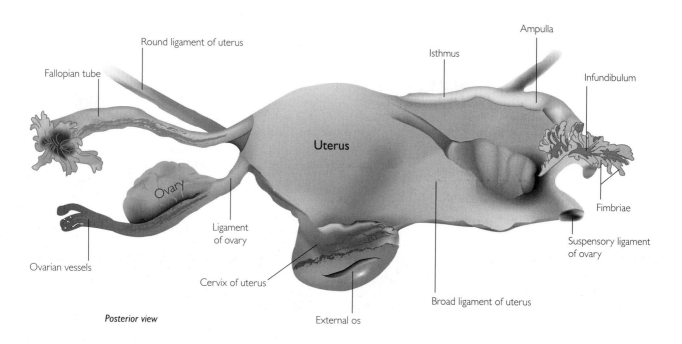

Fig. 6.40 Diagram of the uterus and its relationship to the fallopian tubes and the ovaries.

Fallopian tubes

The fallopian tubes have four parts:
(1) the uterine
(2) the isthmus which is the long, narrow tube
(3) the ampulla which is the dilated outer end
(4) the infundibulum where the fimbriae extend into the peritoneal cavity over the ovary beyond the confines of the broad ligament.

Ovaries

- The ovaries measure 4 × 2 × 1 cm. Ovarian volume is more accurate for assessing ovarian size and the two ovaries should be roughly equal in volume. Cysts larger than 1 cm are excluded from this measurement. Volume decreases from puberty to after the menopause, decreasing from 14 ml in adolescence to 2.5 ml at the menopause and 0.5 ml a decade after the menopause.

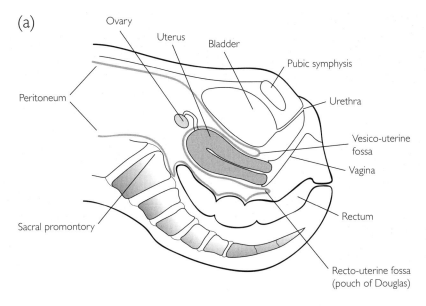

Fig. 6.41 Anatomy of the uterus with a filled bladder as: (a) a sagittal diagram and (b) an axial diagram.

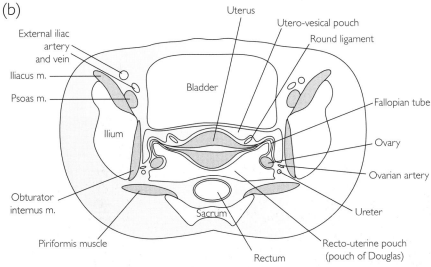

- The ovaries are closely related to the pelvic sidewall and commonly lie anterior to the internal iliac vessels, but are extremely mobile (Fig. 6.42).
- Once ovulation has occurred the follicular cyst becomes a corpus luteum.

Imaging of the female pelvis

Ultrasound of the female pelvis

Indications
- Ultrasound is the initial method for assessing the uterus and can be performed transabdominally (TA) or transvaginally (TVS).
- It is also used to assess the ovaries for masses, diagnosis of ovarian cancer, ovarian cyst assessment, family history screening for ovarian cancer, infertility treatment assessing follicular size and in diagnosis of ectopic and early

pregnancy. The diagnosis of ovarian cancer still involves clinical examination and CA-125 levels.

Technique
- The uterus and ovaries are better resolved with a transvaginal scan using a high-frequency transvaginal probe (5–10 MHz). The high resolution is at the expense of depth penetration and often both TVS and TA ultrasound are complementary for visualization of both the uterus and the ovaries. Visualization of small endometrial lesions is better with TVS and also a retroverted uterus is best assessed with TVS.
- The transabdominal route uses the full bladder as an acoustic window. Large masses arising from the adnexae or pelvis may be missed using the transvaginal probe only. The patient drinks a litre of fluid 1 hour before the study, which fills the bladder and pushes the bowel upwards and out of the way (Fig. 6.43).

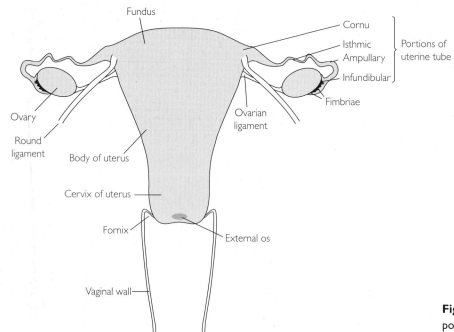

Fundus

Cornu

Isthmic

Ampullary

Infundibular

Portions of uterine tube

Fimbriae

Ovary

Round ligament

Body of uterus

Ovarian ligament

Cervix of uterus

Fornix

External os

Vaginal wall

Fig. 6.42 Diagram showing the position of the ovary in relationship to the fallopian tube.

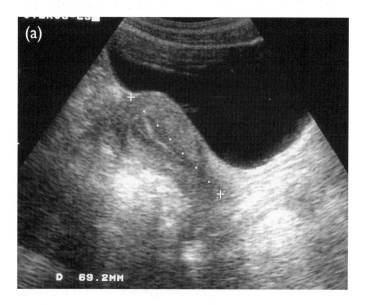

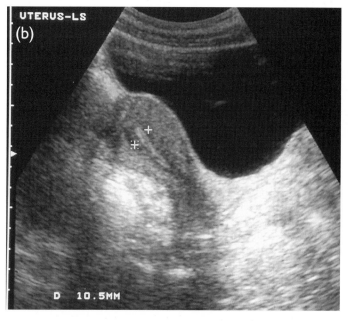

Fig. 6.43 Transabdominal ultrasound of the uterus in the sagittal plain showing (a) the normal length which is normally within 8 cm and (b) normal endometrium and that shown on day 10 of a cycle.

- The bladder should be empty for TVS. A protective sheath is used to protect the TVS probe. The patient normally lies on a cushion to raise the pelvis for TVS providing increased latitude for the probe (Fig. 6.44).
- The ovaries are found anterior to the iliac vessels at the pelvic side wall, although their position is extremely variable.

- Colour flow Doppler ultrasound is helpful in assessing tumour vascularity in the ovary.

Findings
- The uterus should measure a maximum of 7–8 cm in length. The parous uterus is longer than the nulliparous uterus.

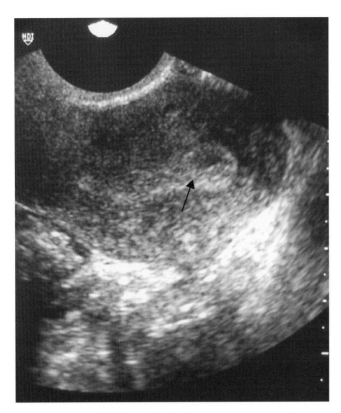

Fig. 6.44 A transvaginal scan of the uterus showing the better resolution of the endometrium (marked by arrow).

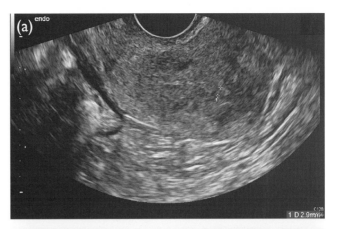

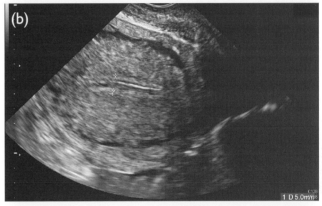

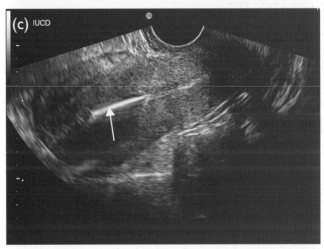

Fig. 6.45 Transvaginal ultrasound of the uterus showing the different appearance of the endometrium: (a) a normal very thin endometrium in a woman on an oral contraceptive; (b) an endometrium following menstruation; and (c) the appearance of an intrauterine coil device as very echogenic band (arrow).

- The uterus may be flexed posteriorly, i.e. retropositioned. This causes a difficult ultrasound image.
- The normal myometrium is relatively hypoechoic.
- Between the endometrium and the myometrium on ultrasound, the junctional zone or subendometrial halo can be seen as a thin echo-poor line.
- The appearance of the endometrium varies with the cycles and is seen as an echogenic band of varying width. After menstruation only a thin cavitary echogenic line is visible.
- A trace of fluid may be visible in the endometrial cavity at the time of ovulation for about 24 hours. A thin fluid space of 1–2 mm may also be present in the endometrial cavity at menstruation.
- The normal endometrium in a menstruating female can measure up to 12 mm in thickness.
- In a normal postmenopausal woman the endometrium should be <3 mm thick. In a woman on HRT a measurement of <10 mm is satisfactory (Fig. 6.45).
- Women on the oral contraceptive have a single line of endometrium.
- The cervix is a midline structure, but the uterus can often lie to one side of the midline and its position varies according to bladder filling.
- The uterus has a fundus and from the cornua of the fundus run the fallopian tubes. The tubes cannot be seen on a transabdominal scan, but can sometimes by seen on transvaginal imaging.
- At the end of the fallopian tubes are fimbriae or fingers which attach to the ovary that is in close proximity.
- The ovaries are extremely mobile and may be found behind the bladder.

- In young children under age 5 years the ovaries have a very small volume of about 1 ml and may be hard to find, reaching 3 ml by age 5–9 years.
- As each cycle progresses the ovaries develop more and more follicles and one becomes dominant – a follicular cyst. Midcycle the dominant follicle measures 20–25 mm and ovulation occurs. A follicular cyst can sometimes measure up to 4 cm in diameter. This will however spontaneously regress and repeating the study at 6–8 weeks will confirm this (Fig. 6.46).
- Free fluid can be detected normally in the pouch of Douglas midcycle in menstruating females.
- A corpus luteal cyst measures about 1 cm in diameter with almost isoechoic reflectivity to the normal ovary. It can, however, be larger and look irregular and very vascular, and cause confusion. If there is doubt repeating the scan at 2–6 weeks is helpful to look for resolution.

CT of the female pelvis

Indications

- Transvaginal scanning and MRI have gradually replaced CT in the investigation of uterine and other gynaecological malignancy, although CT is used for assessing lymphadenopathy. CT cannot define the structures of the uterine wall (Fig. 6.47).
- CT is the investigation of choice in staging ovarian cancer for bowel, peritoneal and liver involvement.

Technique

- Multislice post-intravenous contrast scans are taken. Oral contrast to opacify bowel is essential starting at least 45 min before scanning.
- Moderate filling of the bladder is required and rectal contrast may be used in some institutions.
- A vaginal tampon may be helpful in defining the vaginal vault.

Findings

- In the female patient the uterus undergoes normal enhancement on CT. The uterine cervical ratio is normally reversed in a girl. In a girl the uterus:cervix ratio is 1:2 whereas in an adult the uterus:cervix ratio is 2:1.
- The uterus can normally lie to one side and normally enhances after contrast.

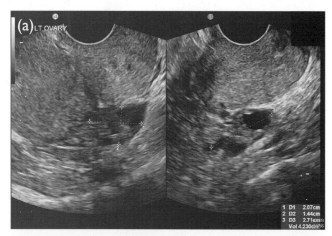

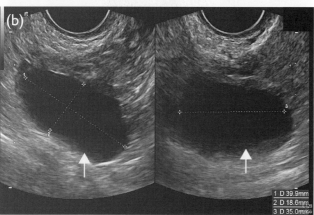

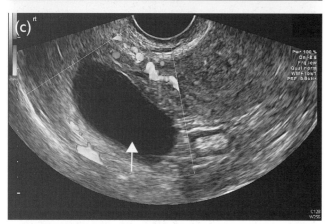

Fig. 6.46 TVS of the ovaries shows the appearance of the normal ovaries: (a) a normal left ovary containing follicles; (b) a simple follicular cyst (arrows), measuring 4 cm which is at the upper limit of normal. No septa and no vascularity are seen in relation to a simple follicular cyst. (c) No vascularity in the ovarian follicular cyst (arrow).

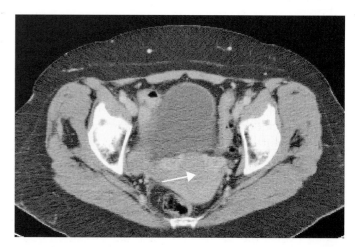

Fig. 6.47 Axial CT of the pelvis showing a normal enhancing uterus on CT (arrow).

- CT does not show the zonal anatomy of the uterus or cervix.
- The ovaries are usually identified on multislice CT, but a review of the adnexal regions for any masses is important.
- The vagina is seen as an oval structure of soft-tissue density anterior to the rectum.
- The uterine round ligament is a band of soft tissue that runs anterolaterally forward that gradually tapers from the uterus (Fig. 6.48).

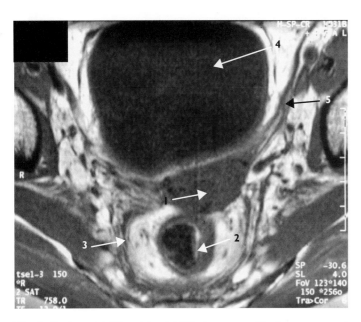

Fig. 6.48 An axial T1-weighted MRI: the uterus (1) shows no zonal anatomy. The rectum (2) can be seen with surrounding mesocolon (3). The bladder contains low signal urine (4). The round ligaments (5) can be seen running anteriorly.

MRI of the female pelvis

Indications

MRI is used to diagnose, stage and follow up cervical cancer and endometrial cancer. Congenital abnormalities and fibroids are well visualized. Ovarian masses can be characterized on MRI.

Technique

- The patient should be fasted to minimize bowel motion and the bladder should be moderately full. An antiperistaltic agent such as glucagon will reduce peristaltic activity.
- The patient is examined supine.
- A phased array pelvic coil is used.
- A combination of T1-weighted and T2-weighted images is taken with sagittal and axial planes angled along the long axis of the uterus or angled images can be taken through he cervix. The correct plane is critical depending on the indication and suspected pathology.

- Intravenous contrast is not usually helpful.

Findings

- The uterus and cervix are best visualized with MRI.
- The zones of the uterus and cervix are seen on T2-weighted and not T1-weighted imaging.
- The uterus and cervix have three zones of signal intensity on T2-weighted imaging on MRI. The endometrial cavity is high signal on T2-weighted imaging, a low-signal line represents the junctional zone, and an intermediate signal zone for the myometrium. (Fig. 6.49).
- T1-weighted images show the ligamentous structures well, but no intrinsic zonal anatomy in the uterus.
- On axial T2-weighted imaging the weighting of the examination can be assessed by looking at the signal of the urine within the bladder. T2-weighted imaging has bright urine. T1-weighted imaging will have dark urine.
- On T2-weighted imaging the bladder wall can be clearly seen as a thin black line. (Fig. 6.50).
- The uterus can be clearly seen on T2-weighted imaging with the junctional zone and zonal anatomy within it. The round ligaments are seen projected anterolaterally from the uterus. Posterior to the uterus the rectum can be

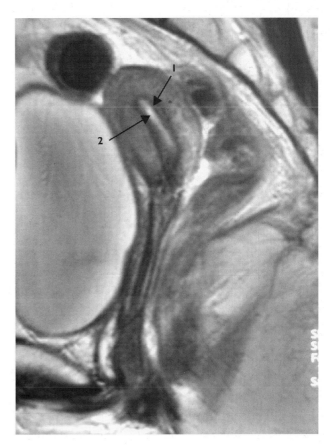

Fig. 6.49 Sagittal T2-weighted MR image of the pelvis showing the uterus posteriorly to the bladder with the junctional zone (1) well seen on the T2 image. The junctional zone is identified as a low-signal band adjacent to the endometrium (2).

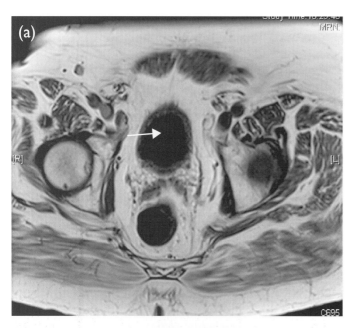

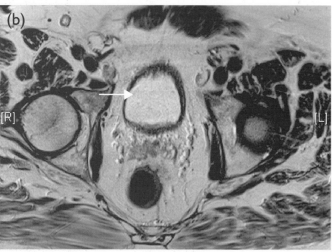

Fig. 6.50 The bladder on MRI: (a) axial T1-weighted when the bladder wall and urine cannot be separated clearly (arrow) and (b) axial T2-weighted MRI when the low-signal bladder wall is easily separated from the bright urine (arrow).

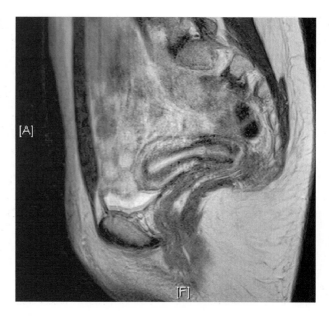

Fig. 6.51 Sagittal T2-weighted uterus showing the zonal anatomy of the uterus.

seen and the mesocolon. This is the fascia that contains the rectum and is important to analyse when interpreting rectal carcinoma. The anatomy is the same as CT and therefore note the piriformis muscle extending through the greater sciatic foramen.

- On sagittal imaging the uterus and cervix are well seen. Cervical tumours show up as areas of low-signal intensity within the cervix.

- The MR appearance of the normal uterus is influenced by hormonal changes. In women of reproductive age, the central high-signal zone, i.e. the endometrial cavity, is thin immediately after menstruation and of maximal thickness midcycle. In women taking the oral contraceptive, or premenarchal or postmenopausal women, the endometrium is thin and atrophic (Fig. 6.51).

- The normal zonal anatomy of the uterus and cervix can be seen on gadolinium-enhanced T1-weighted imaging. The myometrium usually enhances more than the endometrium.

- The ovaries are well visualized on MRI and the presence of fat or haemorrhage in a cyst can be evaluated. MRI can characterize ovarian cysts (Fig. 6.52).

HSG (hysterosalpingogram)

Indication
HSG is performed to assess for patency of the fallopian tubes in infertility. HSG can also assess congenital and acquired abnormalities of the uterus and tubes. The test is contraindicated in pregnancy, infection or contrast allergy.

Technique
- The bladder is emptied before the procedure.
- The patient lies supine in the lithotomy position.
- The optimal time to perform is day 4–10 of a regular cycle when the tubes are most easily distensible.
- One technique is to use a Cusco speculum to visualize the external os of the cervix and vulsellum forceps to grasp the anterior lip of the cervix. A cannula is inserted in to the cervical canal and 20 ml of warmed contrast is injected, excluding any air bubble, while fluoroscopically screening.
- A smooth muscle relaxant such as Buscopan or glucagons may be used for cornual spasm if non-filling of the tubes occurs.

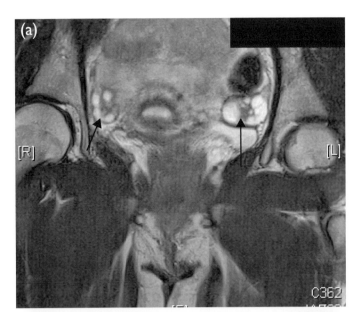

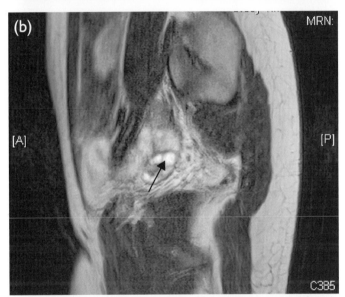

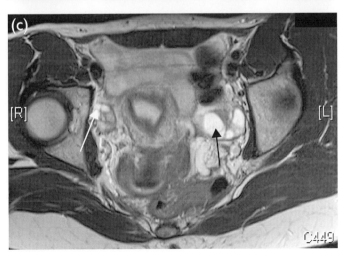

Fig. 6.52 (a) Coronal, (b) sagittal and (c) axial T2-weighted MRI showing the normal ovaries (arrows). The follicles are well visualized. Characterization of ovarian masses is possible with MRI.

- Tube filling occurs most easily at the end of the first week of the cycle (Fig. 6.53).

Findings
- Free spill from the dilated ampulla into the peritoneal cavity concludes a normal tube.
- The normal endometrial cavity is smooth and triangular.
- The cornu of the uterus leads to the tubes which are each 5–6 cm long.

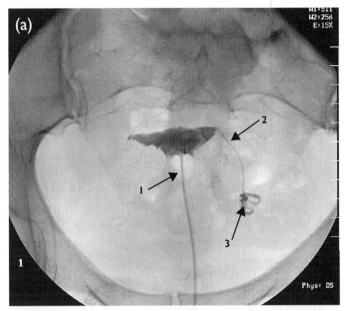

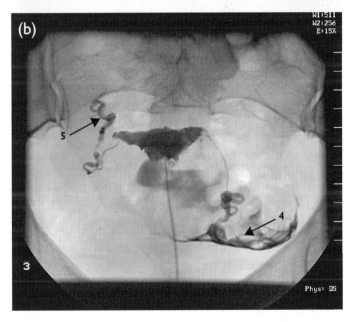

Fig. 6.53 Hysterosalpingogram: (a) the catheter in the endometrium cavity (1). Contrast is seen filling the left fallopian tube (2) and the ampulla (3). (b) Free spill into the left peritoneal cavity on the left side (4). Contrast fills the right fallopian tube and on the right ampulla (5).

CASES

Case 6.1

A patient presents with right renal colic at midnight. Urinalysis confirms microscopic haematuria.

Investigation

A plain KUB is taken (arrow on Fig. 6.54a).

Findings

- Calcific opacities are seen in the right hemipelvis. These may represent phleboliths or a distal ureteric calculus (arrow (1) on Fig. 6.54a).
- An IVU is requested. The patient has no allergy to iodine or history of asthma.
- A full-length film at 10 min is taken. It is customary to perform a limited IVU series for renal colic.

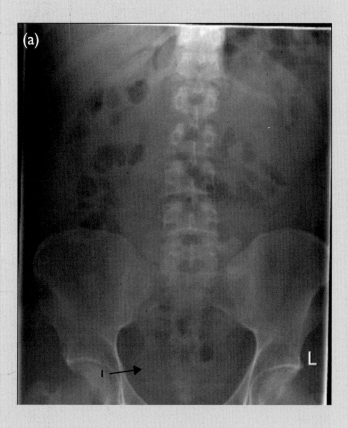 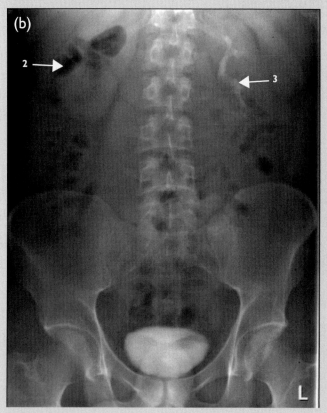

Fig. 6.54 IVU series: (a) unenhanced KUB. (b) 10-min film. (c) A delayed film of 1 hour. (d) A postmicturition film. Phleboliths (1), dense right nephrogram (2), left urogram (3) and right ureter (4).

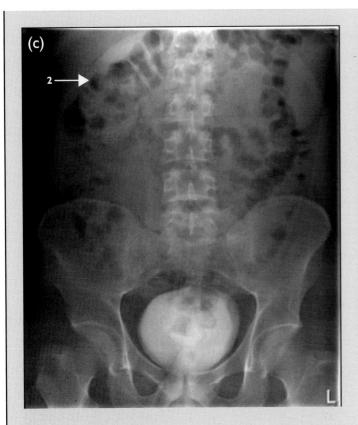

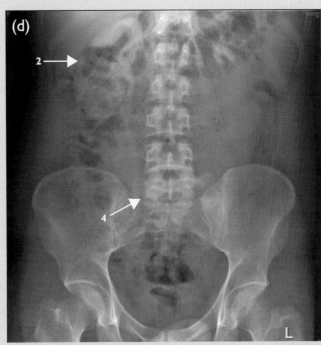

Interpretation of IVU

When looking at an IVU use the following principle – SOC:

- Size of kidney: assess the size first using the control film or first film. Renal size should be up to a maximum of three and a half vertebral bodies.
- Outline: the renal outline is visible due to the fat outlining the kidney, i.e. perirenal fat. Bulges in the contour of the kidney, absence of a kidney or masses arising from the kidney may all be seen on the outline assessment.
- Calyces: the calyces are visualized on the urogram phase. If each calyx is not clearly filled, a compression band should be applied to the iliac crest. Every calyx and minor calyx should distend with a sharp infundibulum and sharp fornices.
- On the full-length 10-min film, the renal size and outlines appear normal. On the left side the calyces are visible and appear normal. On the right there is a dense nephrogram (arrow), a feature of acute renal colic and no calyces are seen (Fig. 6.54b).
- A delayed film at 30 min shows again a persistent dense right nephrogram and a faint outline of a dilated right ureter. The left side appears normal as the contrast has been excreted (Fig. 6.54c).
- A postmicturition film confirms the dense right nephrogram and the dilated obstructed right ureter forming a standing column down to the bladder (Fig. 6.54d).

Concluding
- S normal
- O normal
- C delayed on right, normal on left.

Diagnosis

Acute right renal colic.

Case 6.2

A patient presents with pain and microscopic haematuria at A&E at the weekend. An IVU is performed as renal colic was considered.

- Size: renal size is normal.
- Outline: the renal outlines appear normal as well as can be seen.
- Calyces: are all normal with no blunting.

The IVU control film shows no renal tract calcification. After contrast prompt bilateral nephrograms are seen. The renal size and outlines are normal. Both calyceal systems appear normal. There is, however, a filling defect within the bladder.

Ultrasound confirms a bladder mass consistent with a papillary lesion (Fig. 6.55). It is important to systematically review the IVU for other pathology as well as the obvious findings.

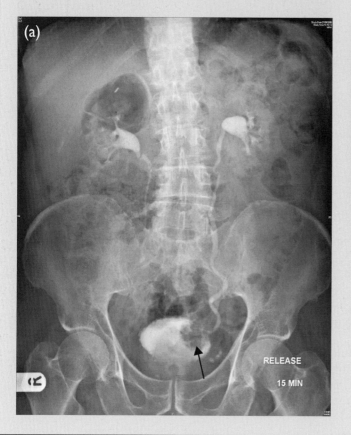

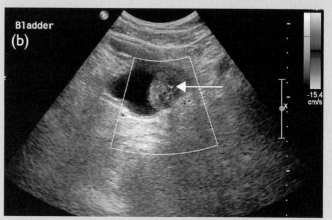

Fig. 6.55 (a) IVU following contrast shows normal upper tract pelvis and ureters. There is, however, a large filling defect in the bladder at the left vesicoureteric junction (marked by arrow). (b) Ultrasound of the bladder showing the mass with marked vascularity within it on Doppler ultrasound (white arrow).

Case 6.3

A patient presents with right loin pain. A CT KUB followed by an enhanced renal CT is performed.

Findings

- On the CT KUB, in order, the liver, spleen, pancreas and gallbladder appear normal. The right kidney shows a cystic lesion related to the pelvis. This is smooth and of fluid density and at first may look like a cyst.
- Coronal images show more clearly the presence of two ureters and that this is an obstructed moiety of the upper pole. A dilated ureter can be seen down to the bladder. No ureterocele was visible. With duplex kidneys the upper pole usually obstructs and the lower pole suffers reflux (Fig. 6.56).

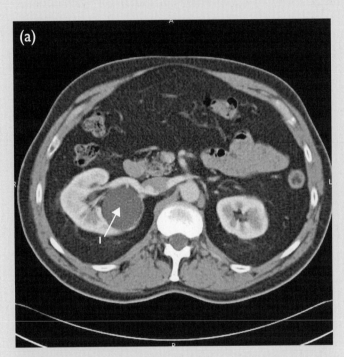 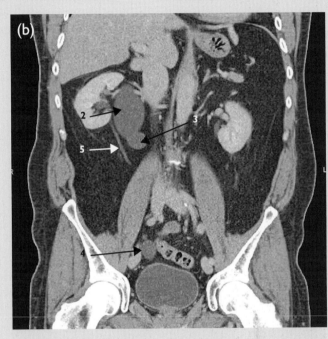

Fig. 6.56 (a) A CT scan showing a dilated upper pole moiety on the right side (1). (b) On the coronal images the dilated renal pelvis (2) and ureter (3) are seen and the dilated distal ureter (4) is seen within the pelvis. The left kidney appears normal. On the coronal images two ureters (3) and (5) can be seen running down to the pelvis.

Case 6.4

A patient presents with right loin pain.

Findings

- An IVU is performed following an ultrasound that shows a prominent right renal pelvis.
- The IVU shows:
  - S normal size
  - O normal outline
  - C the calyces are normal on the left. On the right the calyces are blunted. The right fornices are not present.
- If the interpapillary line is drawn it shows an even band of cortex of equal thickness to the left, so there is no scarring.
- The right ureter is not dilated, suggesting that the obstruction is at the pelviureteric junction, i.e. PUJ obstruction.
- Following micturition there remains contrast in the dilated right renal pelvis.
- A CT IVU shows the right PUJ.
- A dynamic DTPA scan confirms the hold-up of contrast in the right renal pelvis and shows the divided renal function (Fig. 6.57).

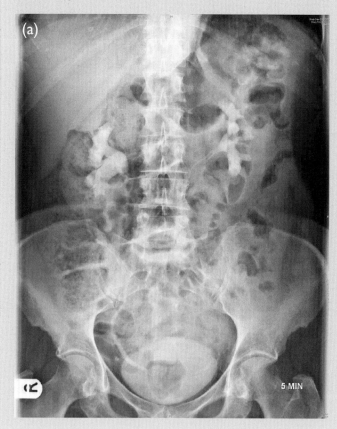
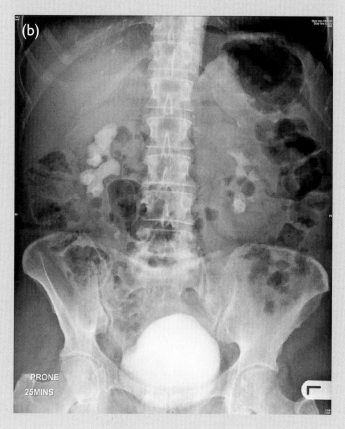

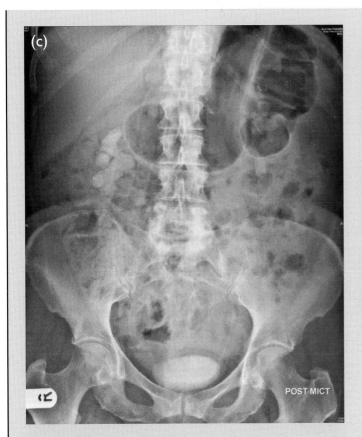

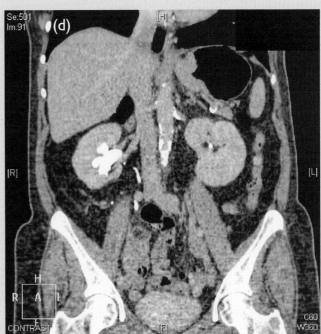

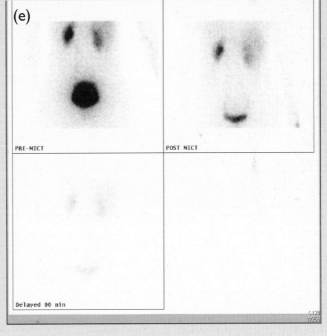

Fig. 6.57 (a) A 5-minute film from an IVU series with the calyces poorly seen. (b) The prone film at 25 min shows the left calyces normal. However, the right calyces are blunted. (c) On the post-micturition film hold of contrast is seen within the right collecting system with dilated blunted calices consistent with a PUJ obstruction. (d) A CT IVU showing a dilated right renal pelvis with hold up of contrast. (e) A series from DTPA scan showing a dense right renal pelvis consistent with a pelvicoureteric junction obstruction.

Case 6.5

A patient presents with hypertension and haematuria and is referred for a renal ultrasound.

Findings

- The renal ultrasound shows large kidneys measuring 19.3 cm on the right and 15.4 cm on the left in length. Initially the normal renal structure is hard to visualize but knowing the anatomical position of the kidneys helps diagnose the large cystic structures as the kidneys.
- Multiple renal cysts are seen bilaterally suggesting adult polycystic kidney disease (Fig. 6.58a,b).
- CT kidneys are performed to look for a complication of APCK (adult polycystic kidney) disease, which increases incidence of renal malignancy.
- A three-phase CT is performed.
- The liver and spleen show some cysts, but the pancreas, gallbladder and lung bases all appear normal.
- In the retroperitoneal region huge lobulated masses are seen on the unenhanced CT, and the normal renal outlines are not visible. The kidneys are huge with loss of normal architecture bilaterally.
- Initially some hyperdense renal cysts are seen and some low-density cysts. The renal size is measured on the coronal images. Cysts can undergo haemorrhage and be hyperdense which is appreciated on unenhanced CT.
- Following contrast some normal cortex enhances but there is no feature to suggest malignancy. No septa or masses are seen in association with the cysts (Fig. 6.58c,d).

The diagnosis is adult polycystic kidney disease with no evidence of malignancy.

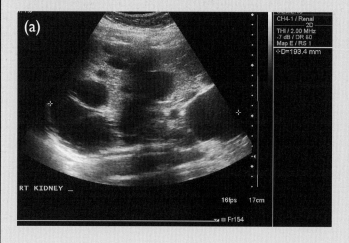
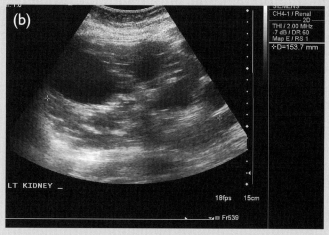

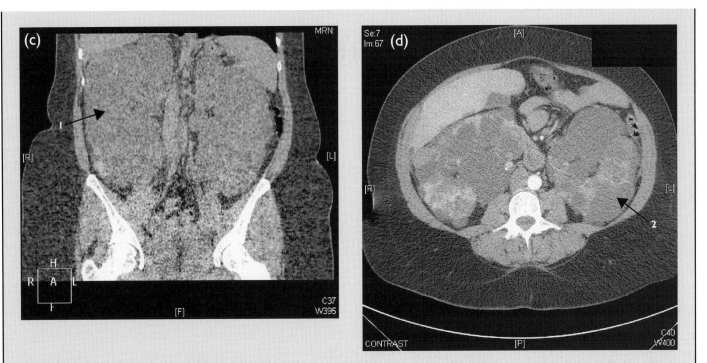

Fig. 6.58 (a,b) Renal ultrasound showing large kidneys (1) with multiple cysts. The normal renal ultrasound size is 9–12 cm. (c,d) Unenhanced and post-contrast CT scans. (c) An unenhanced coronal image through the kidneys showing large multilobulated kidneys (1); (d) an axial enhanced CT of the kidneys showing enhancement of the cortex and the presence of multiple cysts (2).

7 Imaging of the spine

There are 33 vertebral bodies in the spine:
- Cervical: 7
- Thoracic: 12
- Lumbar and sacral: 5 + 5
- Coccygeal: 4.

The vertebrae vary in size and shape according to their anatomical site. A typical vertebra has a vertebral body anteriorly which is connected by pedicles to the lamina posteriorly (Fig. 7.1). The spinous process arises poste-riorly from the lamina. A transverse process arises from the junction between the pedicle and the lamina on either side. There are four articular processes projecting from the lamina, each having an articular facet with the superior facets facing backwards and the inferior facets facing for-wards. The facets restrict different movements in different parts of the spine. The pars interarticularis lies between the lamina and the facets. The cervical and lumbar vertebrae are convex anteriorly whereas the thoracic and sacral ver-tebrae are concave anteriorly.

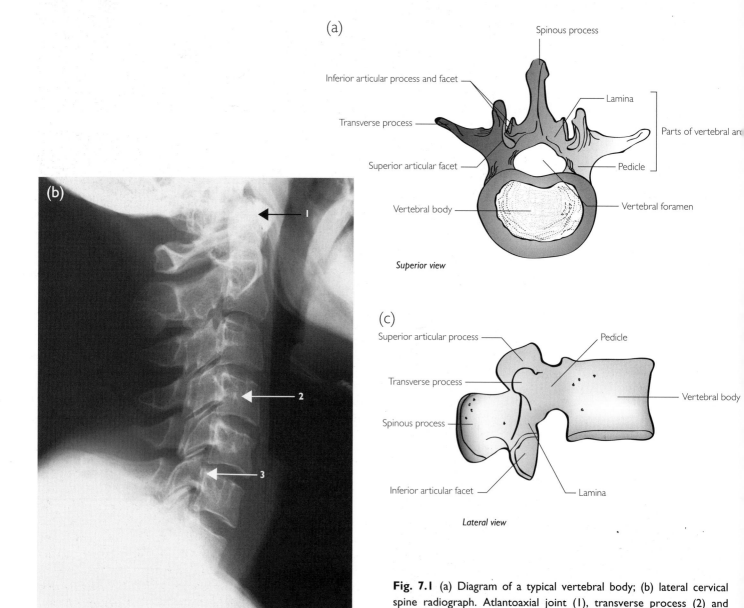

Fig. 7.1 (a) Diagram of a typical vertebral body; (b) lateral cervical spine radiograph. Atlantoaxial joint (1), transverse process (2) and joints of Lushka (3). (c) Diagram of lateral vertebral body.

RADIOLOGICAL ANATOMY

Cervical spine

- C1, C2 and C7 are atypical cervical vertebrae.
- C1 (the atlas) has no vertebral body or spinous process, but lateral masses and a posterior tubercle. Each lateral mass has a tubercle for articulation with the occipital condyles (Fig. 7.2).

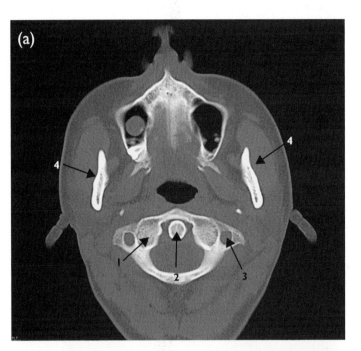

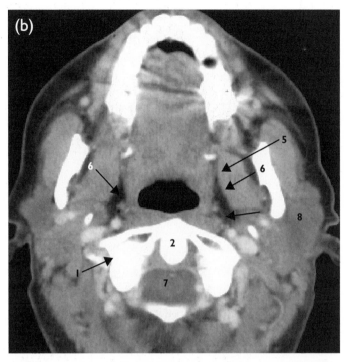

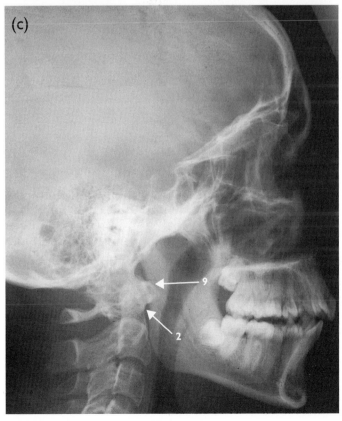

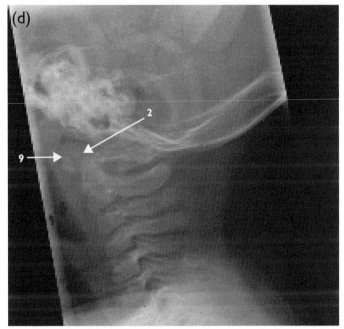

Fig. 7.2 (a) Axial CT C1–2 bony window. (b) Axial CT soft-tissue window of the atlas and odontoid peg. The lateral mass of the atlas (1). The odontoid peg (2) can be seen midway between the two lateral masses of the atlas. The atlas has no spinous process. Foramen transversarium (3), masseter muscle (4), pterygoid muscle (5), lateral pharyngeal fat space (6), theca (7) and parotid gland (8). Lateral cervical spine radiographs of (c) an adult and (d) a child. The adult shows the normal atlantoaxial distance in an adult of <2 mm; the anterior arch of the atlas (9). A child has a wider normal limit of the atlantoaxial distance of 5 mm. Odontoid peg (2).

- C2 (the axis) comprises a body and the odontoid peg or the os odontoideum which appears at age 3–6 years and fuses by 12 years. The peg represents the body of C1. In a few individuals it may remain unfused mimicking a fracture (Fig. 7.3). C2 has the longest bifid transverse process.
- There is a facet on the posterior aspect of C1 that articulates with a facet on the odontoid peg. This is a synovial joint and hence the peg can be destroyed by an erosive arthropathy such as rheumatoid arthritis. Review should be made of the C1–2 articulation routinely to assess for such destruction.

- C7 has a large non-bifid spinous process which is palpable called the 'vertebra prominens'. The foramina transversaria are small or even absent on C7.
- The foramina transversaria are small holes in the transverse processes, which are peculiar to the cervical vertebrae. The vertebral vessels pass through the foramina of C1–6, but not C7, and then loop back to enter the foramen magnum. When performing Doppler ultrasound of the vertebral vessels, the Doppler signal is found between the acoustic shadows of the foramina transversaria (Fig. 7.4).

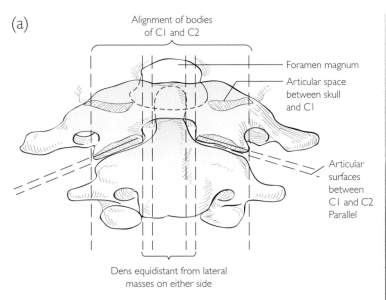
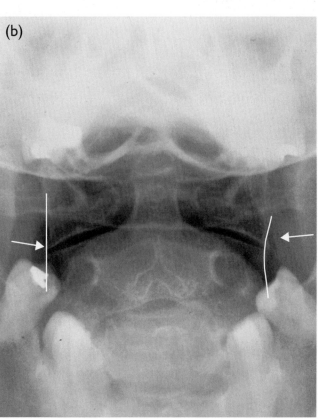

Fig. 7.3 (a) Diagram of peg view and (b) radiograph of peg view. Alignment between the articular surfaces of C1 and C2 laterally is marked with an arrow. The peg should lie equidistant between the lateral masses of C1 and the lateral masses should be aligned with the body of C2 inferiorly.

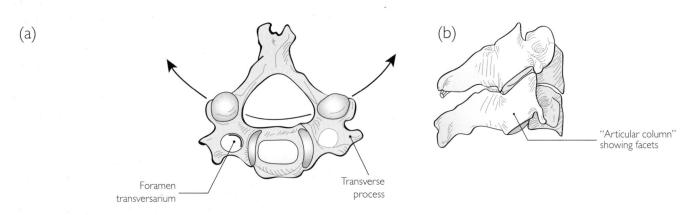

Fig. 7.4 Diagrams of normal cervical spinal vertebrae: (a) axial image showing that the cervical vertebrae have foramen transversarium and (b) the facets form an articular column.

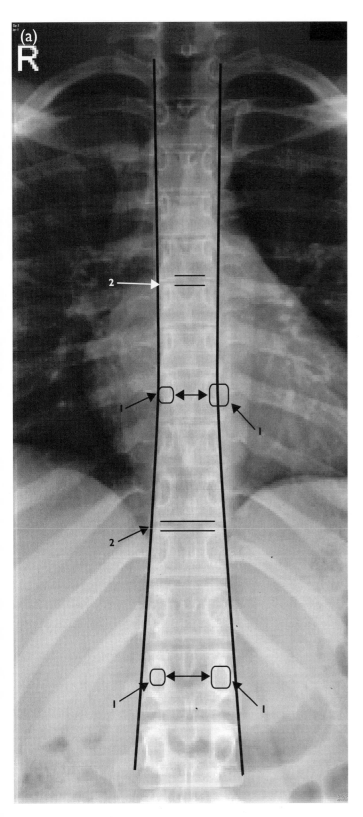

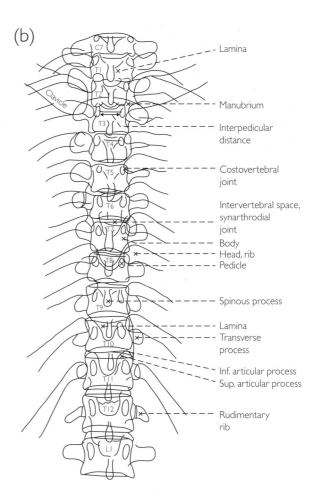

Fig. 7.5 (a) Radiograph of thoracic spine and (b) diagram. The pedicles are marked (1). The interpedicular distance widens on descent from T5 into the lumbar spine, reaching its narrowest level at T5. The endplates of the vertebra can be clearly seen (2).

- The joints of Lushka are articular joints on the superior and lateral surfaces of the lower five cervical vertebral bodies. These are synovial joints and therefore also affected by erosive arthropathies such as rheumatoid arthritis. Due to their strategic position on the posterolateral lip of the vertebral body, hypertrophy of the joints may lead to compression, i.e. narrowing, of the neural exit foramina and hence neural impingement, e.g. narrowing of C5–6 foramen will impinge on C6 exiting nerve root. The joints of Lushka are also known as the uncovertebral joints or neurocentral joints.
- The facet joints or the zygapophyseal joints are synovial and prone to erosion in synovitis. The superior facets face superoposteriorly and the inferior facets inferoanteriorly. The facets permit rotation, flexion, extension and lateral bending. The facet joints are oriented in the coronal plane in the cervical region on CT. They form an articular column in the cervical region.
- The spinous processes of C2–6 are small and bifid.
- The cervical spinal canal is small and triangular in shape.
- There are eight cervical nerves but only seven cervical vertebrae. The cervical nerves exit above the corresponding pedicle and body through the neural exit foramen at 45°. The neural foramina are oriented at 45° obliquely.

Thoracic spine

- The smallest vertebral body is T3 (Fig. 7.5).
- The thoracic vertebrae have facets for rib articulation on the lateral aspect of the body. The upper eight thoracic bodies articulate with two ribs, and the lower four with only one rib.
- The thoracic facet joints are oriented in the coronal plane and permit rotation in the thoracic region, as well as flexion and extension.
- A central defect may be present in the superior aspect of the vertebral body called Schmorl's node. This has no clinical significance, being the result of protrusion of disc material into the endplates and is not associated with collapse of the vertebra (Fig. 7.6).
- The interpedicular distance decreases on descent down the cervical spine to T5, and thereafter increases throughout the lower thoracic and lumbar spine. This is the distance between the inner aspects of the pedicles and represents the transverse diameter of the spinal canal. The pedicles may be eroded in malignancy; an absent pedicle may be the only evidence of bony metastases. Second, long-standing or slow-growing intradural abnormalities within the spinal canal may lead to slow erosion of the pedicles and widening of the interpedicular distance. Achondroplasia leads to congenital spinal stenosis and a decreased interpedicular distance.
- The paraspinal lines can be seen on an AP (anteroposterior) view of the thoracic spine or on a chest radiograph. These lines represent the soft tissue normally present at this level such as nodes, vessels, fat and lymphatics. Widening indicates pathology such as lymphadenopathy or paraspinal soft tissue infection or malignancy. The left paraspinal line is usually <10 mm and the right <2 mm. The left is usually wider due to presence of the aorta (Fig. 7.7).

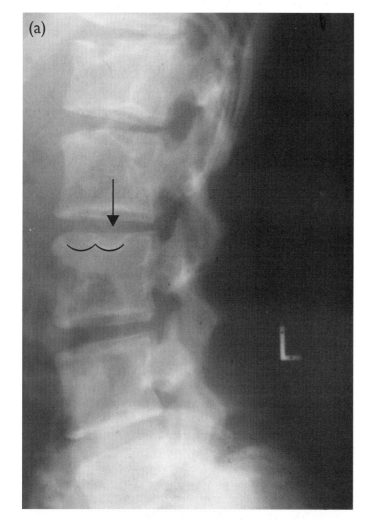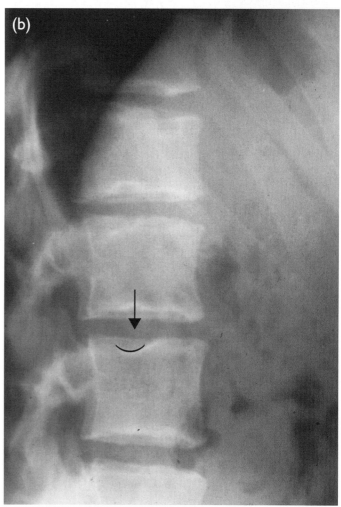

Fig. 7.6 Lateral thoracolumbar spine views: (a,b) central depressions in the endplates of the vertebral, called Schmorl's nodes (arrows), due to herniation of disc material into the body.

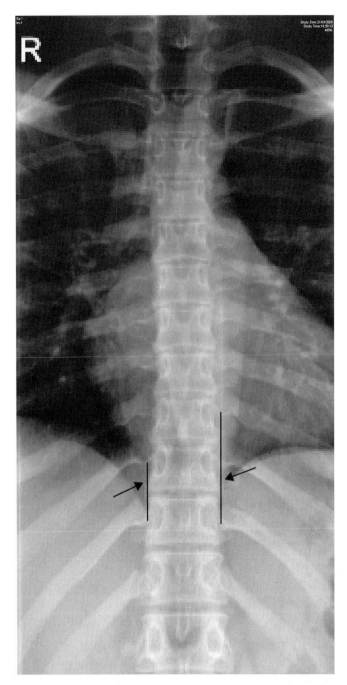

Fig. 7.7 AP view of the thoracic spine: the paraspinal lines can measure 2 mm on the right and 10 mm on the left (arrows). On the thoracic or chest radiograph, soft tissues in the paravertebral region can be visualized.

- In the vertebral body the basivertebral veins lie posteriorly, causing a central defect. A Y-shaped defect is visible in the vertebral body on axial CT due to nutrient vessels anteriorly plus the basivertebral vein posteriorly. This normal appearance must be differentiated from a vertebral fracture (Fig. 7.8).
- In a child anterior defects may be seen in the vertebral bodies of the whole spine called Hahn's fissures. These make the primitive vertebral body look like 'hamburgers' and are a normal finding to be differentiated from vertebral body abnormalities seen in mucopolysaccharidoses such as Morquio's, Hunter's, etc. (Fig. 7.9).

The lumbar vertebrae

- The lumbar vertebrae are kidney shaped. L1 and L2 are deeper posteriorly and L4 and L5 are deeper anteriorly. This contributes to lumbar lordosis.
- The intervertebral discs range in height. L5–S1 usually has the narrowest intervertebral disc so a decreased disc height at this level does not always indicate pathology.
- The pedicles are stubby processes that connect the body anteriorly to the arch posteriorly. The distance between the pedicles, the interpedicular distance, increases on descent through the lumbar sacral spine (Fig. 7.10).
- The facet joints are synovial and oriented sagittally; they interlock in the lumbar region. Flexion and extension movements and lateral bending are permitted in the lumbar region, but not rotation. The facets can be assessed with arthrography. The facet joints lie at the level of the discs in the lumbosacral region.
- The nerves exit underneath their corresponding pedicle, e.g. the L2 nerve roots exits under the L2 pedicle. An L2–3 posterior or posterolateral disc protrusion will most likely impinge on the L3 nerve root. This is because the second nerve root has already exited and passed underneath the pedicle just above the disc. A very lateral disc protrusion can affect the nerve root above if the protrusion extends far enough laterally (Fig. 7.11).
- The pars interarticularis is the part of the lamina between the superior and inferior articular processes. There may be a defect in the pars that can lead to slipping of the vertebra anteriorly or posteriorly, i.e. spondylolisthesis.
- There may be variations in segmentation of the vertebra of the spine leading to transitional vertebra. The sacral vertebrae may be 'lumbarized', i.e. S1 shows lumbar features and is not fused to the sacrum but separate, or the lumber vertebrae 'sacralized' when L5 fuses with the sacrum mimicking S1. This is important when naming the vertebral bodies or the discs for spinal surgery because it can lead to confusion about the relevant level for intervention. The variation in length and shape of the transverse processes is used to differentiate the vertebrae, i.e. L3 is longest (Fig. 7.12):
  - L3 has the longest transverse process.

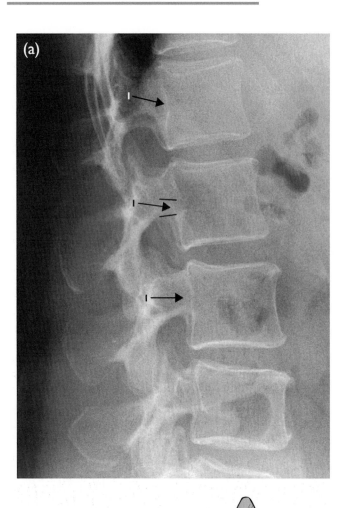

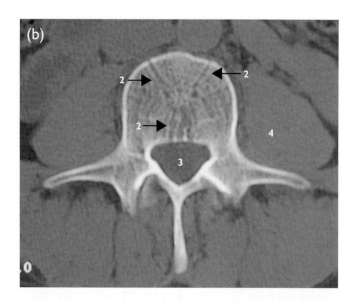

Fig. 7.8 Lateral lumbar spine radiograph (a) showing the slight defect posteriorly due to the basivertebral veins, marked with a black arrow (1). (b) Bony windows CT showing the classic 'Y' shape (2) in the vertebral body due to the basivertebral vein, not to be confused with a fracture. Theca (3) and psoas muscle (4). (c) Diagram of the venous and arterial circulation to the vertebra, accounting for the defects.

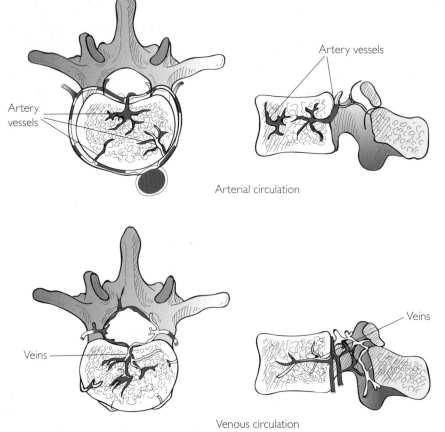

Artery vessels

Artery vessels

Arterial circulation

Veins

Veins

Venous circulation

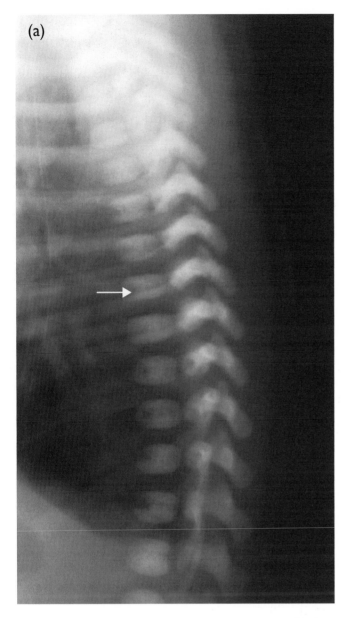

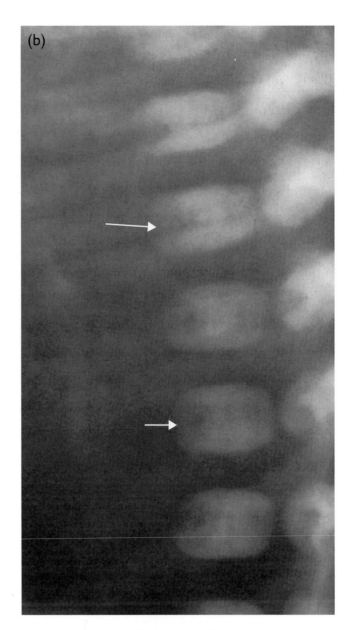

Fig. 7.9 Lateral thoracic spine infant (a) and zoomed view (b). In the infant spine anterior defects are present, called Hahn's fissures, which may persist into adult life (arrows).

– L4 has a transverse process pointing slightly upwards.
– the L5 transverse processes are shorter and pyramid shaped (Fig. 7.12b).
- The basivertebral vein is a nutrient channel found posteriorly in the vertebral body which causes a central posterior defect (Fig. 7.13).
- The lateral recess is the recess anterolaterally in the spinal canal in which the descending nerve root sits. The root may be impinged on by a disc bulge or facet joint disease at this site (Fig. 7.14).
- The spinous processes extend inferiorly in the lumbar region down to the level of the disc below.

The sacrum and sacroiliac joints

- The sacrum consists of five fused vertebrae with four foramina on each side. It is a triangle-shaped bone that is concave anteriorly. The lamina and spinous processes are fused to form a medial sacral crest. There is one large facet laterally on each side, called the auricular surface because it is shaped like an ear, which forms the sacroiliac joint with the ilium of the pelvis. The sacral foramina should not be confused with lytic bone lesions.
- The sacrum can be seen on an AP view of the lumbar spine. It may be absent congenitally or as a result of destruction, so, when reporting a radiograph of the spine

(a)

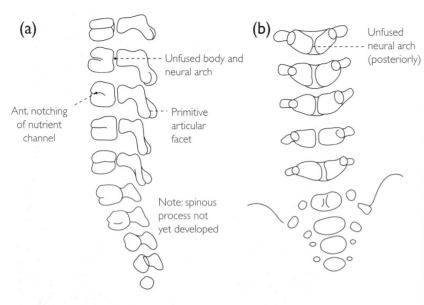

Unfused body and neural arch

Ant. notching of nutrient channel

Primitive articular facet

Note: spinous process not yet developed

(b)

Unfused neural arch (posteriorly)

(c)

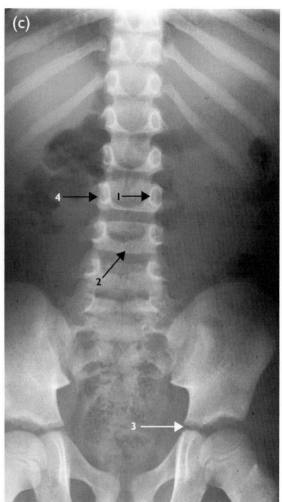

Fig. 7.10 (a,b) Diagram of the spinal column at birth in the lateral and AP projections, showing the primitive body and neural arch. (c) The AP lumbar spine radiograph shows the increase in the interpedicular distance (1) on descent and the unfused neural arches posteriorly marked, which is normal at this age (2). (3) The triradiate cartilage and (4) pedicle.

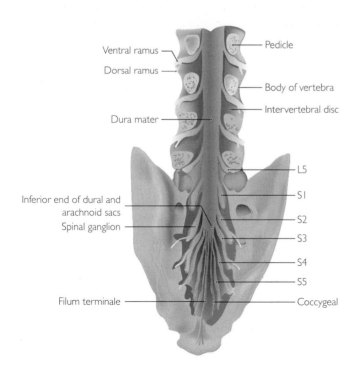

Ventral ramus

Dorsal ramus

Dura mater

Inferior end of dural and arachnoid sacs

Spinal ganglion

Filum terminale

Pedicle

Body of vertebra

Intervertebral disc

L5

S1

S2

S3

S4

S5

Coccygeal

Fig. 7.11 The diagram shows the pedicle and its relationship with the nerve root, which exits underneath the pedicle, but above the intervertebral disc below.

(a)

(b)

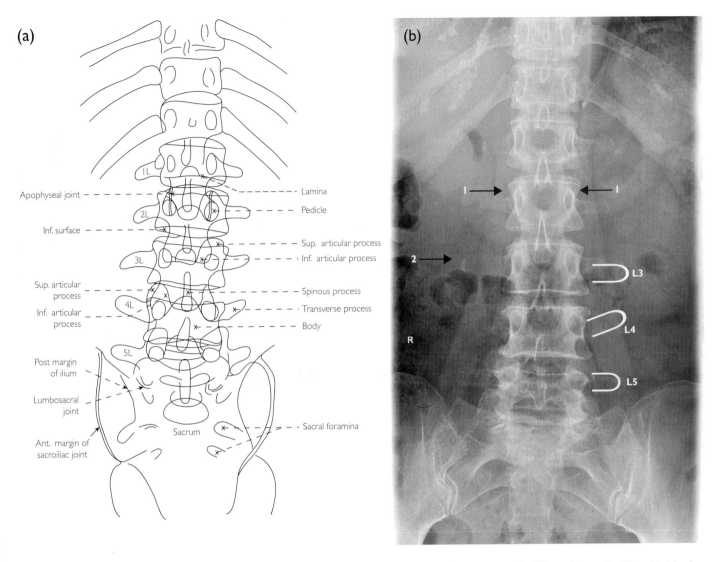

Apophyseal joint

Inf. surface

Sup. articular process

Inf. articular process

Post margin of ilium

Lumbosacral joint

Ant. margin of sacroiliac joint

Lamina

Pedicle

Sup. articular process

Inf. articular process

Spinous process

Transverse process

Body

Sacral foramina

1L

2L

3L

4L

5L

Sacrum

L3

L4

L5

R

Fig. 7.12 (a) Diagram of lumbar spine; (b) AP radiograph of spine and diagram showing the psoas muscle (1) on either side. The third lumbar vertebra has been marked (2). This has the longest transverse process. L4 transverse processes are short and point slightly upwards.

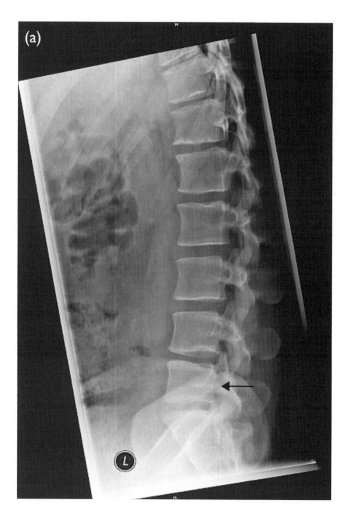

(a)

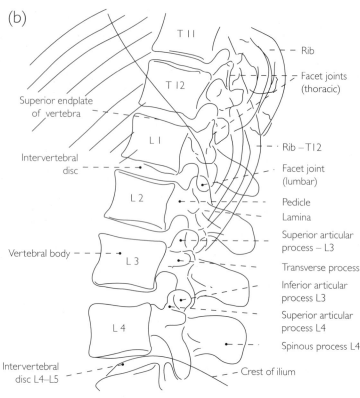

(b)

Fig. 7.13 (a) Lateral lumbar spine radiograph and (b) diagram showing the normal appearance and normal narrowing posteriorly of L5 (arrow).

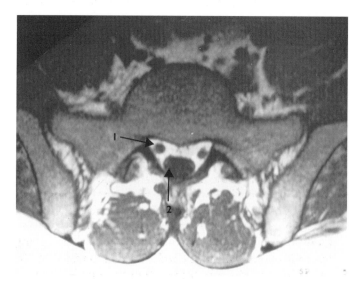

Fig. 7.14 Axial T1-weighted MRI shows the first right sacral nerve root (1) in the lateral recess. (2) The theca.

or an abdominal radiograph, checking that the sacrum is present is an important review area. Overlying bowel gas shadows may mimic lytic lesions in the sacrum.

- The inferior two-thirds of the sacroiliac (SI) joints are synovial, hence sacroiliitis occurs and is radiographically visualized in the inferior two-thirds. The upper third of the joint is not synovial, hence erosions will not be detected at this site (Fig. 7.15).
- The sacral promontory is the most superior and anterior part of the sacrum and contributes to the true conjugate diameter of the pelvis.
- The SI joints lie at 25° to the oblique. The left SI joint is visualized by obliquing to the opposite side, i.e. a left oblique is taken to visualize the right SI joint. This is the opposite direction to rotate the spine to image the facet joints (Fig. 7.16).

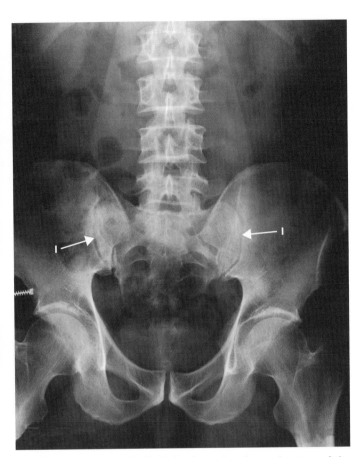

Fig. 7.15 AP radiograph of the lumbar spine shows the view of the sacroiliac joints (1). These lie at an angle.

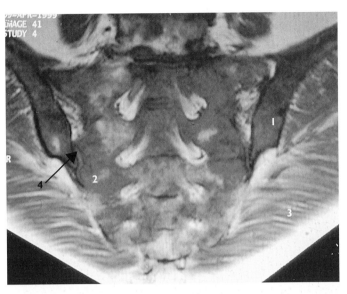

Fig. 7.17 MRI of the sacrum: angled views through the sacrum, T1-weighted images showing the sacral foramina and the sacroiliac (SI) joints. The inferior two-thirds of the SI joints are synovial. Iliac bone (1), sacrum (2) gluteal muscles (3) and SI joints (4).

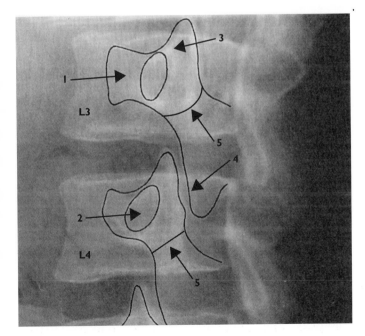

Fig. 7.16 Diagram oblique view of lumbar spine; the Scotty dog has been drawn on. The nose corresponds to the transverse process (1), the pedicle (2) is the eye, the ear is the superior facet (3) and the leg is the inferior facet (4); the collar for the Scotty dog is the pars (5).

- MRI is superior to plain film for assessing the SI joints. Angled coronal STIR and T1-weighted images are more sensitive in detecting early changes of sacroiliitis (Fig. 7.17).
- Sclerosis can happen on one side of the SI joint, called condensans ilii, which mimics sacroiliitis. This condition can be painful.
- The true conjugate diameter of the pelvis can be a limiting factor in a spontaneous vaginal delivery. This is the AP diameter from the sacral promontory to the superior and posterior aspect of the symphysis pubis (Fig. 7.18).

The spinal cord

The spinal cord extends from the medulla in the posterior fossa to the conus in the lumbar region (Fig. 7.19).

- The conus medullaris, or conus for short, is the terminal cord and should have a tapered appearance. In an adult the conus ends between T12 and the disc between L2 and L3 in 97.8%. The conus may extend to L3 in an infant, which is almost the length of the canal. However, by the age of 20 years the cord termination or conus apparently rises, and the lower limit possible in an adult for the inferior limit of the cord is the intervertebral disc between L2

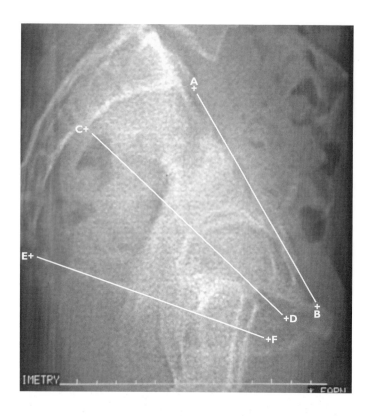

Fig. 7.18 CT pelvimetry: A–D, the true conjugate diameter which is from the sacral promontory to the back of the symphysis pubis; C–D, mid-pelvis; E–F, pelvic outlet.

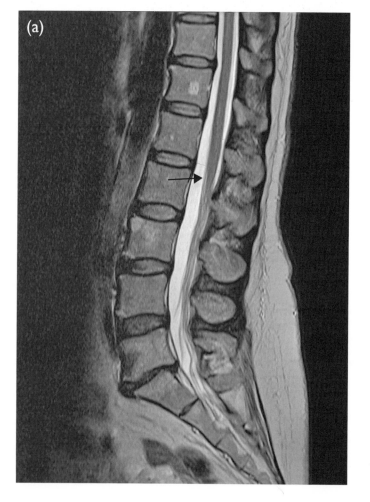

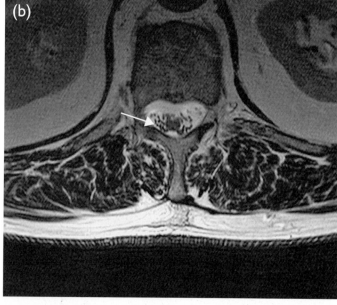

Fig. 7.19 (a) Sagittal T2 MRI showing the conus (arrow) which can extend down to the disc of L2–3. (b) Axial T2-weighted images through the conus, which has a 'crab' appearance (arrow). Sagittally the conus has a slightly triangular appearance.

and L3. If the conus extends to L3 in an adult, i.e. there is a low lying cord, this may imply pathology such as a tethered cord or diastematomyelia (Fig. 7.20).

- The filum terminale, a continuation of the pia and conus that looks like a glistening thread, continues inferiorly or caudad from the conus to attach to the first coccygeal segment C1 (Fig. 7.21).
- Within the spinal canal below the conus lie the cauda equina, the descending lumbosacral and coccygeal nerve roots and the filum.

- The subarachnoid space continues inferiorly to S1–2, S2 or even lower. The filum continues below the subarachnoid space.
- The spinal cord, in axial imaging or in cross-section, is an elliptical shape with a notch anteriorly. The notch is called the anterior median sulcus and the anterior spinal artery runs in it (Fig. 7.21b).
- Within the spinal cord centrally is the central canal which transmits cerebrospinal fluid (CSF) and communicates with the fourth ventricle.

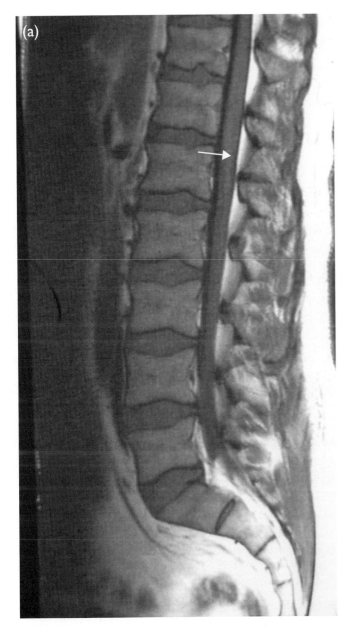
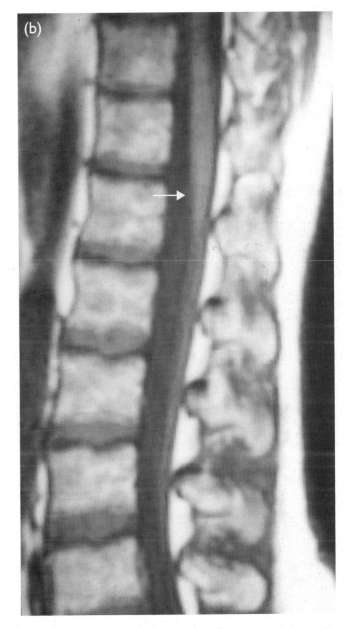

Fig. 7.20 (a,b) Two examples of T1-weighted images sagittal showing the conus (arrows). Abnormalities within the conus are appreciated on T2-weighted imaging.

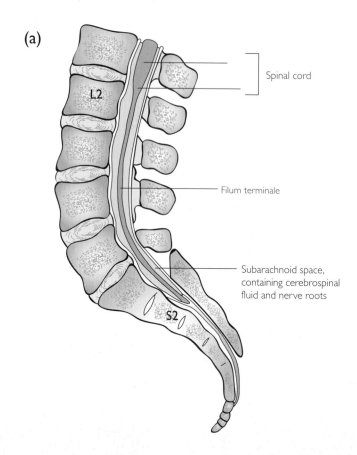

(a)

Spinal cord

Filum terminale

Subarachnoid space, containing cerebrospinal fluid and nerve roots

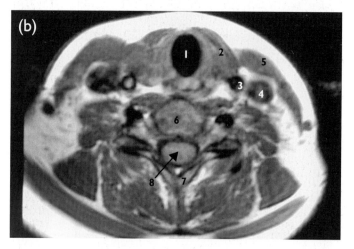

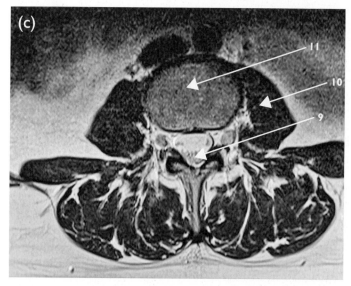

Fig. 7.21 (a) Diagram of the conus and filum showing the continuation of the filum inferiorly from the conus to the S2 level. (b) Axial T1-weighted image through the cervical spine showing the spinal cord surrounded by CSF. Detail of the spinal cord is visible only on T2-weighted imaging. Subglottic region (1), thyroid gland (2), common carotid artery (3), internal jugular vein (4), sternomastoid muscle (5), vertebral body (6), lamina (7) and spinal cord (8). (c) The second image is an axial T2-weighted MRI in the lumbosacral region showing the nerve roots in the cauda equina (9). These should not be clumped. T2 shows the nerve roots in an axial T2-weighted image in the lumbosacral region. Psoas (10) and vertebral body (11).

- Around the central canal within the cord there is an H-shaped area of grey matter. This can be resolved on MRI in the axial plane on T2-weighted imaging and gradient echo imaging at high field strength.
- Two posterior arteries and one anterior artery supply the cord. These arise from the vertebral arteries or their branch, the posterior inferior cerebellar artery (PICA), in the neck. They receive further branches from the intercostals and lumbar arteries as they descend. The largest of these branches and the best known arises at T8–12, called the artery of Adamkiewicz, which is the predominant supply to the thoracolumbar cord. It arises on the left in 75% and makes a characteristic hairpin bend in its course. The upper thoracic cord is poorly supplied with a watershed area at T4.
- The cerebellar tonsils can normally extend through the foramen magnum by 3–6 mm but not more (Fig. 7.22).

Ligaments in the spine

The following ligaments stabilize the spine:
- Anterior longitudinal ligament runs anterior to the bodies, important for post-traumatic stability (Fig. 7.23).
- Posterior longitudinal ligament: posterior to bodies. Demarcates the anterior spinal canal and provides a barrier between the canal and the discs.
- Ligamentum flavum: important in degenerative change when it can thicken and contribute to stenosis. This shows intermediate signal intensity compared with all other ligaments and lies posteriorly within the canal anterior to the lamina.
- Interspinous ligament: not seen on cross-sectional imaging.

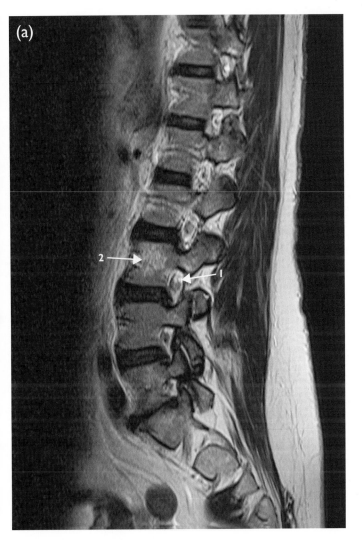

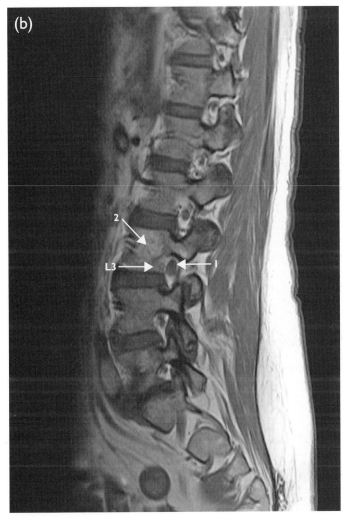

Fig. 7.22 (a) Parasagittal T2-weighted images showing the third lumbar nerve root (1) L3 exiting below the L3 pedicle, which is above the disc L3–4 below. Usually an L3–4 disc does not impinge on the L3 nerve unless the protruded disc extends superiorly. (b–d) Parasagittal T1- and T2-weighted MRI showing a well-circumscribed high signal lesion in the body of L3 consistent with a haemangioma (2).

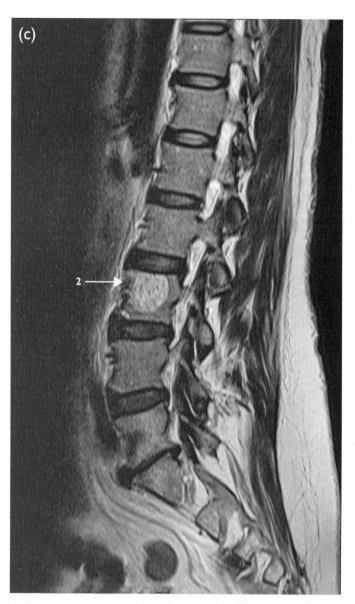

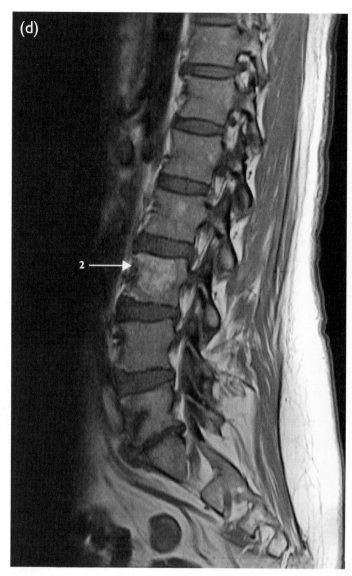

Fig. 7.22 (c) and (d)

The spine at birth

- The primitive body or centrum is present at birth, with two neural arches making three primary ossification centres (Fig. 7.23b).
- The neural arches fuse together posteriorly from 1 year to 2 years starting in the lumbar vertebrae. Fusion then ascends to the cervical region, with the sacrum fusing last at approximately 7 years. This is important for assessing for spina bifida as the lamina will not fuse normally until at least age 7 in the sacral region.
- The posterior arches fuse with the centrum at 3 years in the cervical region and is complete in the lumbar region at 6 years (Fig. 7.23c).
- There are five secondary ossification centres that appear at puberty: two transverse processes, one spinous process, and the superior and inferior epiphyseal end-plates. These remain unfused into adult life and can cause confusion with fractures. Fusion usually occurs at age 25 years (Fig. 7.23d,e).
- The lower vertebrae may be absent in caudal regression syndrome or sacral agenesis, so in infants it is important to check that all the vertebrae and sacrum are present.
- Scoliosis in children may be due to hemivertebra or butterfly vertebra, which is a congenitally abnormal body. A hemivertebra, or 'half' vertebra, is more likely to cause a scoliosis than a butterfly vertebra, which is balance of two halves with a midline cleft. When present consider other anomalies as part of the VATER (**v**ertebral, **a**norectal, **t**riacheal, o**e**sophageal, **r**adial/**r**enal) anomaly (Fig. 7.23f).

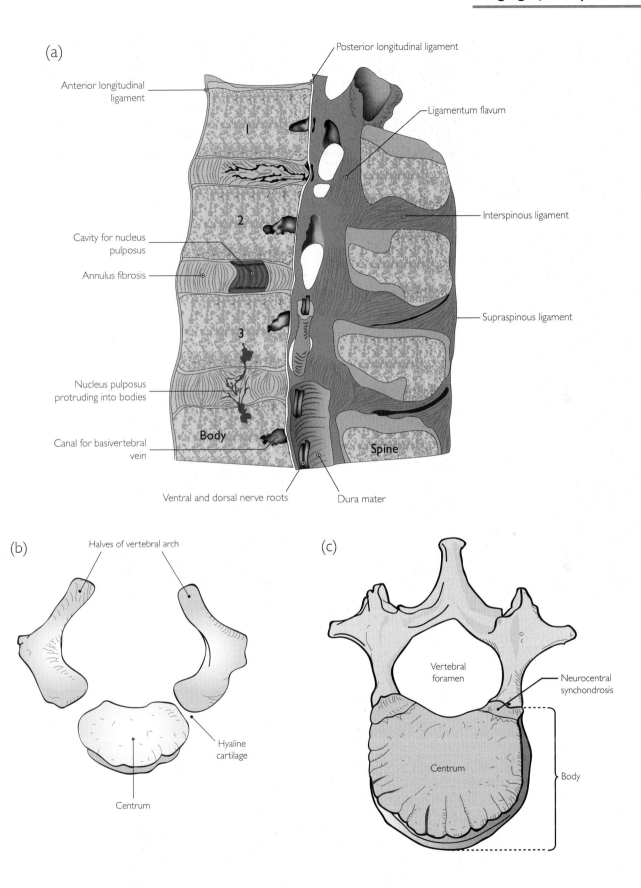

(a)

Anterior longitudinal ligament

Posterior longitudinal ligament

Ligamentum flavum

Interspinous ligament

Supraspinous ligament

Cavity for nucleus pulposus

Annulus fibrosis

1

2

3

Nucleus pulposus protruding into bodies

Canal for basivertebral vein

Body

Spine

Ventral and dorsal nerve roots

Dura mater

(b) Halves of vertebral arch

Hyaline cartilage

Centrum

(c) Vertebral foramen

Neurocentral synchondrosis

Centrum

Body

Fig. 7.23 (a) Diagram showing the normal supporting ligaments of the spine. The ligamentum flavum can encroach on the theca if hypertrophied. (b) Diagram of the primitive body and neural arches at birth. (c) Diagram showing how, at age 6 years, fusion has commenced forming the pedicle.

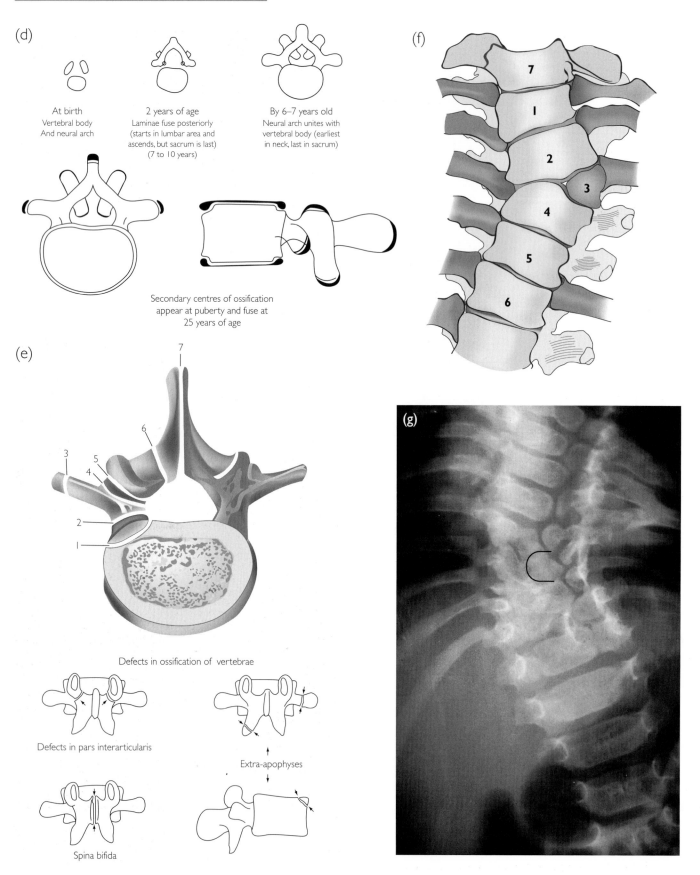

(d)

At birth
Vertebral body
And neural arch

2 years of age
Laminae fuse posteriorly
(starts in lumbar area and
ascends, but sacrum is last)
(7 to 10 years)

By 6–7 years old
Neural arch unites with
vertebral body (earliest
in neck, last in sacrum)

Secondary centres of ossification
appear at puberty and fuse at
25 years of age

(e)

Defects in ossification of vertebrae

Defects in pars interarticularis

Extra-apophyses

Spina bifida

(f)

(g)

Fig. 7.23 (d) Diagram showing the secondary apophyses that appear at puberty. Two endplates, a spinous process, the transverse processes and the ends of the facets appear at puberty and fuse by age 25. (e) Diagram showing how failure of an apophysis to unite can mimic abnormalities such as fracture. Possible sites for a failure of apophysis to unite: (1, 2) pedicle, (3) transverse process, (4, 5, 6) lamina, (7) spinous process. (f) Diagram of hemivertebra. (g) Radiograph of a hemivertebra. A hemivertebra can be lead to a scoliosis.

- The neonatal spine has just a primary curve. Two secondary curves develop in the cervical and lumbar regions as the upright position is adopted.
- Hahn's fissures are midline anterior defects seen normally in the primitive vertebral body on a lateral view.

IMAGING

Imaging modalities

- Plain films are usually the first-line investigation in spinal trauma and degenerative change.
- CT is the mode of choice for the further assessment of spinal trauma, including cortical bone, bony alignment and comminuted fractures.
- MRI is best for assessing spinal cord pathology and bone marrow abnormalities.
- Myelography has been completely superseded by MRI. If MRI is contraindicated a CT myelogram may be performed

Plain film: cervical spine

There are three standard neck views in trauma in the cervical spine. The peg view is usually omitted in cervical spondylytic change.

Lateral c-spine
- 70% of injuries are seen on the lateral, which must include the top of the first thoracic (the T1 vertebra).
- AP c-spine must include as far down as possible, usually assessing C3–7.
- Odontoid peg view for C1–2: the peg view is taken through an open mouth and autotomography may aid peg visualization.

C-spine view 1: lateral cervical spine

Plain films are performed after trauma. If the patient cannot be mobilized and is wearing a neck collar the horizontal beam lateral may be used (Fig. 7.24).

C7–T1 must be adequately visualized. Formerly a swimmer's view and now CT are performed as supplementary tests to see C7–T1. CT is performed in trauma if there is difficulty obtaining adequate views of any level.

The most common site of injury is C1–2, C5–7. On a lateral cervical spine view assess the following.

Alignment

The integrity of these lines must be present on all lateral views and their loss aids detection of injury. There may be ligamentous injury in the absence of a visible fracture (Fig. 7.25a and b).

- Spinolaminar line: a line demarcating the junction of the lamina and spinous processes.

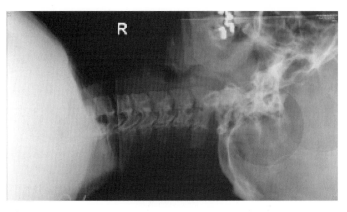

Fig. 7.24 Radiograph, horizontal beam lateral view, taken in the trauma setting. The normal lines should be reviewed.

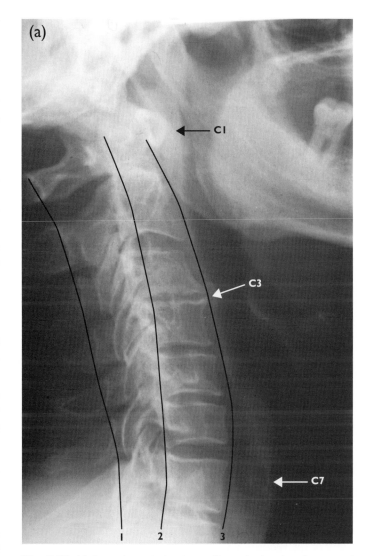

Fig. 7.25 (a) Lateral cervical spine radiograph showing the normal prevertebral soft tissues: C1 (3 mm), C3 (7 mm) and C7 (21 mm). Spinolaminar line (1), posterior vertebral line (2) and anterior vertebral line (3).

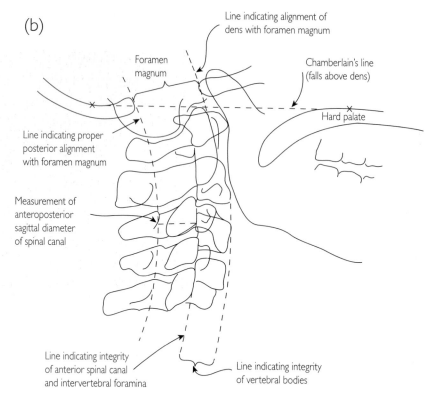

(b)

Line indicating alignment of dens with foramen magnum

Foramen magnum

Chamberlain's line (falls above dens)

Hard palate

Line indicating proper posterior alignment with foramen magnum

Measurement of anteroposterior sagittal diameter of spinal canal

Line indicating integrity of anterior spinal canal and intervertebral foramina

Line indicating integrity of vertebral bodies

Fig. 7.25 (b) Diagram of the lines indicating integrity of the vertebral bodies: anterior vertebral line, posterior vertebral line, spinolaminar line and the pillar line.

- Anterior vertebral line: a line along the anterior vertebral bodies.
- Column line: assesses the facets for unilateral or bilateral facet dislocation.
- Posterior vertebral line: a line drawn along the posterior limit of the vertebral bodies.

The soft tissues

Soft-tissue swelling suggests a prevertebral haematoma in trauma cases or infection(s) or mass in non-trauma cases. It points to the site to assess carefully for a fracture/dislocation or pathology.

The following measurements can be used to assess the prevertebral soft tissues giving a maximum thickness for normality:
- C1: 3 mm
- C3: 7 mm
- C7: 21 mm.

Alternatively at C4 the soft-tissue thickness can measure half the diameter of the C4 vertebral body, and at C7 the soft tissues can measure up to the diameter on the lateral view of the whole C7 vertebral body.

The atlantoaxial distance

This is the distance between the anterior limit of the C2 vertebral body and the posterior limit of the anterior ring of C1 on a lateral view. It should be less than 3 mm in an adult and 5 mm in a child. Flexion and extension views in the lateral position are used to check for integrity of C1–2 articulation (Fig. 7.26).

Vertebral body height

A compression fracture of a vertebra may only be visible as some anterior wedging of the body. Note that the C5–6 vertebral bodies may normally be slightly narrower anteriorly than other the bodies.

AP canal diameter

The AP spinal canal diameter is the distance on a lateral view between the posterior limit of the body and the spinolaminar line; 13 mm is the minimum in the cervical region. The neural canal is disproportionately larger in infants.

The disc spaces

The intervertebral disc spaces should be uniform in the cervical region and all the endplates present. Infection such as discitis may decrease the disc space and destroy the endplates.

Chamberlain's and Macgregor's lines

Chamberlain's and McGregor's lines are lines drawn on a lateral view to assess for basilar invagination or softening

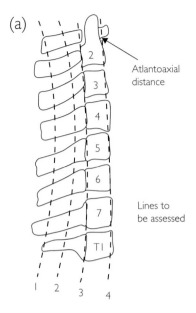 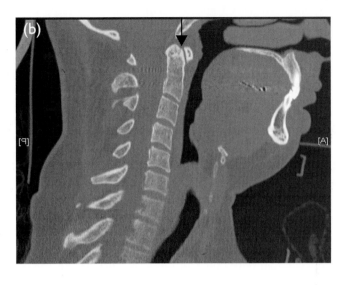

Fig. 7.26 (a) Diagram and (b) sagittal reconstructive image of the atlantoaxial distance (arrow). In an adult this should be 2 mm.

of skull base, which occurs in conditions such as Paget's disease and osteomalacia. Chamberlain's line is drawn from the posterior limit of the hard palate to the inner table of the skull vault and <2 mm of the tip of the odontoid peg should lie above the line. Macgregor's line runs from the hard palate to the outer table of the occiput and <5 mm of the peg should lie above this line (Fig. 7.27).

Rules and variants in the lateral neck
- In a child pseudo-subluxation can occur at C2–3; this is the point of maximum movement and is seen if the lateral view is taken in flexion. It can be confused with pathological subluxation.
- The interspinous distance, i.e. the distance between the spinous processes, is greatest in a normal individual at C2–3.

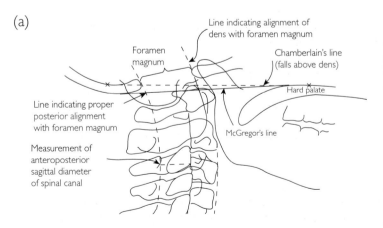 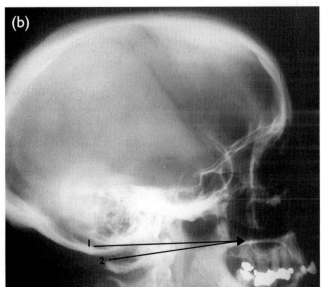

Fig. 7.27 (a) Diagram and (b) radiograph showing the position of Chamberlain's and McGregor's lines. Chamberlain's line (1) lies above McGregor's (2) line. The line is taken from the hard palate to the inner and outer table of the skull.

- C1 may be incorporated into the skull base due to segmentation anomalies. Other anomalies such as articulations between C1 and the skull base may occur, or even the absence of the anterior or posterior arch of C1. These variants must be differentiated from pathology and it is always worthwhile looking up in the *Atlas of Normal Roentgen Variants that may Simulate Disease* by Keat T. and Anderson M. (London: Mosby, 2006).
- Rotated, flexed or extended lateral spine views may give false signs of trauma so assess if a true lateral has been taken.
- Failure of segmentation can occur where bodies are fused. The fused vertebra is narrower in the AP diameter if congenitally fused (Fig. 7.28).

Supplementary views

Swimmer's
This is taken with one arm raised by the ear and the other arm down. The beam is centred though the axilla. It has now been largely superseded by CT in trauma settings (Fig. 7.29).

The oblique cervical spine
Taken with the patient erect and at oblique 45° to the midline. To see the left neural exit foramina the patient looks to the right side. If the chin is pointing to the right then the left foramina are visualized. Narrowing of the left C5–6 foramen will impinge on the left C6 nerve (Fig. 7.30).

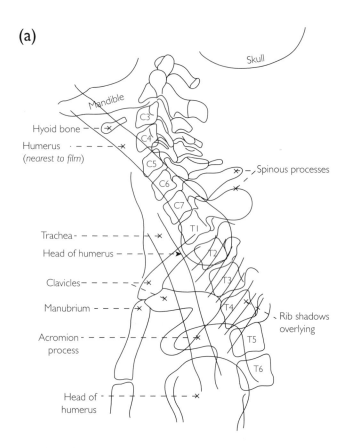

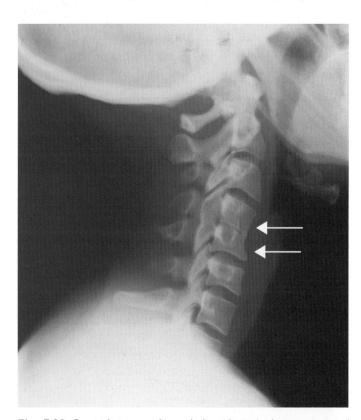

Fig. 7.28 Cervical spine radiograph lateral view: shows congenital fusion of C4 and C5, which are narrower in the AP diameter (arrows).

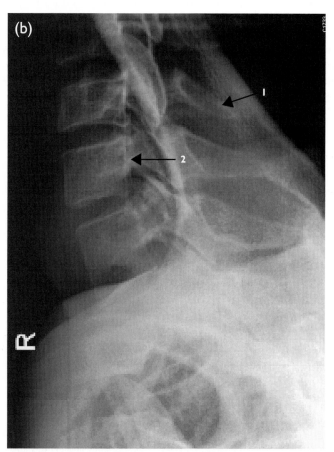

Fig. 7.29 (a) Diagram and (b) swimmer's views. This last view can still be performed but CT has mainly replaced it. Humerus (1) and facets (2).

(a)

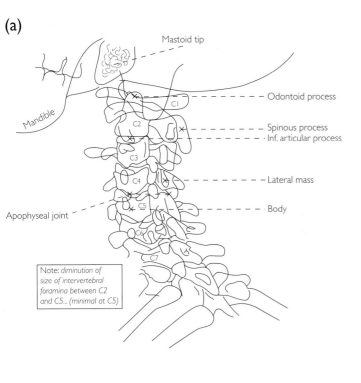

(b)

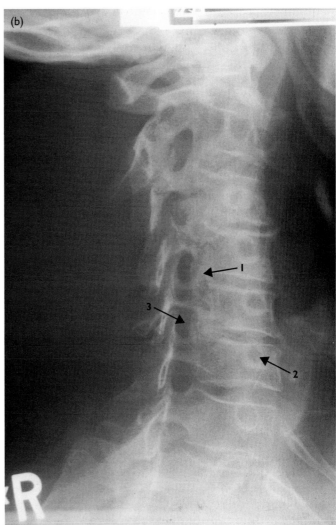

Fig. 7.30 Oblique cervical spine: (a) diagram and (b) radiograph showing the neural exit foramina. There are eight cervical nerve roots and the nerves exit above their corresponding pedicle. Joint of Lushka (1), transverse process (2) and neural exit foramen (3). The patient is looking to the left so this is a right foramen.

Flexion and extension views

These are still performed with medical supervision to look for ligamentous damage. Even if an MRI is normal, if there is strong suspicion of ligamentous trauma then these views are performed.

C-spine view 2: AP view for cervical spine

- Taken using an angled beam.
- The lamina of the thyroid cartilage can be seen projected over the cervical bodies. This can be wrongly interpreted as calcification of the vertebral arteries (Fig. 7.31).
- The spinous processes must be aligned in the midline and have even interspacing. Loss of this may point to a unilateral facet joint dislocation. The distance between the spines should not be less than 50% of adjacent interspinous distance (Fig. 7.32a,b).
- This view does not visualize C1–2.
- The joints of Lushka can be seen on the posterolateral corner of the vertebral body on an AP view.
- The interpedicular distance is the distance between the inner aspects of the pedicles; it reflects the spinal canal

dimensions and the width of the spinal cord. This is greatest at C5–6 due to the brachial plexus expansion.
- The transverse processes point upwards for thoracic vertebrae and downwards for cervical vertebrae. This can be useful when the assessing for cervical ribs. If a 'rib' articulates with a body with a downward-facing transverse process, then it is a cervical rib (Fig. 7.33).

Odontoid peg view

- This is taken through an open mouth (Fig. 7.34).
- The Mach effect may be seen where the shadow of the tongue or the inferior cortical margin of the posterior arch of C1 or the occiput crosses the dens on an AP view and may simulate a fracture. A gap in between the front teeth can be seen projected over the peg, again simulating a fracture.
- Peg should lie midway between lateral masses of C1.
- Lateral masses should align with body of C2.
- Autotomography may be used – opening and closing of the mouth to blur the lips.
- An os odontoideum may simulate a fracture.

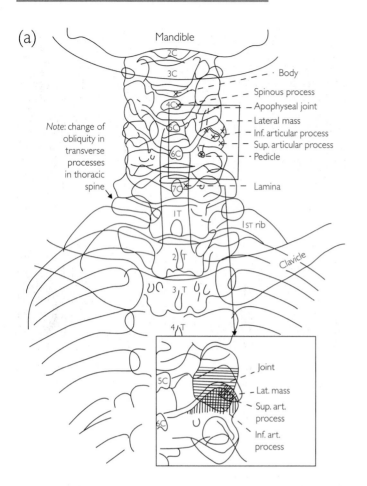

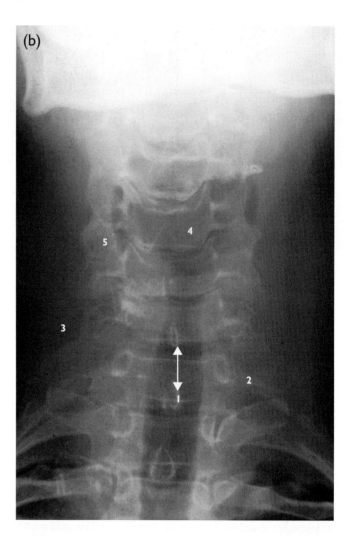

Fig. 7.31 (a) Diagram and (b) AP radiograph of the cervical spine. The interspinous distance (1) should be roughly equal throughout the cervical spine and alignment of pedicles is important to assess. Left transverse process T1 (2), right transverse process C7 (3), joint of Lushka (4) and facet joints (5).

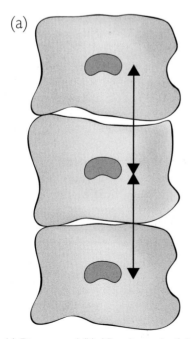

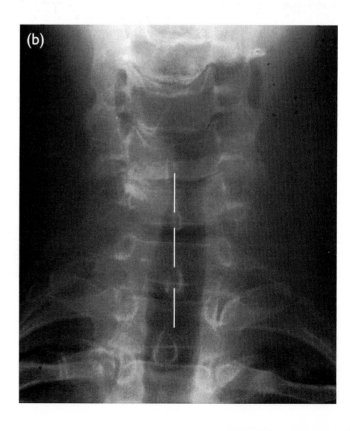

Fig. 7.32 (a) Diagram and (b) AP radiograph of the spine showing the interspinous distance on an AP cervical spine (lines).

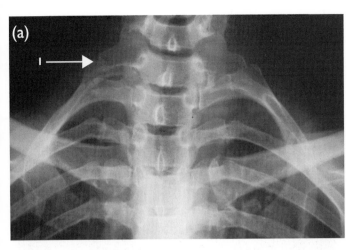

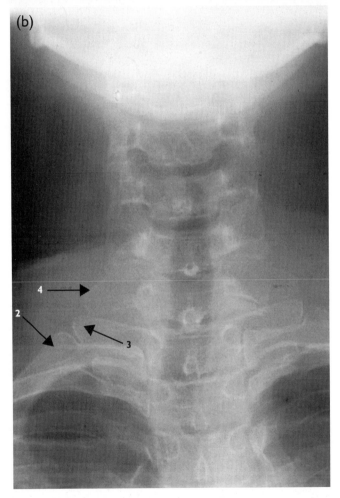

Fig. 7.33 Radiograph of cervical rib: (a) a cervical rib (1) arising from a downward pointing transverse process. (b) The normal thoracic rib (2) articulating with an upward pointing transverse process (3). The downward pointing cervical transverse process above has no rib (4).

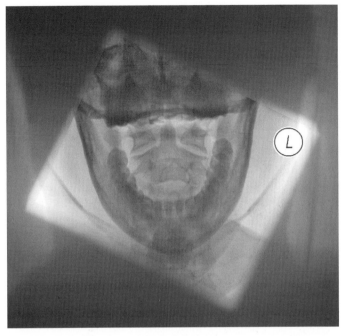

Fig. 7.34 Radiograph of C12 taken AP open mouth. The odontoid peg should lie midline between the lateral masses. The lateral masses should be aligned with the lateral aspect of the body of C2.

Soft-tissue neck lateral

This is done to assess for prevertebral soft-tissue swelling or for foreign body ingestion, i.e. swallowed fish bone (Fig. 7.35a).

- Lower kilovoltage to 55 kV is used for this.
- The epiglottis is yellow cartilage so this does not calcify. There should be no calcified structures at the tongue base, a common site for fish bones in the valleculae.
- All the other cartilages in the neck are hyaline cartilage and therefore these undergo calcification.
- The hyoid bone is U shaped and lies at C3. There should be no calcification above the hyoid at C3 as structures above do not calcify. If there is calcification behind the tongue base suspect a foreign body.
- The triticea cartilago is a small calcified structure representing a calcified thyrohyoid ligament. It lies just above the tip of the superior aspect of the lamina of the thyroid cartilage.
- The thyroid cartilage is V shaped and the notch lies at C4.
- The cricoid cartilage lies at C6 and is a reverse signet ring.

The normal calcified structures in the neck must be identified on a soft-tissue lateral neck radiograph so that foreign bodies can be identified.

Paediatric soft tissue

Lymphoid tissue in children widens the prevertebral soft tissues to C4 5 mm, C6 12 mm.

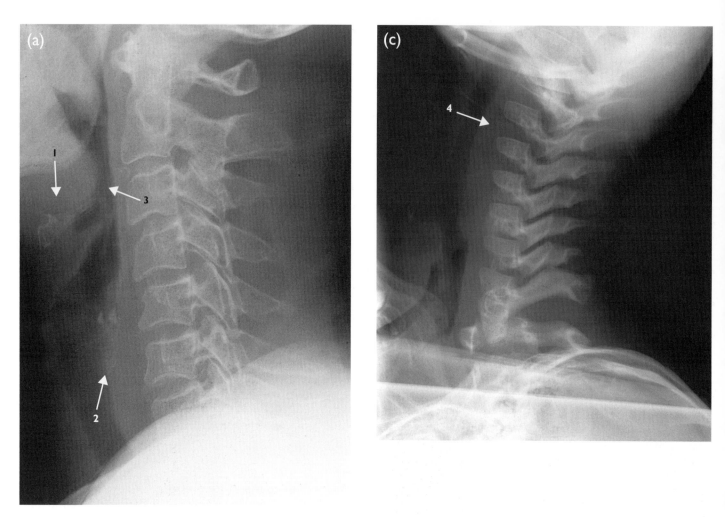

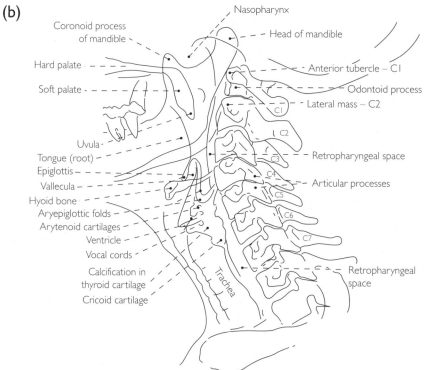

Fig. 7.35 (a) A soft tissue lateral view shows the hyoid bone (1), the thyroid and cricoid cartilage (2) and the soft tissue of the epiglottis (3). (b) Diagram of a lateral c-spine. (c) Paediatric soft tissues (4) are wider than in an adult due to adenoidal tissue.

The adenoids widen the soft tissues in the naso- and oropharynx and may cause a large soft-tissue shadow. In children the retropharyngeal soft tissues may be prominent in expiration and simulate an abscess (Fig. 7.35c).

Plain film: thoracic spine

The standard thoracic spine views are the AP and the lateral views:

- AP view: the pedicles and endplates should be assessed on every spine as should the paraspinal soft tissues (Fig. 7.36).
- Lateral view: the vertebral body height can be assessed. Note that the intervertebral discs are generally flat in this region. This view has a significant radiation dose.
- There is physiological wedging of the lower thoracic spine and the pedicles are thinner at this site.
- The anterior defects caused by venous sinuses, Hahn's fissures, may persist into adult life.
- The young infant spine may have a 'bone within a bone' appearance normally.

- A scoliosis of the thoracic spine may simulate pedicular erosion.
- There is a widening of the interpedicular distance from T9 downwards due to the lumbar expansion.
- There are far fewer rules and lines to review in the thoracic spine compared with the cervical spine as injury is less common.

Plain film: lumbosacral spine

The standard views are:

- AP: to assess paraspinal soft tissues, endplates and pedicles. On standard review transitional vertebrae should be identified. Unilateral 'lumbarization' or 'sacralization' may be symptomatic.
- Lateral: may need dedicated view to see L5–S1.
- Coned lateral of L5–S1: performed for better visualization of L5–S1 (Fig. 7.37).
- Supplementary views: the oblique view is taken to assess for either SI joints or pars interarticularis defect (Fig. 7.38).

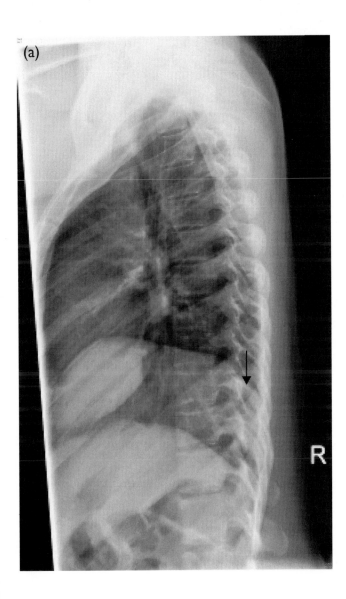

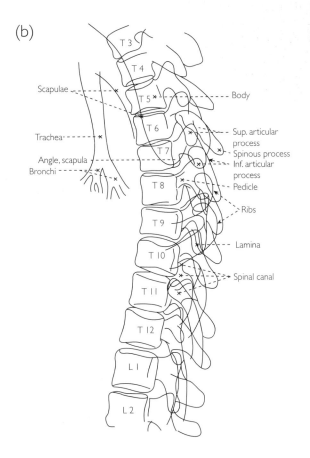

Fig. 7.36 Thoracic spine radiograph: (a) there should normally be an increase in transradiancy down the thoracic spine, i.e. the radiograph should become blacker as the eye descends inferiorly over the spine (arrow). (b) Diagram of the thoracic spine.

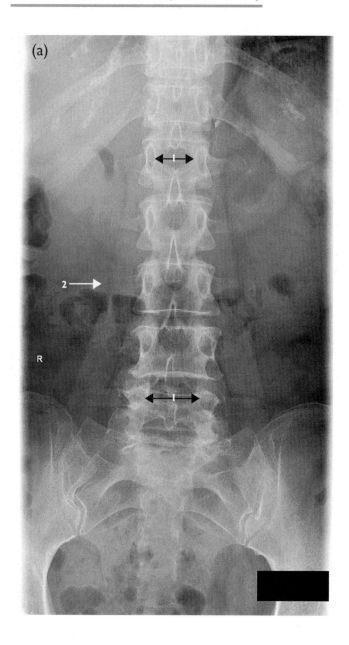

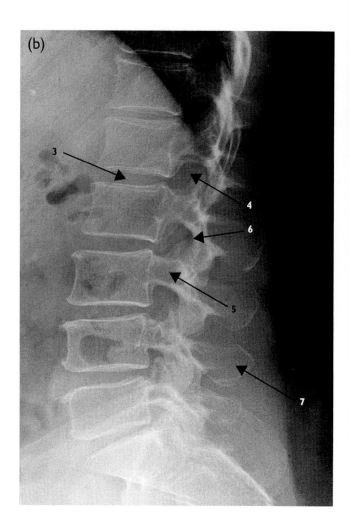

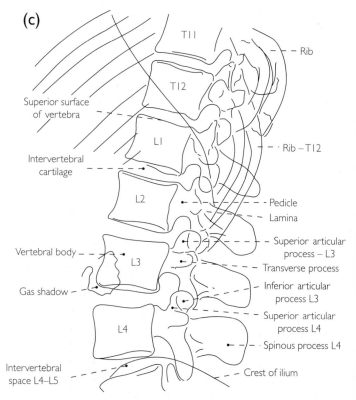

Fig. 7.37 (a) A lumbar spine radiograph showing the normal widening of the interpedicular distance (1) with descent and the psoas shadow (2). (b,c) Lateral lumbar spine radiograph and diagram. Disc (3), superior facet (4), pedicle (5), inferior facet (6) and spinous process (7).

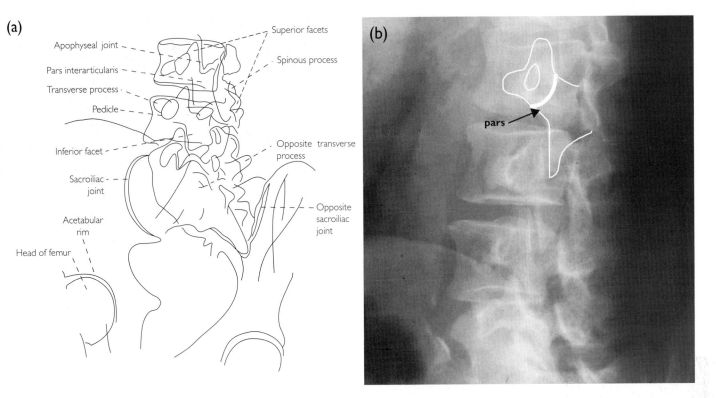

Fig. 7.38 (a) Diagram of the Scotty dog for the oblique lumbar spine radiograph. (b) Oblique view of lumbar spine; the Scotty dog has been drawn on.

To help diagnose and locate pars defects the 'Scotty dog' diagram can be used. The bony structures on an oblique view of the lumbosacral spine simulate a 'Scotty dog'. Identifying this is helpful as the 'neck' of the 'dog' is the site at which a pars interarticularis defect is found, representing the dog's collar.

To visualize the Scotty dog:
- Eye = pedicle
- Nose = transverse process
- Ear = superior facet joint
- Front leg = inferior facet joint.

A pars defect will occur across the neck of the Scotty dog, i.e. where the collar would lie, the pars interarticularis is the neck.

Views of the coccyx
These are not performed even in cases of trauma due to extreme variation in the normal coccyx in segmentation and angulation.

Interpretation of plain spinal radiographs
- Alignment: any slips, check the three lines on the lateral.
- Bones are the vertebrae of normal height, all the pedicles and endplates intact.
- Discs: even disc spaces.
- Soft-tissue swelling in the paravertebral region.

CT of the spine

Indications
- CT is the diagnostic method of choice in spinal skeletal trauma for assessing severity of injury. CT can assess for instability and bony fragments in the spinal canal, enabling surgical planning. It is more sensitive and accurate than plain films.
- Multiplanar reformatting with CT in coronal and sagittal planes with curved angled reformatting in oblique position has revolutionized spinal trauma assessment. In difficult cases when patients cannot lie straight or suspected spinal trauma prohibits movement of the patient, curved reformatting with CT can create the coronal and sagittal plane.

Technique
- A scout or scanogram shows the angulation and level imaged.
- The standard settings are soft tissue 40/350 and bony windows 350/2000. A high-resolution bone algorithm is applied (Fig. 7.39).
- There is a significant radiation dose of 5 mSv.

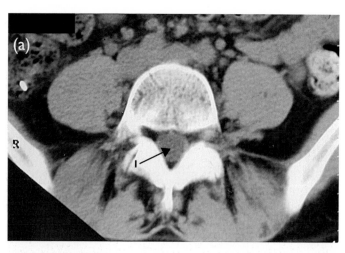
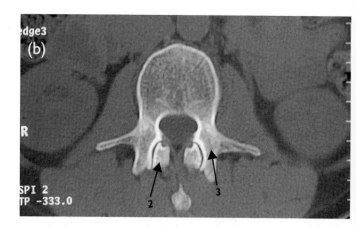

Fig. 7.39 CT of the vertebra: (a) soft-tissue window; (b) bony window. (a) Greater detail in the soft tissues and fat in the retroperitoneum. The theca can be identified. (b) Less detail in the surrounding soft tissues, but greater detail on the bony window in the vertebrae themselves. (1) Theca, (3) superior facet from vertebra below and (2) inferior facet from vertebra above.

Findings and variants

The bones
- Nutrient channels supplying the vertebrae such as the basivertebral vein and unfused apophyses can be mistaken for fractures. The basivertebral veins make a typical 'Y' shape in the body. The rich venous connection is the source of haematogenous metastases to the spine (Fig. 7.40).
- The anatomical level scanned can be established approximately by looking at the surrounding soft tissues, e.g. in the retroperitoneum, the psoas muscles, division of the aorta at L4 and formation of the inferior vena cava (IVC) at L5 or the renal veins at L2 enable the level to be established.
- Transitional vertebrae are difficult to interpret on CT or MRI and plain film correlation is recommended in the presurgical context when reporting, to give the level of abnormality accurately.

Soft tissues
- The spinal cord terminates between L1 and the disc of L2–3 in normal individuals. It is therefore inappropriate to call the canal appearances 'the spinal cord' at the L5–S1 level. It is best to call it the theca.
- The spinal canal dimensions can be narrow due to congenital narrowing, encroachment by disc disease, facet joint hypertrophy or ligamentous thickening. The ligamentum flavum is one of the strengthening ligaments in the spine that covers the lamina posteriorly in the canal. This can thicken in degenerative change and lead to canal stenosis.
- The intervertebral disc can be recognized by its soft-tissue density of 70 ± 30 HU. The disc is made up of a soft watery central portion, the nucleus pulposus, and the fibrous outer portion, the annulus fibrosus. The anterior and posterior longitudinal ligaments attach to the annulus. On axial CT the discs are bean shaped with a concave posterior border. L4–5 may have a flattened posterior border and there may even be a slight convexity to the disc of L5–S1.
- MRI is superior to CT in the evaluation of disc and nerve root pathology (Fig. 7.41).
- The nerve roots exit caudad, i.e. below the corresponding body and pedicle.

Spinal canal dimensions
Narrowing of the spinal canal dimensions can lead to impingement of the cord or the nerves as they exit the cord or pass through the lateral recess. The cause of stenosis, the number of levels affected and whether it is the whole spinal canal at a level, the neural exit foramina or the lateral recesses that are affected should be included in a report because the management differs according to the site and cause. Spinal stenosis may be due to:
- disc disease
- facet joint hypertrophy affecting the lateral recess
- ligamentum flavum hypertrophy in degenerative change
- a congenitally small canal (Fig. 7.42).

Commonly it may be a combination of several of these. Surgical intervention will be based on imaging findings and symptoms. To purely perform a discectomy when there is gross ligamentous and facet joint hypertrophy will fail to treat the symptoms in some cases and lead to the 'failed back' syndrome.

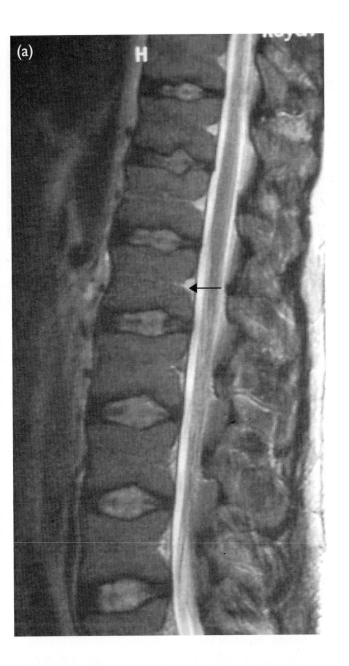

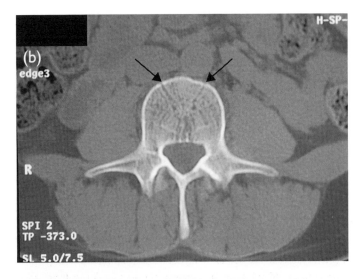

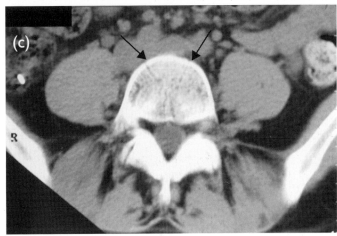

Fig. 7.40 (a) An MRI sagittal T2W of the spine, (b) axial CT bone windows and (c) axial soft-tissue windows with the normal findings from the basivertebral veins, which can form a 'Y' shape on axial imaging, and the posterior defect on sagittal imaging (arrows).

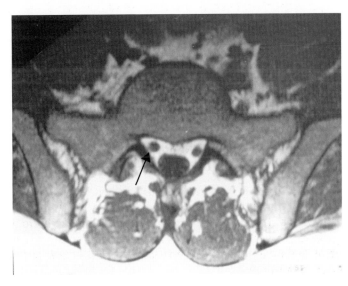

Fig. 7.41 MR axial T1-weighted image of the nerves shows nerve S1 in the lateral recess (arrow).

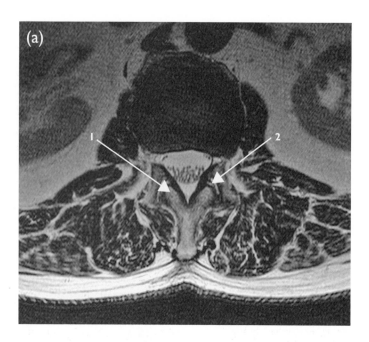

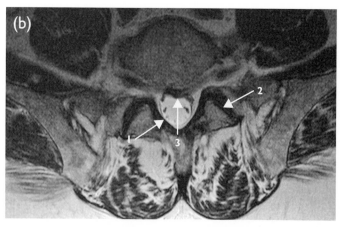

Fig. 7.42 Axial T2-weighted imaging (a) showing the ligamentum flavum slightly hypertrophied (1). The facet joints are hypertrophied (2) and (b) a left-sided disc protrusion displacing the left nerve V root (3).

MR of the spine

Indication
MRI is the current investigation of choice for bone marrow disease and the spinal cord.

Technique
To image the whole spine along its length, two surface coil placements are required because the coils have a limited field of view. The whole spine is imaged by moving either the tabletop or the patient. Image resolution is improved using the dedicated surface posterior neck coil in the cervical region (Fig. 7.43).

- The whole spine should be imaged to assess for cord compression and not just one level because there may be multiple level involvement.
- The patient has to remain absolutely still for each series. Any movement will degrade the images so they may become uninterpretable. The examination needs to be

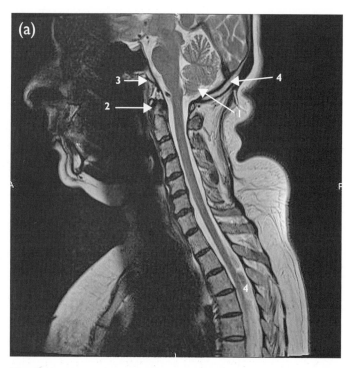

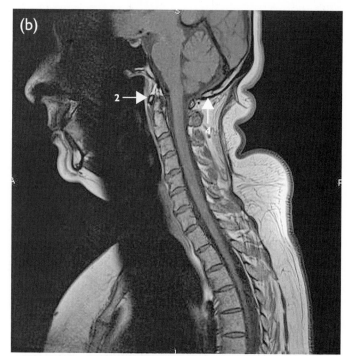

Fig. 7.43 MRI: (a) T2- and (b) T1-weighted images of the cervical spine. The cerebellar tonsils (1) can be assessed at the foramen magnum for descent. The atlantoaxial distance (2) can be seen on MR. Clivus (3) and basiocciput (4).

adapted to the patient and the most important series should be the first one. A standard spine protocol includes T1-weighted and T2-weighted sagittal images of the spine.

- Both patient and physiological movement obscure detail. Sedatives and adequate analgesia can help the patient with a painful back to remain still. Presaturation pulses or bands are applied to decrease motion artefact from the beating heart and aorta, chest wall and abdomen. CSF pulsation can lead to artefact in the CSF in the spine on T2-weighted images which can mimic an arteriovenous malformation.
- The most common scanning planes in the spine are the axial and sagittal.
- There is a weight limit on the MRI table and some larger patients may not fit into the gantry of the magnet.
- In severe scoliosis, standard sagittal and axial images are not possible and a mixture of coronal images is taken to ensure complete coverage.
- T1-weighted imaging provides the best anatomical detail and can detect bone marrow pathology. The CSF is normally dark grey on T1. Normal bone marrow is composed of fat which is bright on T1, i.e. high signal. The discs are low signal on T1 due to their water content. Cortical bone has no signal on MRI because there is no proton spin, i.e. cortical bone gives a signal void. T1-weighted imaging assesses for vertebral bone marrow disease. The vertebral bone marrow should be brighter than the intervertebral discs on T1-weighted imaging. If this ratio is lost, i.e. the discs are brighter than the bodies on T1, diffuse malignancy should be suspected.
- T2-weighted imaging provides the image with the best intrinsic spinal cord detail and can detect meningeal pathology. The CSF is normally bright, i.e. white on T2-weighted imaging. The marrow is normally fatty with a high signal and so marrow metastases that also have a high signal due to their water content may be missed because there is no contrast between normal and abnormal marrow.
- MR contrast, e.g. gadolinium, with T1-weighted imaging is used for problem-solving. Contrast is given in suspected cases of spinal infection and to detect meningeal deposits, intramedullary spinal cord tumours, inflammatory cord lesions and in 'failed back' post-surgical cases. The dose is 0.2 ml/kg administered as a bolus. A maximum of 20 ml is administered.
- The investigation of choice for sacroiliitis is MRI with angled coronal STIR (short T1 inversion recovery) and T1-weighted imaging.

Findings and variants
- The signal intensity of the vertebra normally depends on the tyre of marrow present. Normally there is more red marrow than yellow marrow and the bodies are medium-to-high signal on T1 and intermediate signal on T2. After radiotherapy the marrow fat increases and the bodies become brighter (Fig. 7.44).

- Haemangiomas in the vertebra can mimic pathology.
- The MR appearance of the discs varies according to their water content. Normal discs are low signal on T1 and high signal on T2-weighted and gradient echo. With normal ageing dehydration change occurs within the disc and it gradually loses signal on T2 weighting, becoming desiccated and degenerate (Fig. 7.45).
- In the lumbosacral region the nerve roots should run from posterior to anterior as they descend within the theca/canal itself.
- The individual nerve roots are identified on T2- but not T1-weighted images.
- On axial T2-weighted image the nerve roots can be identified individually and should not be clumped together. Clumping posteriorly is seen in arachnoiditis.
- In the lumbar sacral region the nerve routes run underneath the pedicle, e.g. the third route will run under the pedicle and would therefore probably miss any disc disease at the L3–4 level.
- On a parasagittal MRI on T1-weighted imaging, the nerve can be seen in the upper or cranial portion of the neural foramen. Compare the shape with a keyhole.
- The nerve roots pass through the lateral recess of the canal and emerge from the neural foramen in a root sheath. Epidural fat surrounds the sheath in the neural foramen; this can be seen on sagittal T1-weighted imaging. A normal variant that is rare is for two nerve roots to emerge from the same foramen, called a conjoined nerve root. This is larger than usual and decreases the amount of surrounding epidural fat (Fig. 7.46).
- The inferior two-thirds of the SI joints are synovial (Fig. 7.47).
- In the spinal canal in the sacral region Tarlov's cysts can mimic pathology (Fig. 7.48).

Artefacts on MR of the spine
Gibb's artefact
This is a central high-signal linear abnormality running through the cervical spinal cord, which is a truncation artefact and occurs at high-contrast boundaries such as the cord/CSF interface. It is an artefact and should be differentiated from pathology, such as a cord infarct or a syrinx. A real signal abnormality in the cord is present in a constant position on two perpendicular planes of imaging, usually axial and sagittal.

Flow artefacts may be seen in the spinal canal on T2-weighted imaging particularly in the thoracic region. These can simulate an arteriovenous malformation (Fig. 7.49).

Easy guide to MR sequences
It is important not to become bogged down with sequences when reporting MRI but to use anatomy and first principles:
- T1W: good for anatomical detail of the spine and to assess for marrow deposits in metastatic disease. The CSF is dark and fat is bright. The sequence is used after intravenous contrast enhancement.

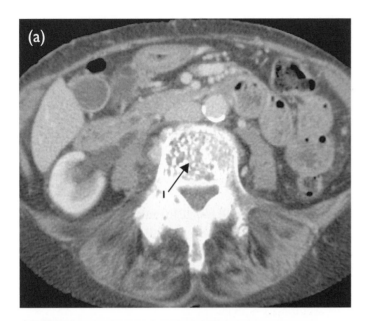

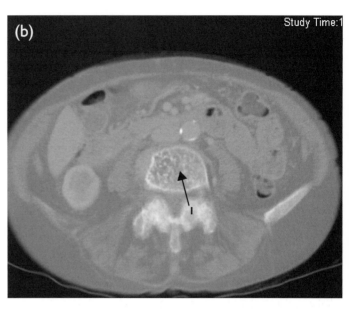

Fig. 7.44 (a) Axial CT soft-tissue window, (b) bony window and (c) MRI of haemangioma. Haemangioma can mimic pathology. On CT it gives a sunburst speckled appearance (1) and on MRI, on T1, a high-signal abnormality (2).

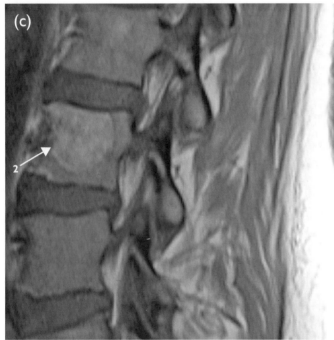

- T2W: shows oedema and CSF as bright fluid. The best sequence to assess spinal cord pathology. Fat is bright.
- STIR inversion recovery: nulls out fat so only fluid shows up brightly. A time-consuming sequence and not routinely used.
- Gradient echo imaging: speeds up imaging times by decreasing the radiofrequency (RF) pulse angle from 90° to less. An angle of around 30° is usually a T2-weighted image; an angle of 45° is usually proton density and an angle of 60–70° is usually T1W. Spinal cord detail in the cervical region is visible as an 'H' shape in the cord in the axial plane.

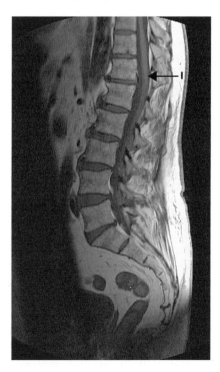

Fig. 7.45 T1W MRI of the lumbosacral spine. The marrow on the T1W normally shows a higher ratio of signal of the body to the disc. The body should be brighter than the disc. Conus (arrow).

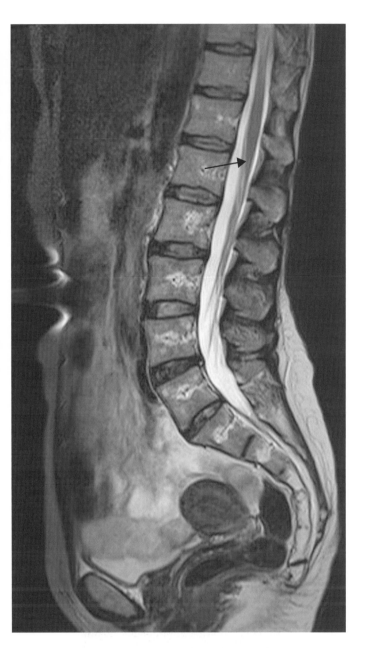

Fig. 7.46 T2 MRI of the lumbosacral spine. The conus (arrow) is evaluated on T2-weighted imaging. It should have a slightly pointed appearance. The nerve roots should then extend from posterior to anterior within the theca.

- Turbospin imaging: decreases the scanning time by sending in more RF pulses at once and receiving more echoes at a time. It does not alter the angle of the RF pulse.

Interpretation of spine MRI and application of anatomy

Similar to all radiology it is important to develop a system for reviewing images. It can be overwhelming having so many MR images but a methodical review will simplify this. The A, B, C, D, E guide is helpful. Look for signs of abnormality with:

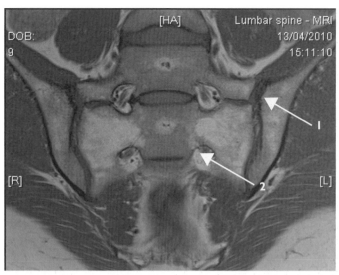

Fig. 7.47 MRI of the sacroiliac joints and sacrum – T1W. SI joint (1) and sacral foramina (2).

- A for alignment: assess vertebral alignment on sagittal and coronal images if taken. Are there any sudden steps in the vertebral alignment, i.e. retro- or spondylolisthesis? In the lumbar region this slip of vertebra is usually due to a pars defect, which leads to spondylolisthesis = slip forward or retrolisthesis = slip back. Is there a scoliosis?

- B for bones: use T1-weighted images to assess marrow. Always check that the vertebrae are brighter than the discs on T1.

- C for cord: use T2-weighted images to look for cord pathology, which will show up as high signal in the cord. If there is a real cord signal abnormality, rather than an artefact, it should be visible on all planes or imaging on T2, i.e. axial, sagittal or coronal. Is the conus at an acceptable level with a normal shape?

- D for discs: assess hydration of discs on T2W. In young people the discs should be bright on T2W because they contain water. This decreases due to age and the discs become low signal, i.e. dark on T2. Look for disc bulges and prolapses. Disc space narrowing may be a sign of abnormality. Are any of the discs extra bright on T2, which may be seen in discitis?

- E for everything else: important to assess the corners of the image. The spinal canal dimensions for stenosis, the bladder for overdistension, the uterus for fibroids and the ovaries for any masses. Check the scout images for renal masses, lung lesions, ovarian masses and aortic aneurysms (Fig. 7.50).

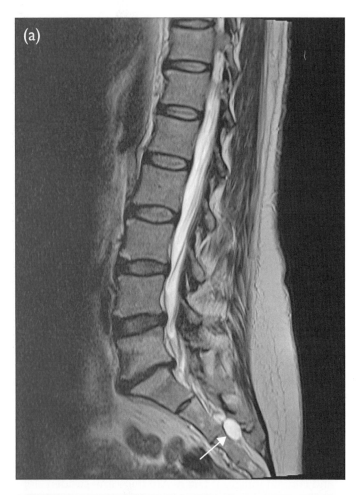

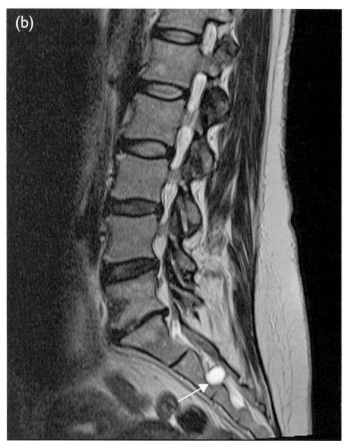

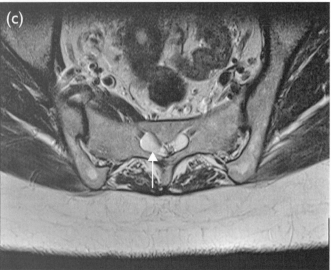

Fig. 7.48 (a,b) Sagittal T2 MRI and (c) axial T2 MRI showing well-defined high signal lesions in the sacral region S2–3, consistent with incidental Tarlov's cysts (arrows).

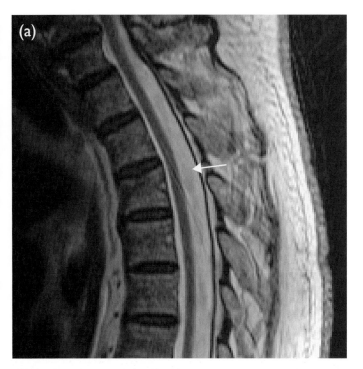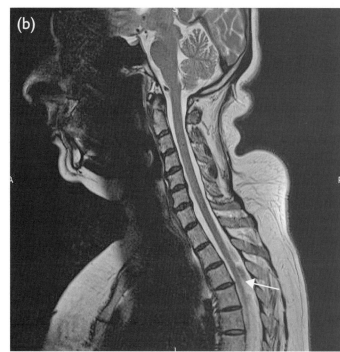

Fig. 7.49 (a,b) Sagittal T2 MRI: two cases shows some increased signal in the theca behind the cord, consistent with flow artefact that can mimic an arteriovenous malformation (arrows).

Myelography

CT myelography is now performed to assess disc protrusions or cord compression only when MRI is contraindicated in specialist centres (Fig. 7.51).
- Contrast enables the individual nerve roots to be seen.
- A short bevelled 22-gauge lumbar puncture needle is used. Ideally L2–3 is punctured as the aim is to use a level below the terminal cord, i.e. L1–2, and above the level where pathology is most common, i.e. L5–S1. Twenty millilitres of water-soluble contrast are used. The patient is in a prone position with the tabletop tipped head upwards. This prevents the contrast from ascending into the ventricles and into the head. The contrast is injected into the subarachnoid space. The water-soluble contrast goes in the nerve root sheath (Fig. 7.52).
- A headache may occur after the procedure.

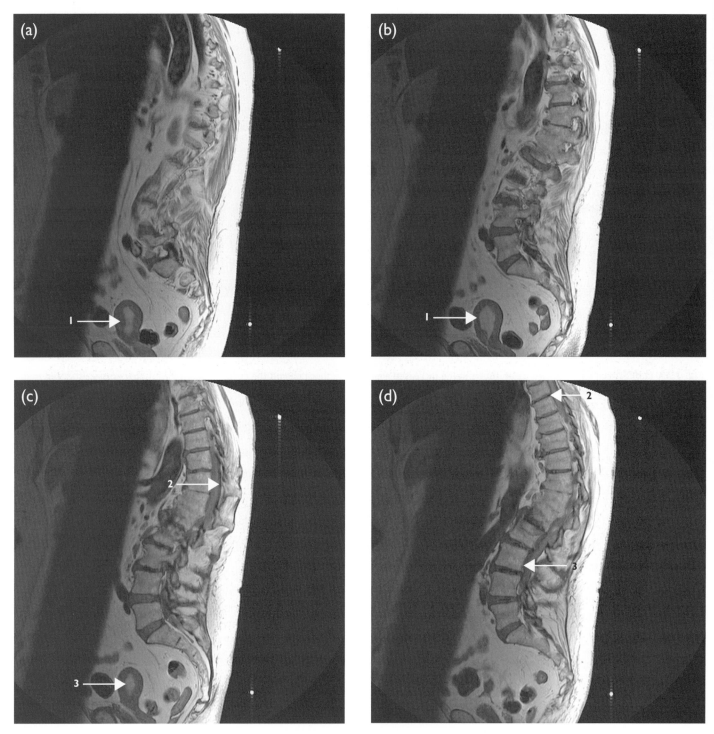

Fig. 7.50 MRI T1-weighted images on a 60-year-old woman with a marked scoliosis. Incidental note is made of a thickened endometrium (1) in the uterus and the pelvis in this postmenopausal woman who is then referred for transvaginal ultrasound. Assessment on scout images should be made of the pelvis, kidneys, aorta and lungs. Scroll through the images in order to visualize the entire spinal cord. Spinal cord (2) and theca (3).

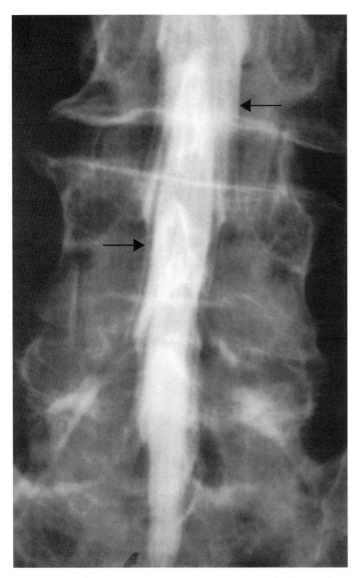

Fig. 7.51 Supine view of the myelogram showing descent of the nerve root underneath the pedicles (arrows).

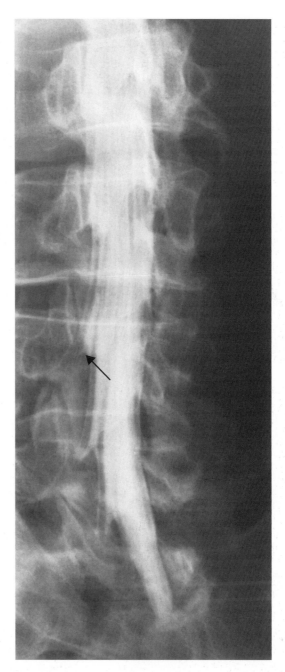

Fig. 7.52 Myelogram oblique view showing the nerve passing under the pedicle (arrow) in the Scotty dog appearance.

CASES

The following cases are given to illustrate the application of anatomy in image interpretation in spinal pathology.

Case 7.1

A patient presents with cauda equina syndrome. To assess for lumbar disc protrusion, MRI of the lumbosacral spine using sagittal T1- and T2-weighted imaging with axial T1-weighted sequences is performed (Fig. 7.53).

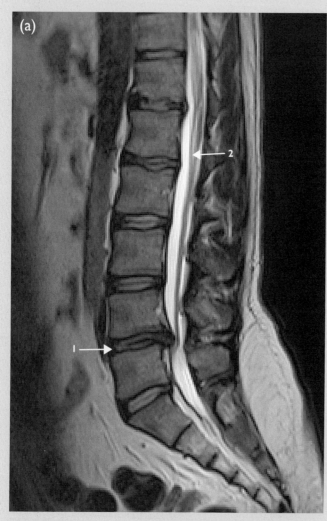

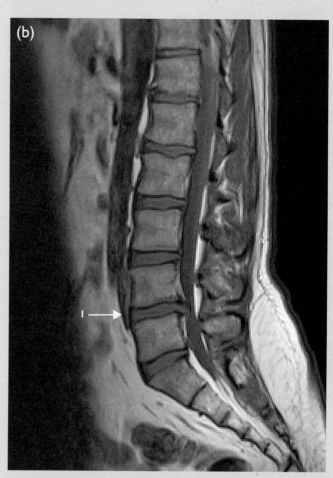

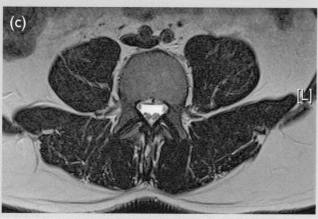

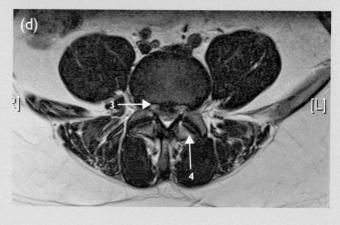

Start using the A, B, C, D and E guide for MRI spine.
- Alignment: in this case the vertebral alignment is normal.
- Bones: are the bodies brighter than the discs on T1W? Yes. This is a normal finding.
- Cord: where is the conus and is there any intracord signal abnormality on T2 sagittal images? If there is a cord signal lesion can it be seen on an orthogonal plane or could it be an artefact? Normal in this case.
- Discs: are there any protrusions or extrusions of the discs on the sagittal plane? Can this be seen on the axial plane? It may contribute to stenosis. Look at the 'keyholes' on T1W parasagittal images to see if there is loss of the normal bright fat around the nerve root in the foramen. Look for canal stenosis due to (1) discs, (2) congenital stenosis, (3) lateral recess narrowing from facet joint hypertrophy and (4) ligamentum flavum hypertrophy. In this case the pathology starts at 'D'.
- Everything else: is the bladder visible? Does it have a normal wall thickness? Are the uterus and ovaries normal?

Here A, B and C are normal which is reflected in the report:
The vertebral bodies are of normal height, alignment and signal intensity. The terminal cord is of normal calibre and signal intensity.
- The pathology starts at 'D' – the discs. Notice the large posterior disc protrusion obliterating both nerve roots and the theca posteriorly. How is a significant impingement assessed? Swelling or displacement of the nerve root is evidence of this.
- Ideally the affected root should be swollen or displaced as firm evidence of significant impingement. If the disc abuts the root alone it may be clinically insignificant. The keyholes on the parasagittal T1-weighted images can show root impingement in the recess.

There is a large central disc protrusion at L4–5 which is causing significant impingement on the both nerve V roots and the theca.
- How is it established which nerve root is involved? The nerve exits underneath the corresponding pedicle, i.e. L4 exits under the fourth pedicle. A disc at L4–5 will therefore not usually impinge on the fourth root unless a very lateral disc lesion because the root had already exited. The L4–5 disc usually impinges on the fifth nerve root.
- The remainder of the series should be reviewed looking at the bladder, the pelvic organs and the aorta for incidental or relevant findings and if negative briefly alluded to in the report.

No other significant abnormality is seen.

Fig. 7.53 MR of the spine: (a) sagittal T2- and (b) sagittal T1-weighted images showing a disc protrusion at L4–5 (1). Conus (2). (c,d) Axial T2-weighted images showing the normal appearance in (c) and on (d) how the normal appearance of theca is obliterated due to the large disc protrusion (3), impinging on both nerve roots. There is also facet joint hypertrophy (4).

Case 7.2

A patient presents with low back pain. Plain films – AP and lateral lumbar spine – are performed initially.

Findings

- The plain films show, on the lateral lumbar spine view, a slip of the L5 vertebra anteriorly relative to the S1 vertebra below (Fig. 7.54a). The AP film was unremarkable.
- Oblique views of the lumbar spine could be performed to show a pars defect that leads to a slip. However, MRI/CT are preferable.
- MRI or CT is performed although MRI is superior for the theca (Fig. 7.54).

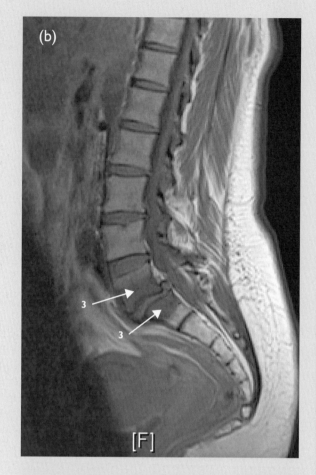

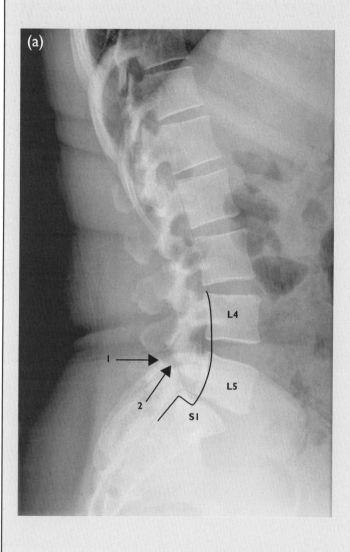

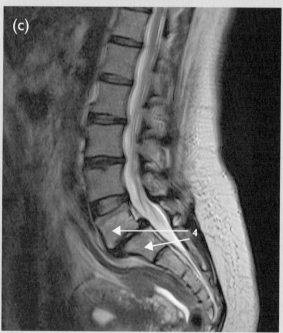

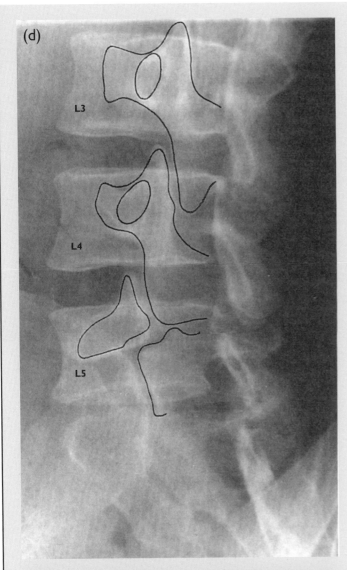

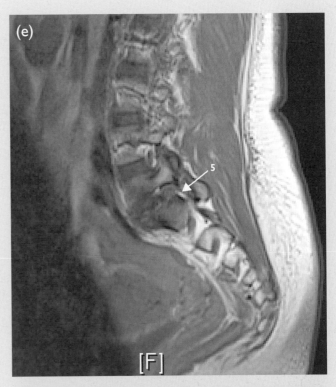

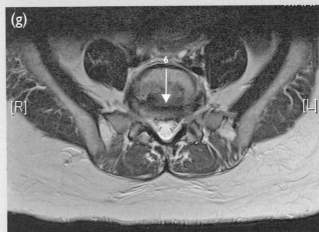

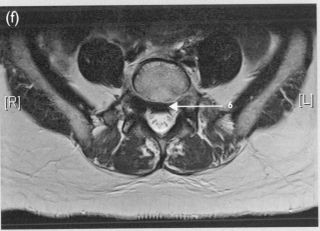

Fig. 7.54 (a) Lateral lumbar spine radiograph showing a 25% slip of L5 on S1 (1). Pars defect (2). (b) Sagittal T1- and (c) T2-weighted imaging confirms the grade 1 spondylolisthesis with endplate signal change at L5–S1 (3). Signal endplates on T2-weighted (4). (d) Diagram showing a pars defect and a slip. The slip occurs across the neck of the Scotty dog. (e) Sagittal MRI of the lumbar spine showing the slip leading to narrowing of the neural exit foramen (5). (f,g) The axial images a little lower confirm the slip, causing a pseudo-disc appearance (6).

Image interpretation of MRI

- Alignment: on the sagittal images the slip of L4 on L5 is 25% of the diameter of the body. The slip severity is compared with the percentage of the total body diameter that it has slipped.
- Bones: remember T1W for marrow change. The remaining vertebrae have normal marrow signal except at L5–S1 where on the T1 images there is endplate low-signal change. Look on the parasagittal T1W images for a pars defect and nerve root impingement. Here the keyhole on the parasagittal image has lost the aft around the root compared with the others, and on the axial images for facet joint hypertrophy.
- Cord: remember T2W for spinal cord or conus abnormality. The terminal cord is normal on the T2W.
- Discs: on axial imaging the relative slip of one vertebra on the adjacent one reveals the intervening disc, giving the impression of a disc bulge which is not real, i.e. pseudo-disc bulge. The sagittal images show the slip and absence of disc protrusion. This is more exaggerated on CT. When assessing discs, the canal dimensions and facets and ligaments must be reviewed. In this case the slip has led to facet joint hypertrophy, which is impinging on the lateral recess at L5–S1. Remaining levels should be reviewed.
- Everything else: normal.

The idealized report in this case would read: The vertebral bodies are of normal height and signal intensity. The terminal cord is of normal calibre and signal intensity. There is an anterior slip forward of L5 on S1 by 25%. This has led to facet joint hypertrophy and ligamentous hypertrophy and is causing significant impingement on nerve V roots bilaterally in the neural exit foramina.

Case 7.3

A patient presents with back pain that causes waking at night and no previous medical history.

Plain film

- Alignment: normal.
- Bones: check height of the bodies and the pedicles; if involved can help differentiate from osteoporotic collapse. No abnormality seen.

MRI (Fig. 7.55)

- Alignment: normal.
- Bones: assess the vertebra on T1W for low signal. The vertebrae should normally be high signal relative to the discs on T1W, i.e. higher signal than the discs. In this case the bodies are diffusely low signal, giving the impression that the discs are high signal on T1W, i.e. reversal of the normal ratio. The height of all the bodies is maintained.
- Cord appears normal.
- Discs are well maintained in height but appear bright.
- Everything else: assess scout image for renal/pelvic masses – clues as to any source of malignancy. If pedicles are involved the process is more likely to be due to malignancy.

In conclusion the bodies are diffusely of low signal on T1W, which is suspicious for diffuse vertebral column metastases.

Note that low signal vertebra may be seen in African–Caribbean individuals as a racial variation rather than being due to diffuse marrow infiltration.

MRI is more sensitive than plain film for marrow replacement, i.e. metastases.

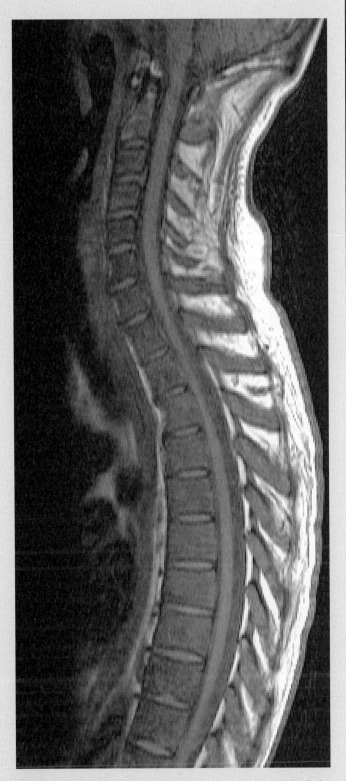

Fig. 7.55 Sagittal T1-weighted imaging showing reversal of the normal disc:body ratio. The discs are higher than the bodies, suggesting diffuse metastases.

Case 7.4

Clinical case for trauma

The patient presents with severe neck pain after a road traffic accident. Initially plain radiographs are taken using a horizontal beam lateral view, if necessary, and an AP view.

- Soft-tissue swelling: is any present in the prevertebral region?
- Alignment: check for slip; if so how much – on both AP and lateral views? Apply the anterior, posterior vertebral line, then the spinolaminar and pillar line for facets (Fig. 7.56).
- Bones: look at posterior border of bodies for loss of concavity. Look for loss of height.
- Disc spaces: are they even (Fig. 7.56)?

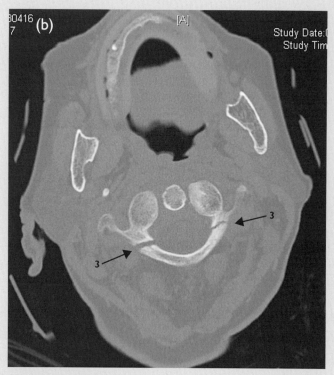

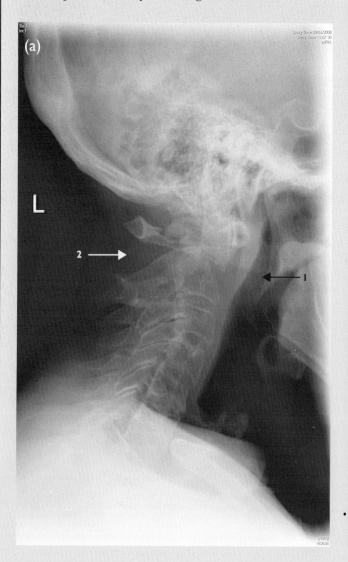

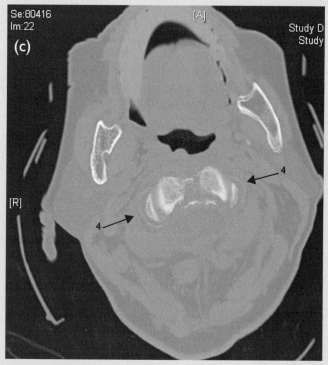

Fig. 7.56 (a) Plain film showing fracture of the posterior arch of C1, fracture of the peg and soft-tissue swelling (1). There is widening of the interspinous distance (2). (b,c) Axial CT scans showing fracture of the posterior arch of C1 (3) and fracture of the body of C2 (4). (d,e) Sagittal reconstructions showing the fracture at the base of the peg (5) and the fracture of the lateral mass of C1 (6).

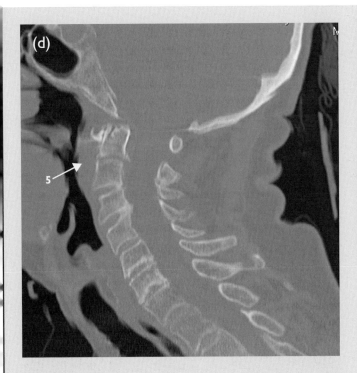

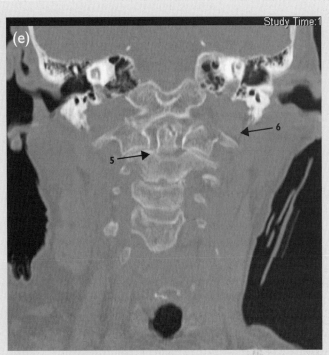

Lateral cervical spine

Findings

- Soft tissues: there is prevertebral soft-tissue swelling at the C1, C2 and C3 levels. The C1 level should normally measure a maximum of 3 mm.
- Alignment: there is loss of the spinolaminar line posteriorly. There is also widening of the interspinous distance between C1 and C2. The posterior vertebral line is lost and the anterior vertebral line is disrupted at C1–2.
- Bones: on close review there appears to be a fracture through the posterior arch of the atlas. A CT scan of the neck was performed of this.
- On the axial images (Fig. 7.56b) a fracture is seen through the anterior arch of C1.
- Fig. 7.56c is an axial CT through the body of C2 showing a comminuted fracture, at the base of the odontoid peg.
- Fig. 7.56d is a sagittal reconstruction through the cervical spine showing a fracture through the base of the odontoid peg, with a minimal amount of posterior displacement.
- Fig. 7.56e confirms the fracture of the base of the peg and disruption to the lateral mass of C1.
- The example shows how using the lines and prevertebral soft-tissue swelling on a cervical spine helps as a guide to the trauma. CT is invaluable in vertebral spinal trauma.

Case 7.5

A patient presents with left sciatica affecting left nerve V root.

Investigations

MRI is performed. Fig. 5.57a–c are images from a T2-weighted sagittal series of the spine; Fig. 7.57d is a sagittal T1-weighted image.
- Alignment: the alignment is within normal limits.
- Bones: on T1-weighted imaging the bones are of higher signal than the disc, which is normal. No abnormality or marrow signal is seen.
- Cord: the terminal cord is of normal calibre and signal intensity.

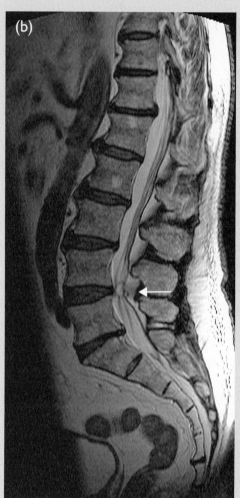

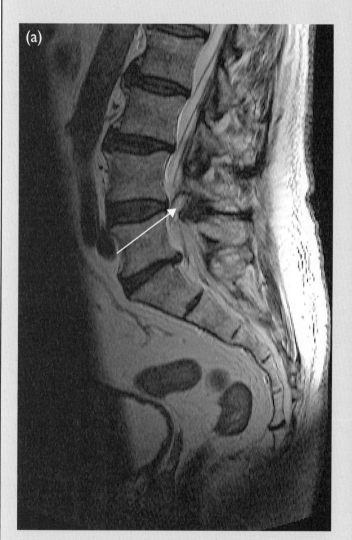

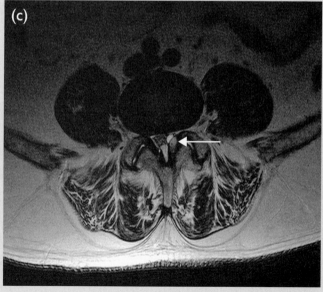

Fig. 7.57 (a) Sagittal T2- and (b) sagittal T2-weighted imaging. A small synovial cyst seen at L4–5 (arrow). (c) Axial T2-weighted imaging showing the synovial cyst (arrow) and obliteration of the theca at the L4–5 level.

- Discs: there is dehydration change affecting multiple disc levels. In addition, at L5–S1, there is narrowing of the disc space, which appears degenerate.
- Everything else: on close review within the theca, on the sagittal T2 images, a small, circumscribed, high-signal abnormality is seen at the L4–5 level.

When an abnormality is seen on one plane, a search for it in the orthogonal plane should be made.

Fig. 5.57e,f shows axial T2-weighted images through the spine. At the L4 level the theca appears normal. However, at the L5 level there is narrowing of the canal dimensions due to a combination of ligamentous and facet joint hypertrophy and a generalized disc bulge. In addition, a small well-circumscribed lesion is seen related to the left facet joint. This is a synovial cyst. The normal root and theca cannot be seen at this level. The loss of visualization of the nerve root is an indication of it being compromised.

This is compatible with a synovial cyst at L4–5, which is leading to left nerve V root symptoms.

8 Imaging of the upper limb

RADIOLOGICAL ANATOMY

The clavicle

- This is the first bone to appear in utero by endomembranous ossification.
- The medial epiphysis is the last to fuse by age 31 years.
- It has a conoid tubercle for attachment of the coracoclavicular ligament (Fig. 8.1).
- It has a rhomboid fossa medially that could be confused with a lytic lesion.

The scapula

- It is a large flat bone with a spine posteriorly and the coracoid process anteriorly.

- It has a large acromion process which is boomerang shaped and runs from posterior to anterior (Fig. 8.2).
- At birth the acromion, glenoid, coracoid and inferior angle are all cartilaginous and not visualized.
- The acromion process may fail to fuse and remain as the os acromiale (Fig. 8.2).

The humerus

- The humeral head has secondary ossification centres. The head should appear by age 1, the greater tuberosity by age 2 and the lesser tuberosity by age 5 (Fig. 8.3).
- The anatomical neck is wide and lies just below the head. The surgical neck is narrow and lies at the proximal end of the shaft.
- Beneath the deltoid muscle and above the humeral head is the subacromial subdeltoid bursa, a hemispherical synovium-lined bursa. This is in close apposition to the supraspinatus tendon and fills with fluid when there is a rotator cuff tear.
- At the distal humerus lie ossification centres for the capitellum, trochlea, and medial and lateral epicondyles. The coronoid fossa lies anteriorly and the olecranon fossa posteriorly in the distal humerus (Fig. 8.4).

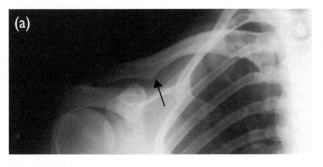

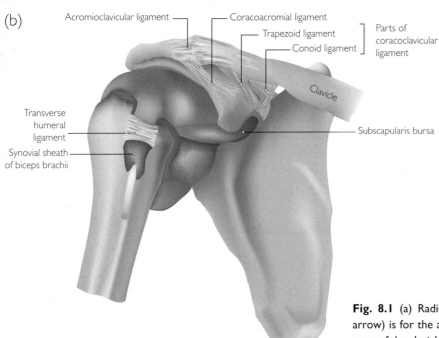

Fig. 8.1 (a) Radiograph of the clavicle. The conoid tubercle (black arrow) is for the attachment of the coracoclavicular ligament. (b) Diagram of the clavicle, scapula and humerus, and the normal glenohumeral joint.

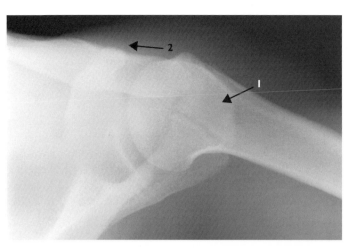

Fig. 8.2 Radiograph of left shoulder showing os acromiale (1); a normal variant of the acromion is seen, which has not fused. This may be symptomatic. The characteristic shape of the coracoid process is seen anteriorly (2).

The radius

- Proximally the circular radial head articulates with the capitellum and the medial notch articulates with the ulna.
- The radial tuberosity lies below the neck.
- The distal radius has a styloid process and the distal radius articulates with the lunate, scaphoid or navicular and distal ulna (Fig. 8.5).

The ulna

- Proximally the ulna has the coronoid process anteriorly which articulates with the trochlea of the humerus, and posteriorly the olecranon process of the ulna.
- The distal ulna does not articulate with the carpus but with the triangular fibrocartilage complex.

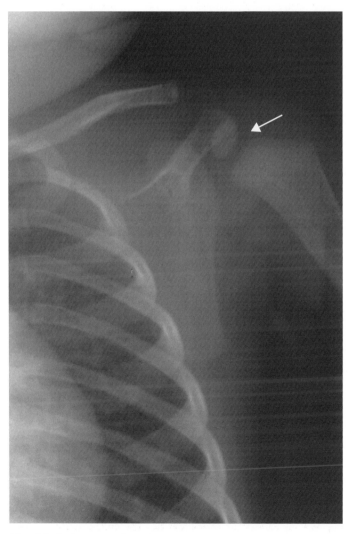

Fig. 8.3 Radiograph of the humerus in an infant. The humeral head (arrow) on the left side has appeared, indicating that the child must be aged 1. The lesser and greater tuberosities have not appeared.

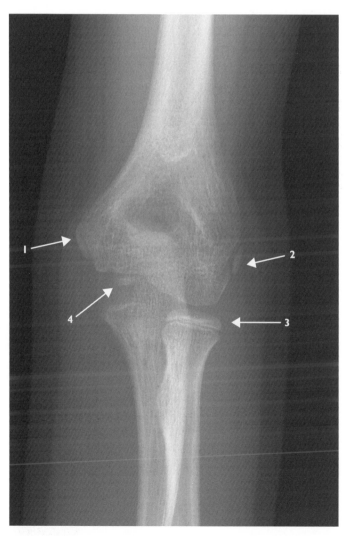

Fig. 8.4 Radiograph showing the ossification centres of the elbow. The medial (1) and lateral (2) epicondyles are seen. The radial head (3) ossification centre is noted and the trochlea (4).

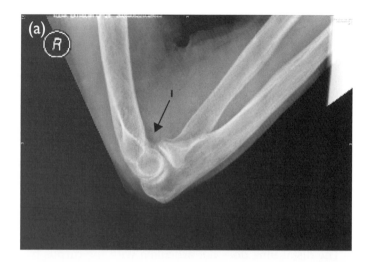

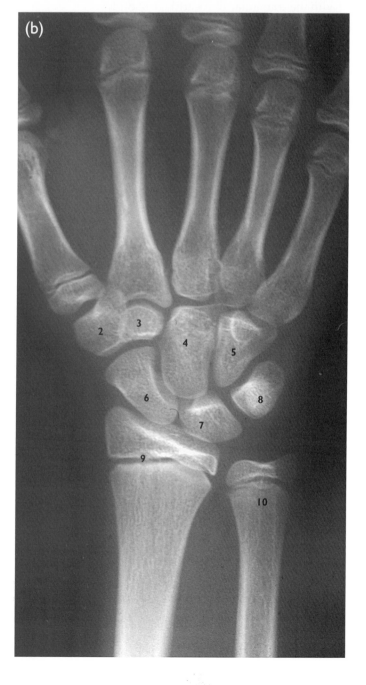

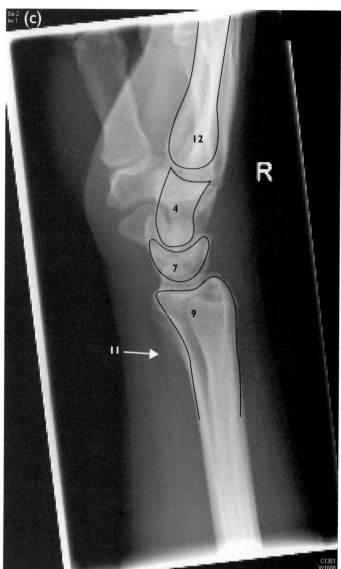

Fig. 8.5 (a) Lateral radiograph elbow: normally a fat pad (1) is seen anteriorly which should not be elevated. There should not normally be a posterior fat pad: AP view (b) of the wrist showing the radius articulating with the scaphoid and the lunate, but the ulna does not articulate with the carpus. The triangular fibre cartilage complex articulates with the ulna. Trapezium (2), trapezoid (3), capitate (4), hamate (5), scaphoid (6), lunate (7), triquetral (8), radius (9) andp ulna (10). (c) Lateral wrist showing the pronator quadratus fat pad (11). Third MCP (12). MCP = metacarpophalongeal joint.

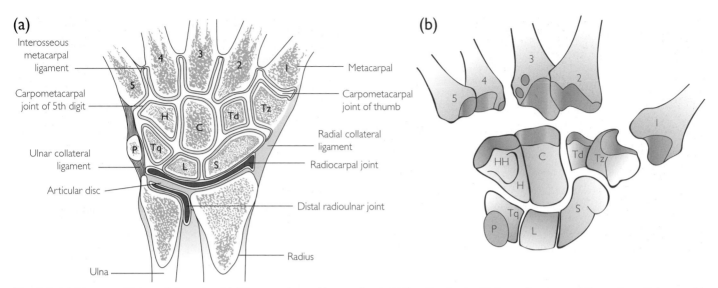

Fig. 8.6 (a) Diagram of joints of the wrist. (b) Diagram of carpal bones. Scaphoid S; radius R; ulna U; lunate L; triquetral Tq; pisiform P; hamate H; capitate C; trapezoid Td; trapezium Tz.

- The ulna has a distal styloid process.
- The long bones of the forearm, i.e. the radius and ulna, are united by the interosseous membrane and as such fracture of one is frequently associated with fracture of the other (Fig. 8.6).

Carpus

- There are eight carpal bones; the distal row are capitate, hamate, trapezium, trapezoid and the proximal row triquetral, lunate, scaphoid, pisiform (Fig. 8.6).
- The carpal bones begin to ossify from birth. There is a definite order of appearance of the carpal bones in the wrist. The first bone to appear is the capitate, followed by the hamate. The ossification then occurs in a definite order in rotation. The scaphoid usually appears by age 6

and the last to appear is the pisiform by age 10–12 (Fig. 8.7).
- Carpal fusion: it is a normal variant for fusion of carpal bones within the same row.
- However, cross-row fusion may be associated with a congenital syndrome.
- Same-row fusion is more common in African–Caribbean individuals. The most common fusion is triquetral lunate. This is more common than capitate hamate (Fig. 8.8).

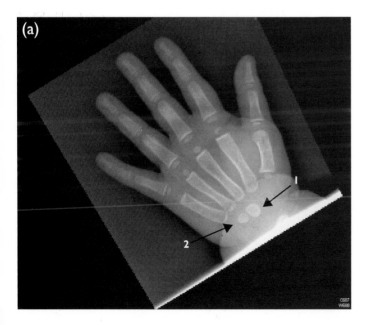

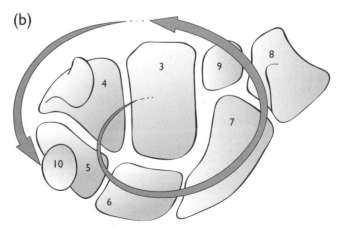

Fig. 8.7 (a) Radiograph of the young carpus. The chronological age of the child can be assessed by looking at the appearance of the carpal bones. The first two carpal bones to appear are the capitate (1) and hamate (2). (b) Age of ossification of carpal bones in childhood. Capitate (3), hamate (4), triquetral (5), lunate (6), scaphoid (7), trapezium (8), trapezoid (9) and pisiform (10).

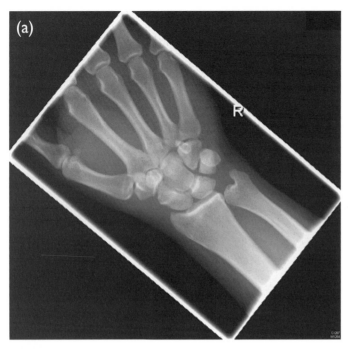

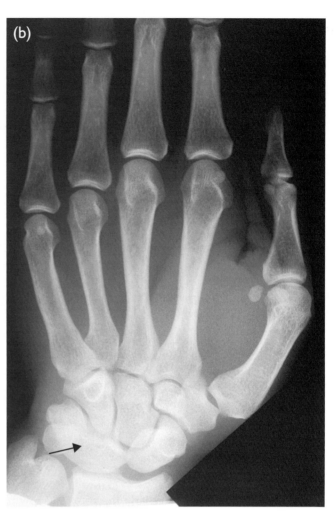

Fig. 8.8 Radiograph of the hand: (a) normal wrist; (b) the triquetral and lunate which have a congenital fusion (arrow).

The shoulder joint

• There are two main articulations in the shoulder region: the glenohumeral joint and the acromioclavicular (AC) joint (Fig. 8.9).

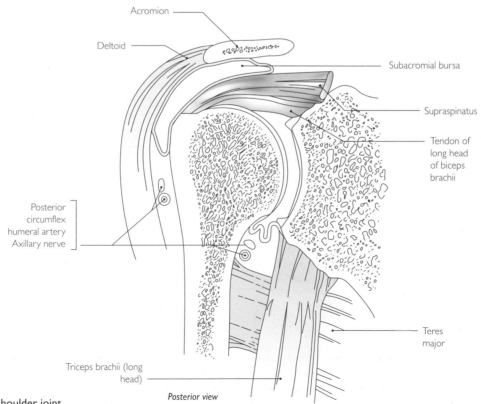

Fig. 8.9 Diagram of shoulder joint.

(a)

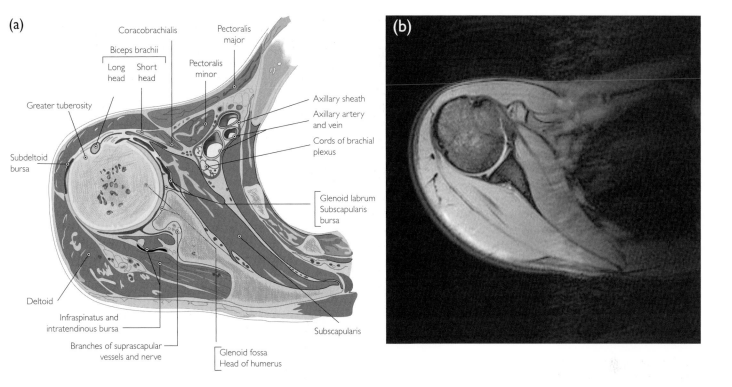

Coracobrachialis

Biceps brachii

Long head | Short head

Pectoralis major

Pectoralis minor

Greater tuberosity

Subdeltoid bursa

Deltoid

Infraspinatus and intratendinous bursa

Branches of suprascapular vessels and nerve

Axillary sheath

Axillary artery and vein

Cords of brachial plexus

Glenoid labrum
Subscapularis bursa

Subscapularis

Glenoid fossa
Head of humerus

(b)

Fig. 8.10 (a) Diagram and (b) axial MRI of the shoulder. (a) The axial MRI of the shoulder shows the glenoid (1). The labium (2) and the long head of biceps tendon are visualized (3). Below the spine of the scapula the infraspinatus muscle is seen posteriorly (4) and a subscapularis muscle (5) anteriorly.

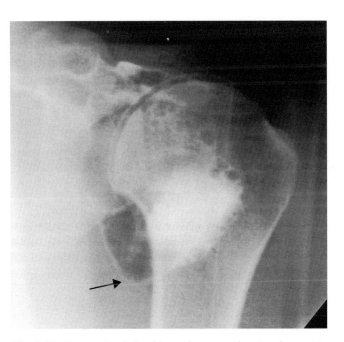

Fig. 8.11 Conventional shoulder arthrogram showing the position of the normal shoulder joint and the deep and prominent inferior aspect of the glenohumeral joint (arrow). Contrast should not normally be seen in the subacromial subdeltoid bursa.

- The AC joint is synovial formed by a capsule around the acromion and distal clavicle. This joint is supported by the AC ligament and the coracoclavicular ligament which runs from the coracoid to the undersurface of the acromion just distal to the AC joint.
- The glenohumeral articulation is formed by the glenoid fossa.
- The glenoid fossa is deepened by the glenoid labrum, which is fibrocartilaginous and appears low signal on MRI, similar to a meniscus.
- The shoulder capsule is lined by synovial membrane.
- The normal glenohumeral joint has a prominent axillary pouch. The fibrous capsule of the shoulder is thickened anteriorly, forming the glenohumeral ligaments. The shoulder capsule extends inferiorly on to the surgical neck of the humerus (Fig. 8.10).
- There are three thickenings of the capsule named the superior, middle and inferior glenohumeral ligaments.
- There are three bursae related to the shoulder joint. The most important is the subacromial subdeltoid bursa which lies between the deltoid and greater tuberosity of the humerus (Fig. 8.11).

- The other two bursae are the subscapular bursa and the coracobrachialis bursa.
- The tendon of the long head of biceps passes through the shoulder joint with a synovial sheath, to lie anteriorly in the intertubercular groove.
- The transverse ligament extends across the intertubercular groove, enclosing the long head of biceps tendon in its synovial sheath.
- The rotator cuff muscles are SITS: S = supraspinatus, I = infraspinatus, T = teres minor, S = subscapularis (Fig. 8.12).
- Supraspinatus arises from the supraspinous fossa and passes underneath the acromion and AC joint to insert into the greater tuberosity of the humerus. It has a broad tendon insertion. Pathology affecting the AC joint and the shape of the acromion can lead to impingement of the supraspinatus tendon and muscle.
- Infraspinatus arises from beneath the spine of the scapula and passes upwards at an angle to insert into the greater tuberosity of the humerus.
- Teres minor follows a more inferior but similar course to insert into the greater tuberosity.
- Subscapularis arises from the anterior surface of the scapula and inserts as a broad tendon into the lesser tuberosity of the humerus.

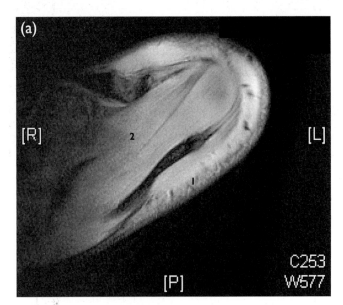

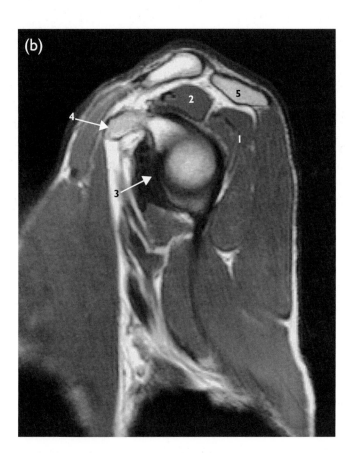

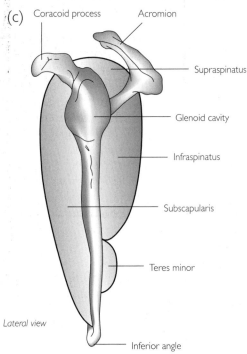

Fig. 8.12 (a) Axial image of the shoulder MRI. The supraspinatus muscle is seen to run superiorly across the shoulder to attach to the greater tuberosity, above and anterior to the spine of the scapular posteriorly. The infraspinatus (1) runs below and posterior to the scapula spine. (b) An oblique sagittal MRI showing the rotator cuff muscles. Supraspinatus (2), subscapularis (3), coracoid process (4) and acromion (5). (c) Diagram of rotator cuff.

(a)

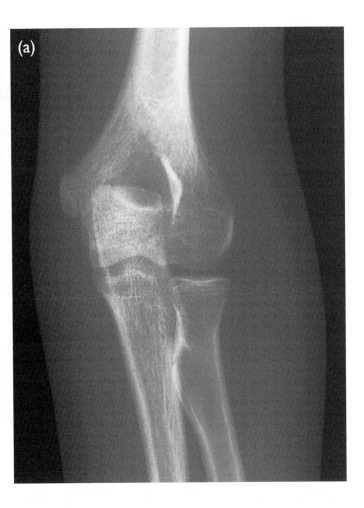

(b)

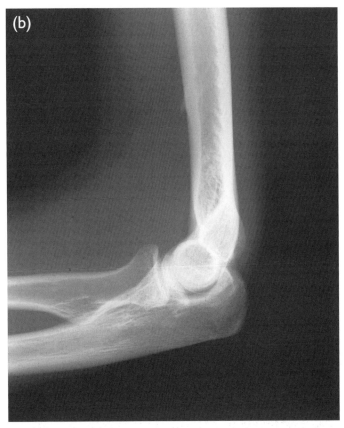

Fig. 8.13 (a) AP and (b) lateral radiographs of the elbow. The normal fat pads of the elbow are visualized.

The elbow joint

- The elbow joint is a hinge joint with the trochlea of the humerus articulating with the ulna, the capitellum of the humerus articulating with the radial head, and the radial head with the radial notch of the coronoid process of the ulna. The interosseous membrane extends between the radius and the ulna.
- The elbow has two or sometimes three bursae of importance called the olecranon bursa, radiohumeral bursa and bursa over the medial epicondyle of the humerus.
- The seven ossification centres of the elbow appear and fuse in a definite age order. At the elbow the following may help: CRITOL: C = capitellum age 1, R = radial head age 5/6, I = internal epicondyle age 5–9, T = trochlea age 10, O = olecranon age 11, L = lateral epicondyle age 14.
- The secondary ossification centres appear in this order, i.e. the capitellum appears first by age 1. The last to appear is the lateral epicondyle age 14 (Fig. 8.13).
- A shortened form may be used: CITE. These appear in this order and fuse in the reverse order and is useful when looking for a common fracture in children, which is fracture of the epicondyle called little leaguer's elbow. The external epicondyle or lateral epicondyle usually fuses before the internal epicondyle. Therefore, if an external

epicondyle is visible but not an internal epicondyle, this most probably represents a supracondylar fracture.
- At the elbow it is usual on the lateral view to have an anterior fat pad but not a posterior one (Fig. 8.14).

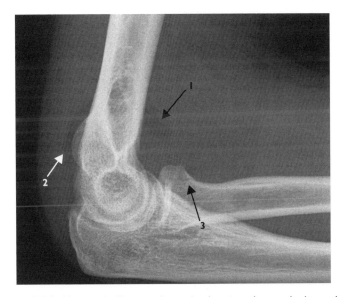

Fig. 8.14 Abnormal elbow radiograph showing abnormal elevated anterior (1) and posterior (2) fat pads. Radial head fracture (3).

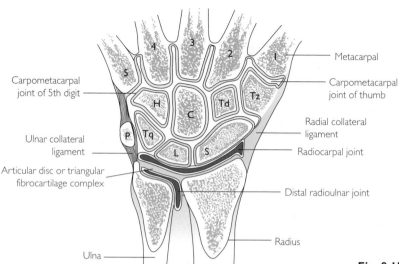

Fig. 8.15 Diagram of the wrist.

The wrist joint

- There are three main articulations in the wrist: radioulnar, radiocarpal and midcarpal.
- The triangular fibrocartilage complex stabilizes the distal radioulnar joint.
- The TFCC is made up of the triangular fibrocartilage, ulnar collateral ligament, ulnocarpal meniscus and distal radioulnar ligaments (Fig. 8.15).

The axilla

- The axilla has three muscular boundaries.
- The anterior wall is formed by the pectoral muscles and subclavius muscle.
- The posterior wall is formed by subscapularis, lattissimus dorsi and teres major.

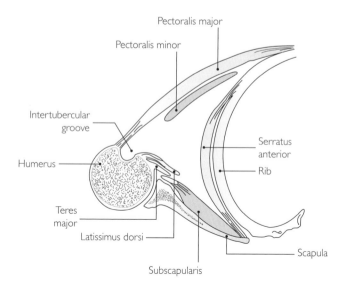

Fig. 8.16 Diagram of the axilla.

- The medial wall is formed by serratus anterior, the bony wall of ribs and intercostal muscles (Fig. 8.16).
- Within the axilla is the axillary sheath enclosing the axillary artery and vein, and the three cords of the brachial plexus forming a neurovascular bundle, surrounded with axillary fat (Fig. 8.17).

Vessels

Subclavian artery

- The subclavian artery arises from the aorta directly on the left and from the brachiocephalic trunk on the right.
- A variant is the anomalous right subclavian artery which may come off the aorta separately and cause a vascular ring and posterior impression of the posterior oesophagus.
- The subclavian artery gives off the vertebral artery as the first branch and then the costocervical and thyrocervical trunks and the internal mammary or internal thoracic artery.
- At the outer border of the first rib the subclavian artery becomes the axillary artery (Fig. 8.18).

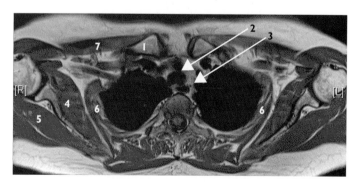

Fig. 8.17 Axillary MRI: axial T1 weighted. Clavicle (1), trachea (2), oesophagus (3), subscapularis (4), infraspinatus (5), serratus anterior (6) and pectoral muscles (7).

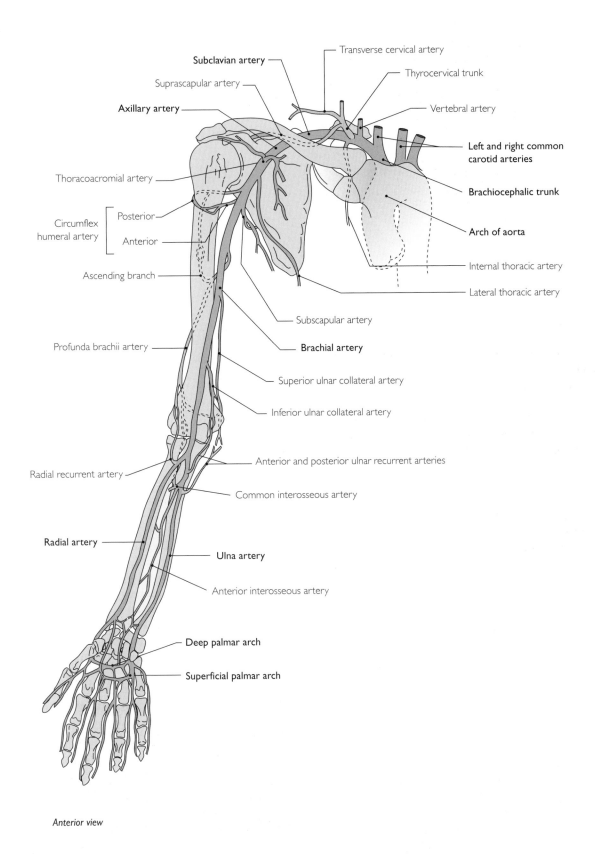

Subclavian artery

Transverse cervical artery

Thyrocervical trunk

Suprascapular artery

Axillary artery

Vertebral artery

Left and right common
carotid arteries

Thoracoacromial artery

Brachiocephalic trunk

Circumflex
humeral artery { Posterior
Anterior

Arch of aorta

Internal thoracic artery

Ascending branch

Lateral thoracic artery

Subscapular artery

Brachial artery

Profunda brachii artery

Superior ulnar collateral artery

Inferior ulnar collateral artery

Anterior and posterior ulnar recurrent arteries

Radial recurrent artery

Common interosseous artery

Radial artery

Ulna artery

Anterior interosseous artery

Deep palmar arch

Superficial palmar arch

Anterior view

Fig. 8.18 Diagram of the arm vessels.

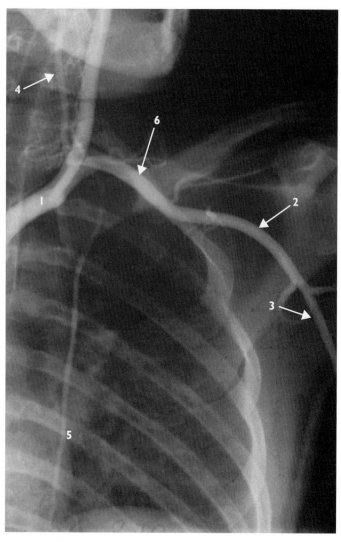

Fig. 8.19 Angiogram of the arm: coronal plane. Conventional angiography shows the normal subclavian artery (1). The origin of the axillary artery at the outer border of the first rib (2), origin of the brachial artery at the lateral border of teres major (3), left vertebral (4) and internal mammary arteries can be seen (5). Thyrocervical trunk (6).

Axillary artery

- Gives off the suprascapular, thoracoacromial and lateral thoracic artery, and circumflex humeral vessels.
- At the lower border of teres major the axillary artery becomes the brachial artery (Fig. 8.19).

Brachial artery

- The brachial artery gives off the profunda brachii artery and continues into the antecubital fossa, where it divides into the radial artery and the common interosseous artery which becomes the ulnar artery in the forearm.
- In the hand the radial artery gives rise to the deep palmar arch and the ulnar artery gives rise to the superficial palmar arch (Fig. 8.20).

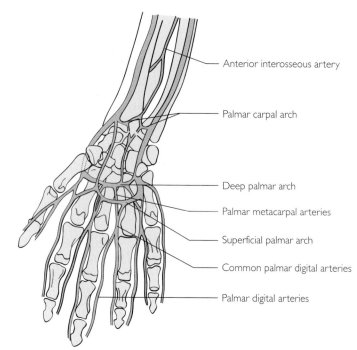

Fig. 8.20 Diagram of hand vessels.

Veins

- In the arm there are deep and superficial veins.
- The cephalic and basilic veins are superficial, with the cephalic vein ascending laterally and the basilic vein ascending medially.
- The cephalic vein pierces the clavipectoral fascia and drains into the axillary vein.
- The deep veins are the basilic vein, which becomes the axillary vein at the outer border of teres major, and this then becomes the subclavian vein at the outer border of the first rib.
- The subclavian vein joins the internal jugular vein to become the brachiocephalic vein posterior to the sternal end of the clavicle (Fig. 8.21).

The brachial plexus

- Nerve roots from C5 to T1 emerge between scalene muscles anterior and medius. These muscles arise from anterior to the cervical spine. The ventral rami of C5–T1 unite to form the three brachial trunks.
- Each of the three trunks divides into two divisions, an anterior and a posterior division, to give six in total (Fig. 8.22).
- The six divisions become three cords which lie posterior to pectoralis minor.

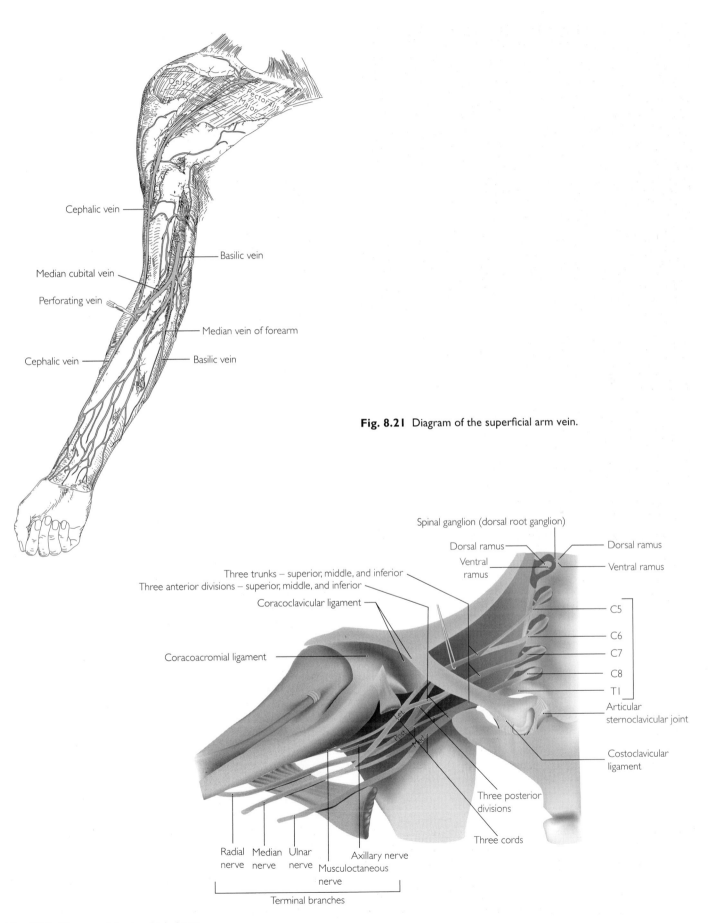

Fig. 8.21 Diagram of the superficial arm vein.

Cephalic vein

Basilic vein

Median cubital vein

Perforating vein

Median vein of forearm

Cephalic vein

Basilic vein

Spinal ganglion (dorsal root ganglion)

Dorsal ramus

Dorsal ramus

Ventral ramus

Ventral ramus

Three trunks – superior, middle, and inferior

Three anterior divisions – superior, middle, and inferior

Coracoclavicular ligament

Coracoacromial ligament

C5

C6

C7

C8

T1

Articular sternoclavicular joint

Costoclavicular ligament

Three posterior divisions

Three cords

Radial nerve

Median nerve

Ulnar nerve

Axillary nerve

Musculoctaneous nerve

Terminal branches

Fig. 8.22 Diagram of the brachial plexus.

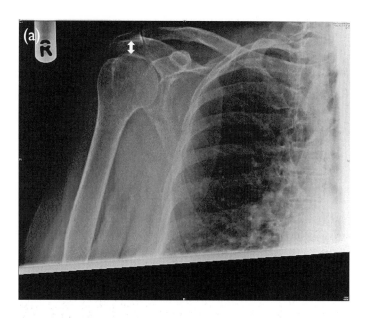

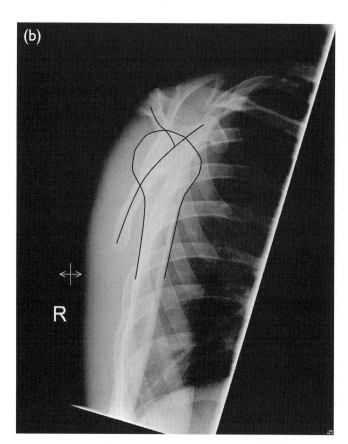

Fig. 8.23 (a) AP view of the shoulder showing the acromiohumeral distance, which should be ≥7 mm (arrow). (b) Lateral scapula view: the humeral head should lie in the middle of the 'Y'.

IMAGING

Plain films of the arm

Shoulder

Indications
Trauma, shoulder pain to look for soft-tissue calcification, arthritis.

Technique
Standard views of the shoulder are AP (anteroposterior), axial and lateral scapula.

Weight-bearing views of the AC joints can be performed and a dedicated clavicular view.

Findings
- A thin radiolucent shadow called vacuum phenomenon can be seen in the shoulder joint (Fig. 8.23).
- The humeral head ossification centres.
- Secondary ossification centres of the acromion process.
- The acromiohumeral distance should be <7 mm.
- The rotator cuff (Fig. 8.24).
- Additional views of the AC joint with weight bearing – the glenoid labrum.

On an axial view orientation can be obtained by observing the coracoid process, which lies more anterior. When

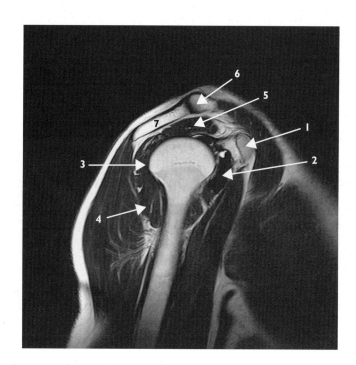

Fig. 8.24 MRI: oblique sagittal image of the rotator cuff muscles. The muscles should appear like a hair on the head around the humeral head. There should not be any gaps. The coracoid process (1) helps ascertain which is anterior. Note: the subscapularis (2) and infraspinatus (3), teres minor (4) and supraspinatus (5) muscles. Clavicle (6) and acromion (7).

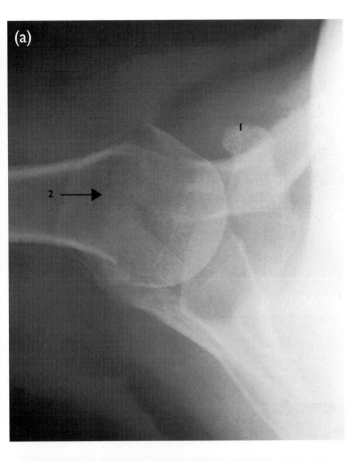

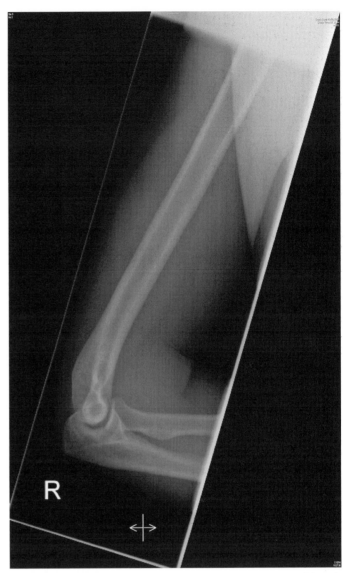

Fig. 8.26 Radiograph of the humerus, lateral view.

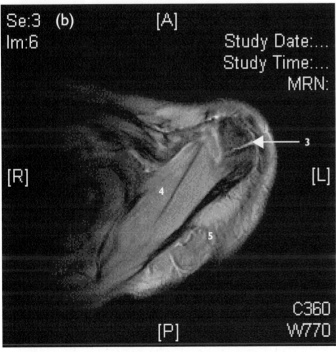

Fig. 8.25 (a) A standard axial image of the shoulder: the coracoid process (1) anteriorly. Views in this position may be limited by the patient being able to abduct the arm. An os acromiale is shown (2). (b) Axial MRI of the shoulder showing an os acromiale (3). Supraspinatus (4) and infraspinatus (5).

assessing for shoulder dislocation two views should be obtained: an AP and either an axial or a lateral scapula. An axial view may not be possible if the patient is unable to abduct the arm (Fig. 8.25).

Observe the normal variant of an os acromiale.

The humerus

Technique

AP and lateral views should include both ends of the humerus and the joints (Fig. 8.26).

Findings

- There may normally be lucency in the greater tuberosity of the humerus.
- There may be some irregularity in proximal humerus due to deltoid insertion.

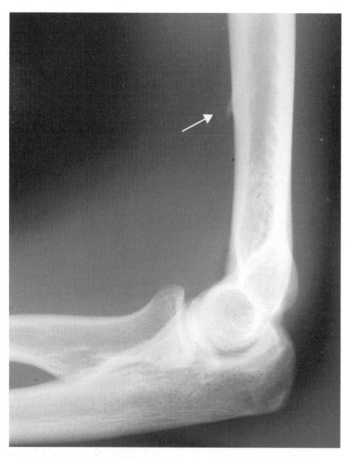

Fig. 8.27 Lateral radiograph of the elbow. A spur (arrow) is noted which points towards the elbow joint.

- A supracondylar spur: usually points towards the joint. The differential is an osteochondroma which points away from the joint (Fig. 8.27).
- On the lateral elbow the anterior humeral line and the midradial line should pass through the middle third of the capitellum.

Elbow and forearm

Indications
Trauma.

Findings

- Both ends of the joint should be included, i.e. the elbow and wrist joint, because a fracture on the end of the radius is associated with a distal ulnar fracture.
- Images should always be taken in two planes, ideally orthogonal to show displacement (Fig. 8.28).

Wrist

Technique
- Standard views of the wrist are lateral and AP. Scaphoid views are taken when suspected scaphoid fracture, i.e.

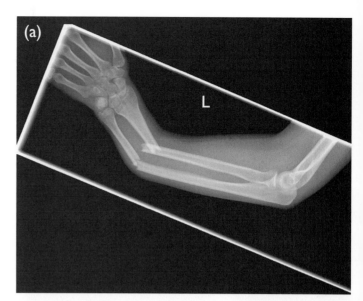

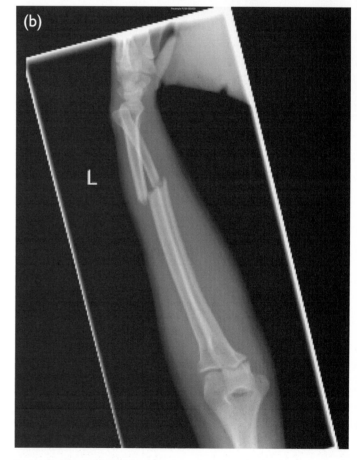

Fig. 8.28 Radiographs: (a) AP view of the forearm and (b) lateral view of the forearm showing a fracture of the radius and the ulna.

anatomical snuffbox tenderness. These are dedicated views of the carpus with ulnar deviation.
- Ball catcher's view: this is good for early osteoarthritis (Fig. 8.29).

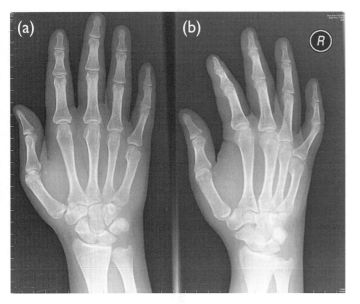

Fig. 8.29 This shows a standard AP: (a) view of the hand and a ball catcher's view; the ball catcher's view is useful for arthritis.

Findings

- The ulnar bone does not articulate with the wrist. The triangular fibrocartilage complex separates the ulnar bone from the carpus.
- The pronator quadratus fat pad is seen anterior to the radius and bulging of this indicates a fracture (see Fig. 8.5b).
- The radius, lunate and capitate should be aligned on the lateral view.
- Triquetral fractures are best seen on the lateral view as a posterior bone fragment.
- On a lateral wrist view the radius, lunate and capitate should all be aligned (Fig. 8.30).

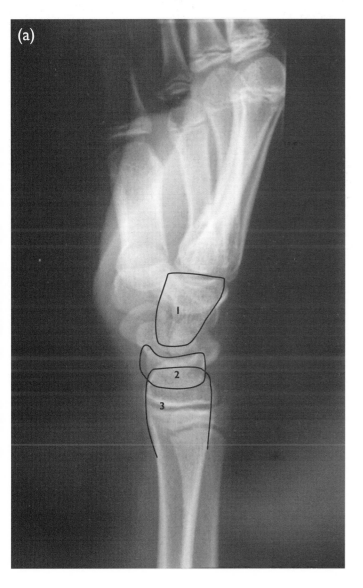

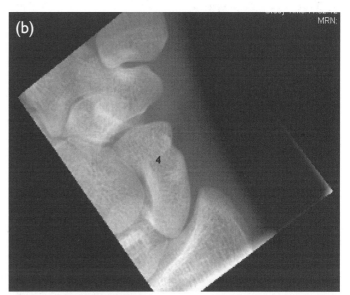

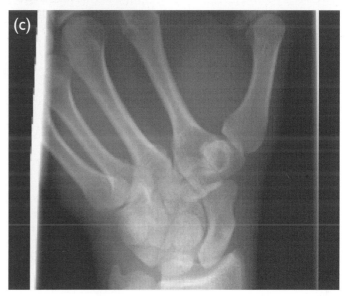

Fig. 8.30 (a,b) Lateral wrist radiograph: the capitate (1), lunate (2) and radius (3) should be in alignment as shown. (c) Scaphoid (4) angled views — one zoomed.

The carpal tunnel

- The flexor retinaculum attaches to the pisiform, hook of hamate, scaphoid bone and trapezium. The median nerve runs through the carpal tunnel. The median nerve supplies the thenar eminence. Patients with carpal tunnel syndrome present with tingling in the fingers of the median nerve distribution, i.e. thumb to radial side of ring finger.
- MRI is the best modality at assessing the carpal tunnel with thin axial images (Fig. 8.31).
- The median nerve lies superficial to the flexor tendons in the canal and deep to the transverse ligaments. Pathology in the canal can lead to sensory symptoms in the median nerve distribution.
- The median nerve normally is elliptical in shape and of higher signal than the tendons (Fig. 8.32).
- The ulnar nerve runs in Guyon's canal, a space at the level of the pisiform between the flexor retinaculum and the volar carpal ligament. Lesions proximal or within the canal can lead to sensory symptoms in the distribution of the ulnar nerve.

Ultrasound of the shoulder

Indication
Mainly one to assess the rotator cuff.

Technique
- Linear-array high-resolution ultrasound.
- For superficial soft tissues.
- Dynamic scanning to assess tendon of long head of biceps for dislocation.

Findings
The superficial supraspinatus tendon is usually convex and flattening or a concave portion implies a tear. Dynamic studies of the shoulder can easily be performed with ultrasound (Fig. 8.33).

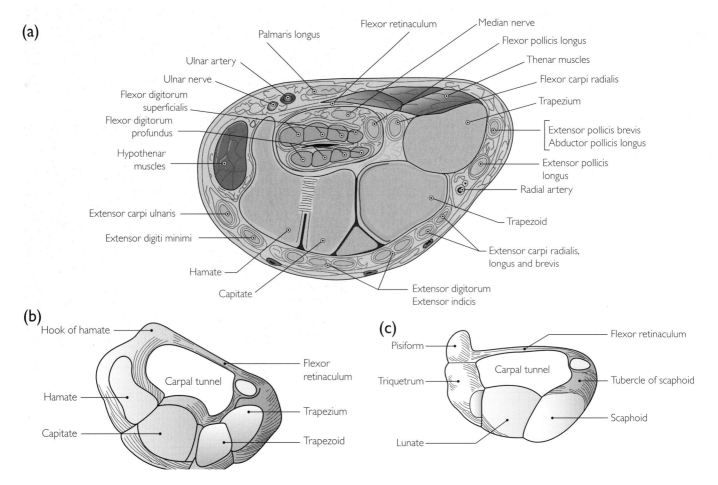

Fig. 8.31 Diagram of the carpal tunnel: (a) contents of carpal tunnel; (b) distal row; (c) proximal row.

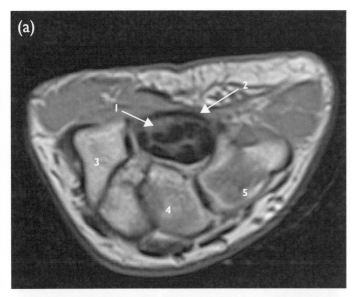

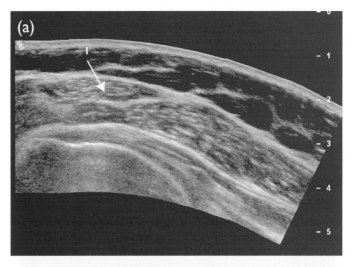

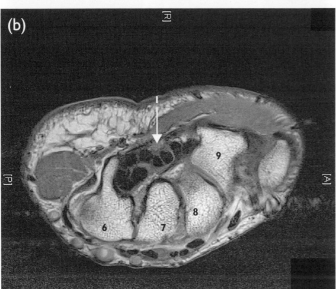

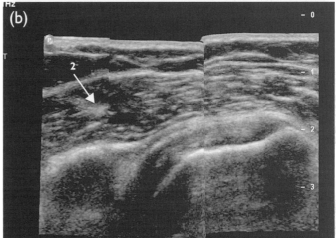

Fig. 8.32 MRI of the carpal tunnel: (a) proximal row; (b) distal row. The median nerve (1) is identified anteriorly underneath the flexor retinaculum (2). There is a slightly increased signal oval structure. The flexor tendons are seen glued to this. The pisiform bone (3) is a triangular bone. Lunate (4), scaphoid (5), hamate (6), capitate (7), trapezoid (8) and trapezium (9).

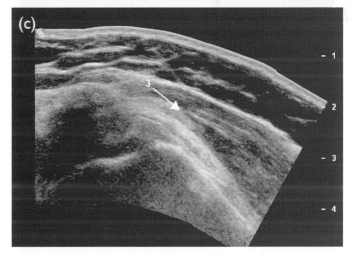

Fig. 8.33 Ultrasound of the shoulder: (a) infraspinatus, (b) subscapularis and (c) supraspinatus. Ultrasound demonstrates the infraspinatus (1), subscapularis (2) and supraspinatus (3) muscles and their insertions.

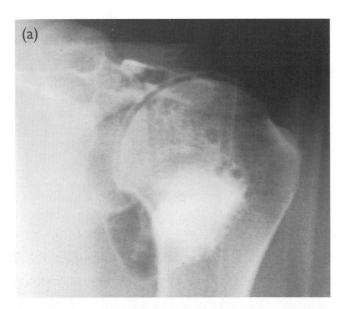

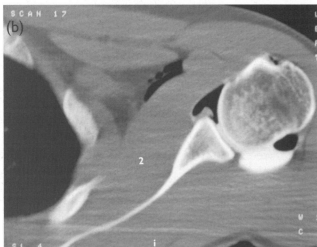

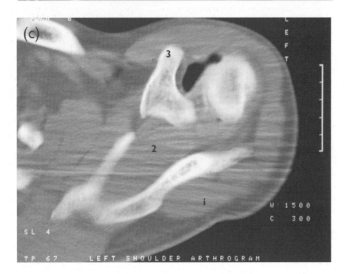

Fig. 8.34 (a) Conventional arthrogram; (b, c) CT arthrogram. Infra-spinatus (1), supraspinatus (2), coracoid (3). The arthrogram is done under fluoroscopy. CT arthrograms are performed when MRI is not possible. This is rare. Supraspinatus is within the V shape of the scapula (c) and infraspinatous lies below the scapula. Note the coracoid (3), projecting anteriorly like a thumb.

CT and MRI of the shoulder

Indications
Rotator cuff disease.

Technique
* The planes used in MRI are oblique coronal, oblique sagittal and axial; MR arthrography is used to assess the glenoid labrum by injecting very dilute into the gleno-humeral joint.
* CT arthrography was formerly used to assess the labrum, but has been superseded by MRI (Fig. 8.34).

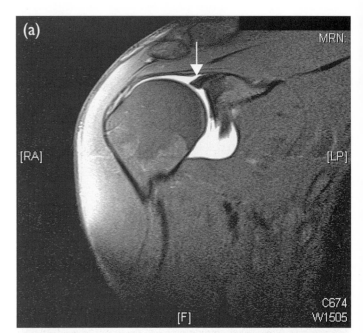

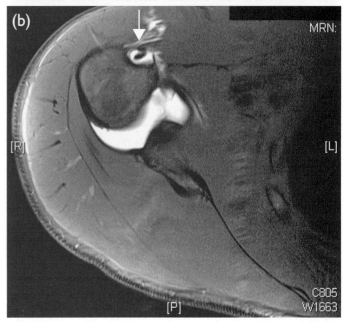

Fig. 8.35 MRI arthrogram of the shoulder in two planes: (a) coronal and (b) axial. The long head of the biceps tendon runs through the joint (arrow). The enhanced synovial sheath of biceps is seen as high signal around the biceps tendon in the bicipital groove.

Shoulder arthrogram

Indications

As part of MR arthrography or CT arthrography to assess the glenoid labrum. Shoulder arthrography is still performed in the setting of MRI or rarely CT (Fig. 8.35).

Technique

- A 22G short-bevel lumbar puncture needle.
- The needle is placed 1 cm below and lateral to the coracoid process under fluoroscopic screening.
- For MRI very dilute gadolinium is used (Fig. 8.36).

Findings

- The long head of biceps normally runs through the capsule (Fig. 8.37).
- The supraspinatus tendon is of low signal and inserts into the greater tuberosity of the humerus. The muscle runs horizontally on the oblique coronal view helping to identify it from the infraspinatus muscle which runs upward obliquely (Fig. 8.38).
- The supraspinatus tendon is also visualized on the oblique sagittal view when the muscle and tendons are seen as 'hair covering a head' – the head being the humeral head. On the oblique sagittal view there should

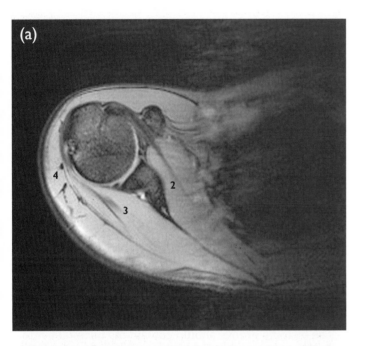

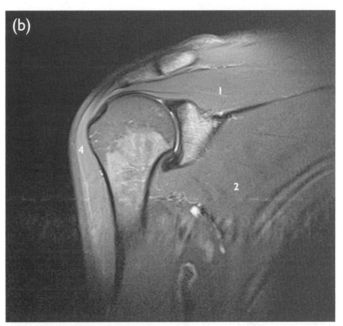

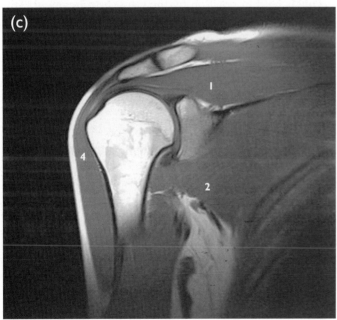

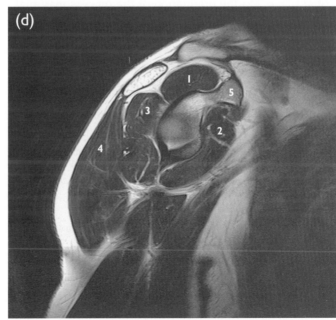

Fig. 8.36 MRI of the shoulder: all three planes. (a) Axial. (b) Oblique coronal. (c) Oblique coronal. (d) Oblique sagittal. Note the coracoid process projecting anteriorly on the oblique sagittal view aiding orientation. Supraspinatus (1), subscapularis (2), infraspinatus (3), deltoid (4) and coracoid (5).

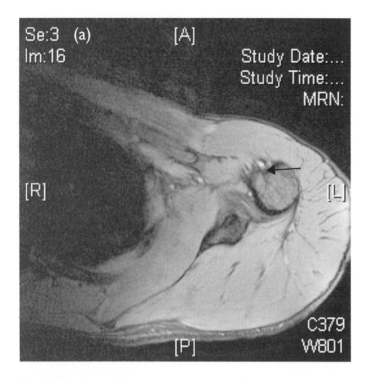

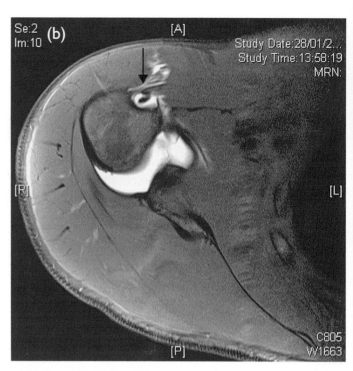

Fig. 8.37 (a) Axial T2-weighted and (b) axial T1-weighted arthrogram of the shoulder. The long head of the biceps tendon (arrow) lies in the bicipital groove on (a) and the enhanced synovial sheath of biceps is seen as high signal around the biceps tendon in the bicipital groove (b) (arrow).

be no large gaps in the muscle overlying the humerus. This could indicate a tear (Fig. 8.39).

- The AC joint is seen on the oblique coronal plane. The shape of the acromion process is seen on the oblique sagittal plane and the orientation of the process may make supraspinatus impingement more likely (Fig. 8.40).
- The subacromial subdeltoid bursae lie under the acromion process. This does not normally communicate with the shoulder joint so fluid in the bursa implies a tear in the rotator cuff. It is easiest to see fluid in the bursa on oblique coronal imaging.
- The glenoid labrum is a low-signal structure best seen on axial grade echo T2 images. There are many anatomical variations in the glenoid labrum and adjacent capsule that can simulate a tear. The most common configuration is a triangular anterior labrum (45%) and posterior labrum (73%). The labrum can be rounded and even absent (Fig. 8.41).
- There is normally a cleft between the anterior labrum and the articular cartilage. The middle glenohumeral ligament can also cause confusion with a tear when it runs close to the anterior labrum called a Burford complex.
- The magic angle is 55°. This may give the impression of tears in the rotator cuff. This occurs when tendons are oriented 55° to the magnetic field and causes intermediate signal intensity on T1 weighting or proton density that does not increase on T2 weighting. This is an area

seen 1 cm proximal to the distal insertion of the supraspinatus tendon of intermediate signal intensity which does not increase signal on T2 weighting.

- The bicipital groove should contain the bicipital tendon. This is held in position by the transverse ligament. This is best seen on the axial view. The long head of biceps usually communicates with the shoulder joints and therefore fluid may be seen around it. The long head of biceps tendon runs through the shoulder joint taking a synovial sleeve with it (Fig. 8.42).
- The shape of the acromion process may affect whether impingement occurs.
- The subdeltoid fat plane must be seen.
- Bursae: the subacromial subdeltoid bursae do not normally communicate with the shoulder joint, so if fluid is seen in bursae this implicates a rotator cuff tear.
- On the most cranial axial images the AC joint is seen and the curved broad shape of the acromion can be appreciated.
- On the axial plane images the supraspinatus muscle lies within the V shape of the scapular, i.e. above the spine. On the most cranial images the supraspinatus can be seen running obliquely and horizontally into the greater tuberosity. Below the V of the scapular spine the muscle seen is infraspinatus. Teres minor lies inferior to this.
- At the level of the spine the coracoid process is seen projecting anteriorly on axial imaging.

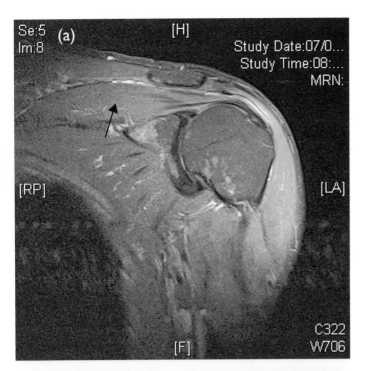

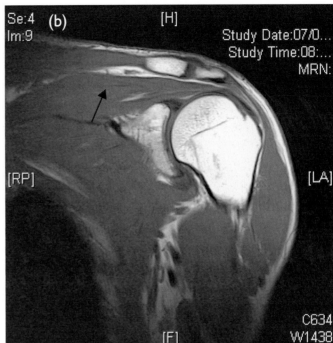

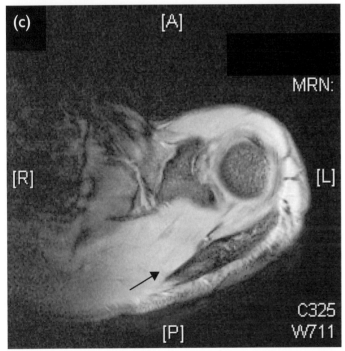

Fig. 8.38 (a) Coronal oblique STIR. (b) Coronal oblique T1 weighted. The coraroid process projects anteriorly. (c) GE gradient echo T2-weighted axial MRI which demonstrated the normal supraspinatus muscle (arrows). Supraspinatus on oblique coronal runs horizontally to attach to the greater tuberosity. T1 is good for the anatomy and the STIR would show abnormal fluid and a tear.

- On the axial plane a defect in the humeral head from a dislocation is seen. In an anterior dislocation a Hill–Sachs deformity is seen with a bony defect posteriorly in the most superior humerus. Narrowing can normally occur posteriorly at the level of the surgical neck normally (Fig. 8.44).
- Deltoid muscle can be seen axially covering the upper arm.

- The amount of red and yellow marrow in the long bones varies, which can cause marked variation in the marrow signal on MRI in the humerus. With age there is generally conversion of red marrow to yellow marrow. The marrow variation can mimic marrow abnormalities and, by comparing with the opposite shoulder, if in doubt this can be differentiated from pathology because marrow patterns are symmetrical (Fig. 8.45).

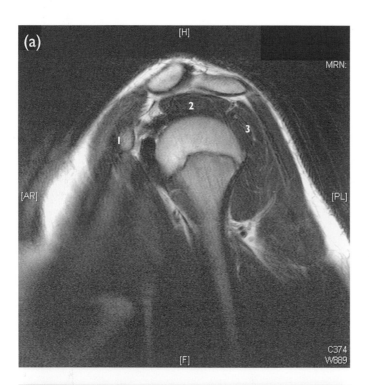

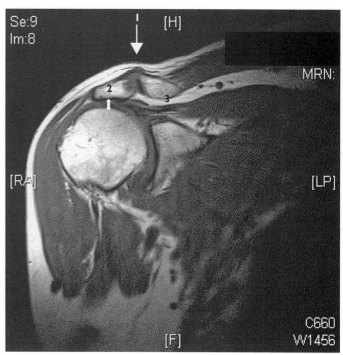

Fig. 8.40 MRI: oblique coronal showing acromioclavicular joint (1). (2) Characteristic boomerang shape of the acromion and clavicle (3). The acromiohumeral distance should be ≥7 mm (double-ended arrow).

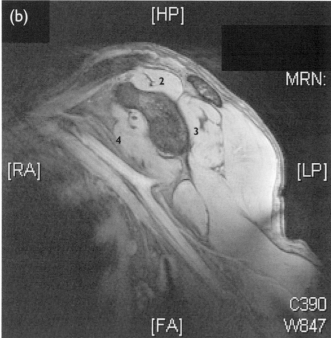

Fig. 8.39 MRI: (a) T1-weighted oblique sagittal views and (b) GE T2-weighted oblique sagittal views. On the oblique sagittal view of the shoulder the supraspinatus muscle is seen superiorly. There should be no defects to suggest any tears around the humeral head. Coracoid (1), supraspinatus (2), infraspinatus (3) and subscapularis (4).

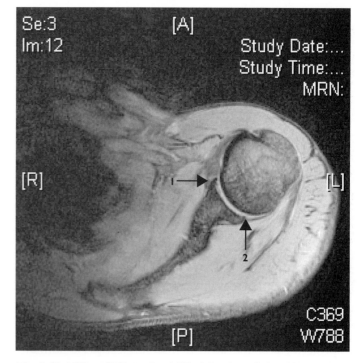

Fig. 8.41 MRI axial T2-weighted GE of the glenoid shows the anterior labrum (1) and the posterior labrum (2). The labrum has many normal variations. MR arthrography shows the labrum to better advantage.

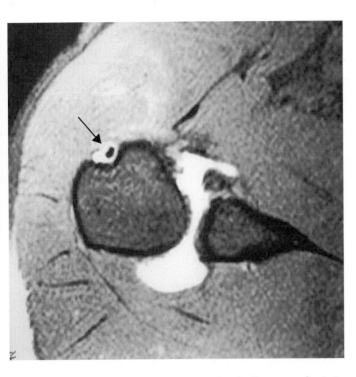

Fig. 8.42 MR arthrogram showing the long head of biceps tendon in its synovial sheath in the bicipital groove (arrow).

- Vacuum phenomenon of air in the shoulder joint can mimic chondrocalcinosis.
- Always locate the coraroid process in all three planes. This aids in orientation, as the coracoid is always anterior. It looks like a 'thumb' projecting anteriorly.
- On the oblique coronal images, the clavicle is more medial than the acromion. If a line is drawn vertically to bisect the humeral head, the clavicle lies medial to the line and the acromion lies lateral to the line.

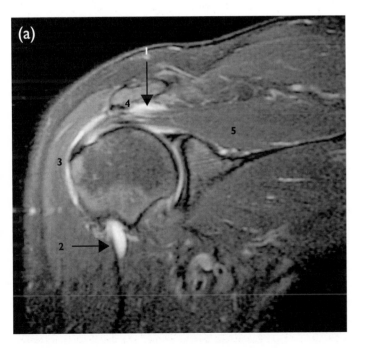
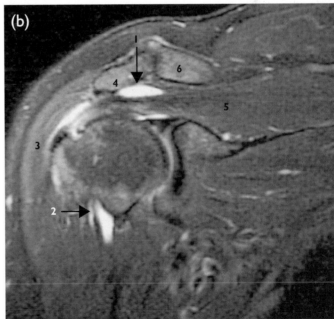

Fig. 8.43 MRI arthrogram: STIR oblique coronal images (a) more posterior and (b) through acromioclavicular joint. It shows fluid in the subacromial subdeltoid bursa, which is abnormal indicating a tear in supraspinatus (1). Long head of the biceps tendon in the intertubercular groove (2), deltoid (3), acromion (4), supraspinatus (5) and clavicle (6).

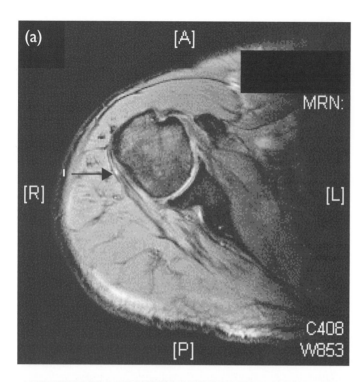

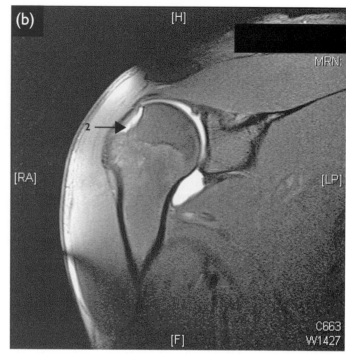

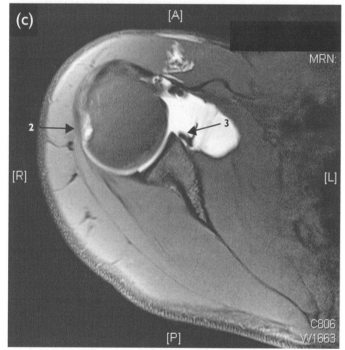

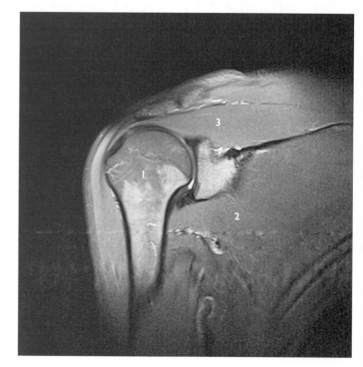

Fig. 8.44 (a) Axial GE T2-weighted normal right shoulder, (b) MRI arthrogram, oblique coronal and (c) MRI arthrogram, axial images of the right shoulder in an abnormal shoulder. (a) (1) shows the normal posterior humerus with a slight normal narrowing seen towards the neck posteriorly. (b,c) An abnormal defect (2) in the superior and posterior humerus called a Hill–Sachs deformity seen after recurrent dislocation. (c) There is also a tear to the anterior labrum associated with recurrent dislocation called Bankart's abnormality (3).

Fig. 8.45 MRI: oblique coronal STIR image of the humerus showing variation in marrow signal (1). Subscapularis (2) and supraspinatus (3).

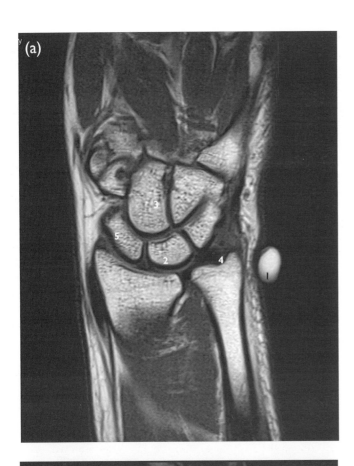

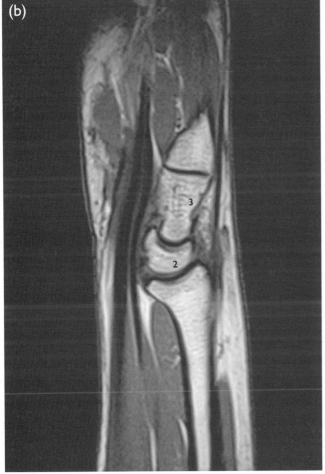

MR of the wrist

Indications
Instability, wrist pain, avascular necrosis, TFCC, carpal tunnel, ligament and tendon injuries.

Technique
- A small field of view with a dedicated wrist coil.
- Usually three orthogonal planes are used: coronal, sagittal and axial.
- A mixture of T1, STIR and T2, either fast T2 or gradient echo to speed things up, is used (Fig. 8.46).
- Wrist arthrography using dilute gadolinium may help visualize the ligaments.

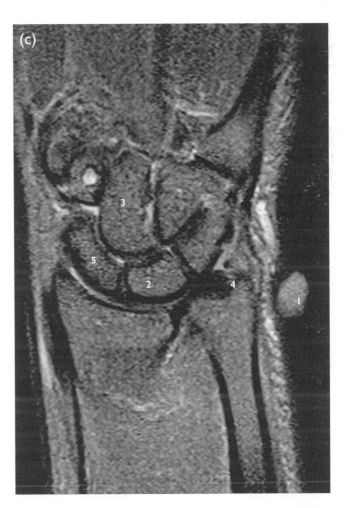

Fig. 8.46 MRI wrist three planes: (a) T1-weighted coronal; (b) T1-weighted sagittal; and (C) coronal STIR. The bright marker is a cod liver oil capsule used to mark abnormalities (1). Lunate (2), capitate (3), TFCC (4) and scaphoid (5).

Findings

- The carpal bones are well seen on coronal T1 and STIR.
- The ligaments supporting the wrist and the triangular fibrocartilage complex are well seen on coronal gradient echo T2-weighted imaging.
- The TFCC and the lunotriquetral and scapholunate ligaments are well seen on coronal imaging (Fig. 8.47).
- The TFCC is low signal on MR.
- The scapholunate ligament is normally triangular in 90% and linear in 10%.
- The lunotriquetral ligament is also linear or triangular and may be of intermediate signal in asymptomatic people.

The hand

- The thenar eminence comprises abductor pollicis brevis, flexor pollicis brevis and opponens pollicis and is supplied by the median nerve.

- The hypothenar eminence consists of abductor digiti minim, flexor digiti minim and opponens digiti minimi. It is supplied by the ulnar nerve.

MRI of the brachial plexus

Indications

This is best visualized with MRI.

Technique

- The nerves are best seen on coronal T1-weighted and STIR images.
- Gadolinium can be helpful in subtle cases or to differentiate fibrosis and scarring from tumour recurrence. Additional series are axial T2-weighted and sagittal T1-weighted images. The sagittal plane enables the nerves to be followed from the neural exit foramina in the cervical spine to the axilla (Fig. 8.48).

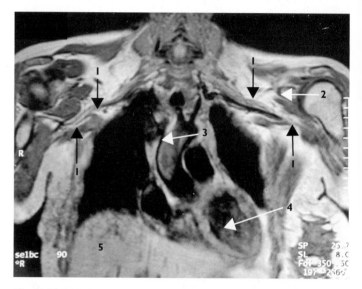

Fig. 8.48 MRI T1-weighted image of brachial plexus showing the nerve roots bilaterally (1). Coracoid process (2), ascending aorta (3), left ventricle (4) and liver (5).

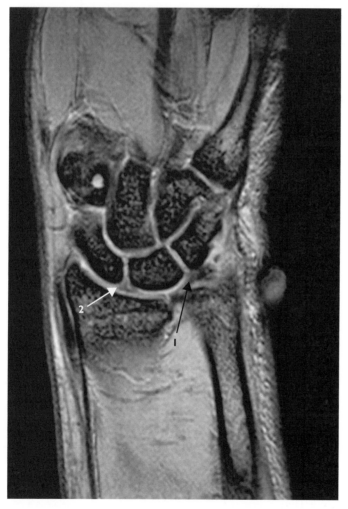

Fig. 8.47 MRI: coronal GE T2-weighted image showing the TFCC (1) and scapholunate ligament (2).

Findings

- Nerve roots from C5 to T1 emerge between scalene muscles anterior and medius. These muscles arise from anterior to the cervical spine (Fig. 8.49).
- The roots become trunks, which then become cords.
- The nerves are closely related to the subclavian vein.
- The nerves are usually low signal on all sequences.
- Observe for asymmetry between the two sides.
- Use T1 to assess for anatomy and STIR to look for pathology.

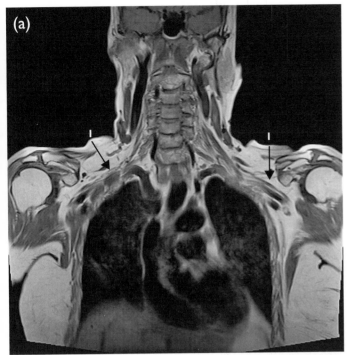

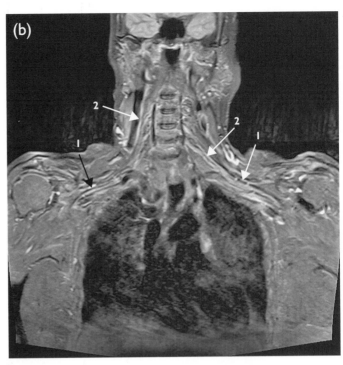

Fig. 8.49 MRI brachial plexus: (a) T1-weighted coronal and (b) STIR coronal images. The T1-weighted images show the anatomy and the STIR images the pathology in the brachial plexus. Cords (1) and trunks (2) of the brachial plexus. The nerves follow the axillary and subclavian vessels.

Angiography

Indications

Brachial angiography is used in cardiac day cases or when femoral cathetherization is precluded. Thoracic outlet syndromes or subclavian steal syndromes may warrant this, or arteriovenous malformations warranting embolization,

It is slightly more difficult than femoral angiography and has an increased incidence of complications. Antispasmodics are required (Fig. 8.50).

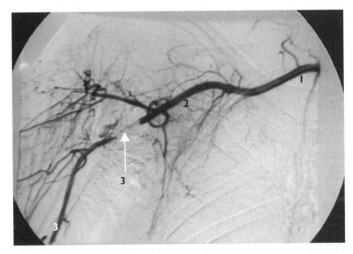

Fig. 8.50 Arm angiogram: (1) subclavian artery, (2) axillary artery and (3) brachial artery. Occlusion in axillary artery (3).

CASES

Case 8.1

A patient presents with shoulder pain after a fall. An AP and an axial shoulder view are performed initially. A plain shoulder AP and lateral scapular view are performed. Two views are required for alignment.

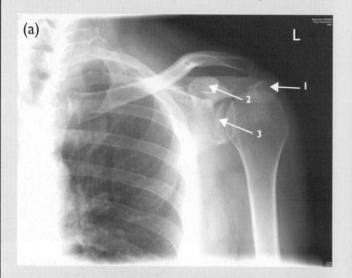

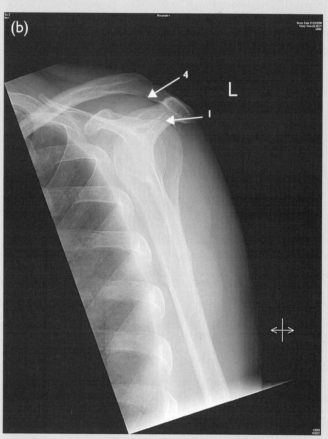

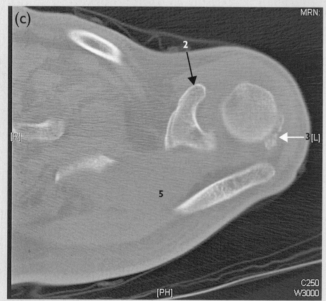

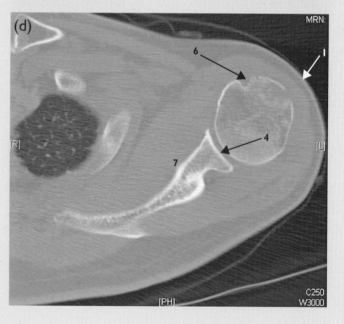

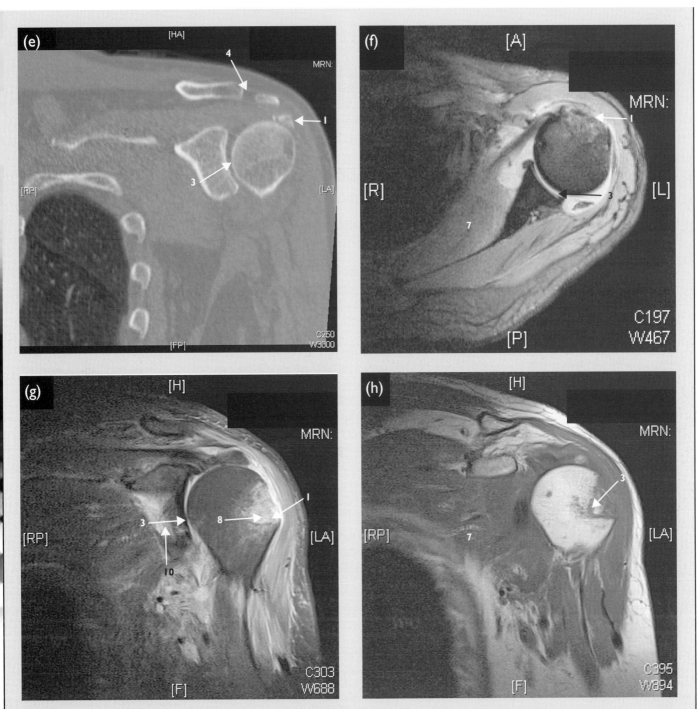

Fig. 8.51 Fracture dislocation of the greater tuberosity: (a) AP view of the shoulder shows a 'light-bulb' appearance to the humeral head, which appears very round suggesting a dislocation and bony fragments. (b) Lateral scapular view showing bony fragments but no dislocation. Two views are always required to assess for dislocation and displacement of bone fragments. (c,d) Axial and (e) coronal reconstructed CT images showing the fracture of the greater tuberosity and the bone fragments. CT shows the bone fragments to advantage. (f) Axial T2-weighted MRI. (g) Coronal STIR MRI. (h) Coronal T1-weighted MRI showing the fracture (1). MRI shows the extensive oedema in the humerus (8) and glenoid (9). It shows bone bruising to advantage and soft tissue trauma. Coracoid process (2) glenohumeral joint (3), acromioclavicular joint (4), supraspinatus (5), bicipital groove (6) and subscapularis (7).

The plain AP shows a defect over the greater tuberosity of the humerus and some bony fragments. The lateral scapular view shows no dislocation. The humeral head should lie in the centre of the 'Y'.

A CT of the shoulder in the axial and coronal planes shows some bony fragments adjacent to the humerus in the glenohumeral joint. Note orientation is obtained by looking for the coracoid pointing anteriorly. The position is well seen on the coronal CT. CT shows the bony fragments to advantage whereas MRI is the modality of choice for soft-tissue injury. The normal intertubercular groove causes a notch anteriorly.

MRI shoulder needs a system of interpretation:
- Start with the oblique coronal T1W images. Identify the coracoid process as the most anterior image. It is then a matter of working more posteriorly. Identify subscapularis anterior to the scapula.
- Work backwards.
- Identify the glenohumeral joint.
- Find the acromiohumeral joint. Is it hypertrophied or impinging on the subscapularis tendon?
- Look at the oblique coronal STIR images. Is there any fluid in the subacromial subdeltoid bursa?
- Are the supraspinatus muscle and tendon intact?
- Look at the axial images. Identify the coracoid anteriorly.
- Then identify the acromion with its boomerang shape superiorly.
- Find the supraspinatus muscle coursing above the spine of the scapula and parallel to the spine of the scapula.
- The infraspinatus is seen below the spine.
- Then identify the glenohumeral joint and the labrum.
- On the third series (not shown) the oblique sagittal finds the coracoid anteriorly. Then find the AC joint. The humeral head should be viewed as a head of hair without any gaps or bald patches.
- On this case look at oblique coronal view first and look from anterior to posterior. The coracoid lies anteriorly and locates the anterior aspect of the shoulder. On the oblique coronal view supraspinatus runs in a true horizontal direction whereas infraspinatus and subscapularis run upwards obliquely.
- On oblique coronal STIR and TIW images, a large defect is seen at the greater tuberosity of the humerus. The axial images show that the labrum and the posterior labrum are abnormal.

Diagnosis

Fracture of the glenoid labrum, abnormal posterior labrum.

The idealized report for the shoulder MRI reads: MR confirms the fracture of the greater tuberosity of the humerus where there is large fracture with bony fragments better seen on the CT and extensive surrounding oedema. There is extensive soft-tissue oedema anteriorly in the subscapularis muscle, in deltoid muscle and inferior to the glenohumeral joint and also within the glenoid itself.

Case 8.2

A patient presents with a history of recurrent dislocation. An MRI arthrogram is performed to show the labrum.

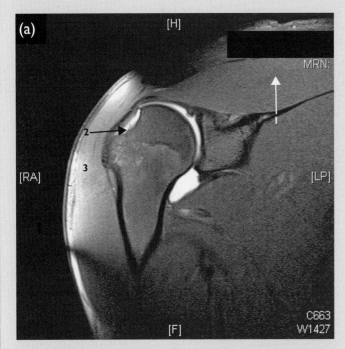 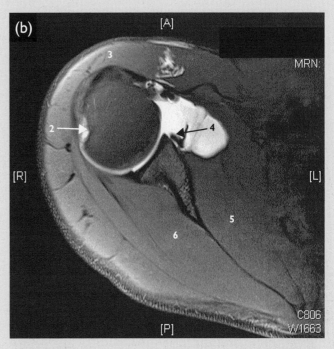

Fig. 8.52 Hill–Sachs/Bankart's: MRI arthrogram. (a) Oblique coronal and (b) axial TI images. (1) Supraspinatus and (2) Hill–Sachs defect in posterior superior humeral head. It is important to check that the defect is on the most superior images in the humeral head. Deltoid muscle (3), Bankart's defect in the glenoid labrum (4), infraspinatus (5) and subscapularis (6).

Findings on this MRI arthrogram

- Use the system.
- Look at the oblique coronal. The supraspinatus muscle is intact.
- There is a defect in the humeral head posteriorly, not to be confused with the slight impression that can be seen in the head at the junction with the neck.
- The axial view shows a defect in the upper posterior humeral head consistent with a Hill–Sachs deformity. There is a defect in the anterior glenoid, indicating Bankart's lesion. The humerus dislocates anteriorly and medially, and the posterior humerus impacts on the anterior glenoid.

Diagnosis

Hill–Sachs and Bankart's abnormality.

Case 8.3

A patient presents after a fall landing on the elbow, which is painful.

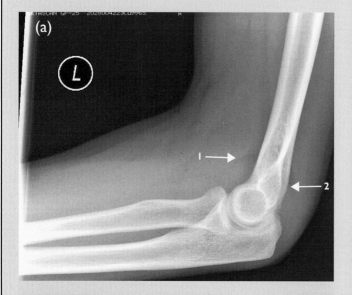

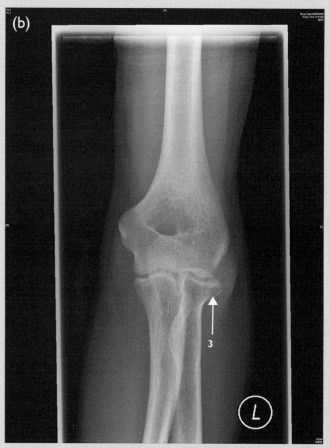

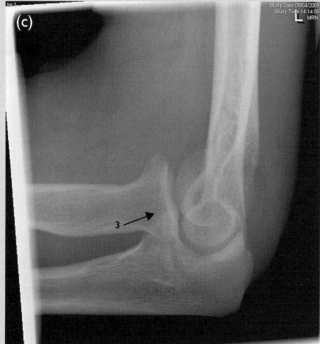

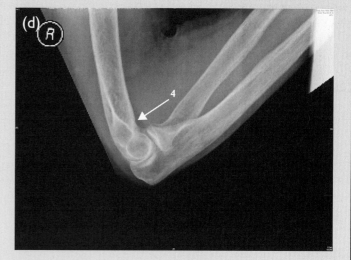

Fig. 8.54 Radial head fracture: (a) lateral elbow radiograph shows raised anterior (1) and posterior fat pads (2). (b) AP view of the elbow suggesting a fracture of the radial head (3). (c) Radial head view confirming a fracture (3). (d) Normal elbow with normal anterior fat pad (4).

A lateral film is taken. It is normal to have a small anterior fat pad but not an elevated one as here. In addition there is a small posterior fat pad which is abnormal. If fat pads are present that are abnormal, commonly there may be an associated radial head fracture. This is seen here and on the radial head view.

9 Imaging of the lower limb

RADIOLOGICAL ANATOMY

Pelvis

Bones

- The pelvis is made of the innominate bone, sacrum and coccyx, which form a bony ring. The innominate bone comprises the ischium, pubis and ilium (Fig. 9.1). The pelvis is a closed ring and trauma to one side of the ring may be associated with an injury to the opposite side. Imaging in trauma should include the whole of the pelvic ring.
- At birth the triradiate cartilage lies between the ischium, pubis and ilium, which fuse in adult life to form the acetabulum.

- The acetabulum articulates with the femur at the hip joint. It is widened by the acetabular fibrocartilaginous labrum.
- The obturator foramen lies anteriorly and is related to the obturator externus muscle externally and the obturator internus muscle internally. It is bound by the pubic rami and ischium (Fig. 9.1c)
- The greater sciatic foramen lies posteriorly between the sacrum and ischial spines.
- The iliopectineal line is a smooth line around the inner surface of the pelvis separating the true pelvis and the false pelvis.

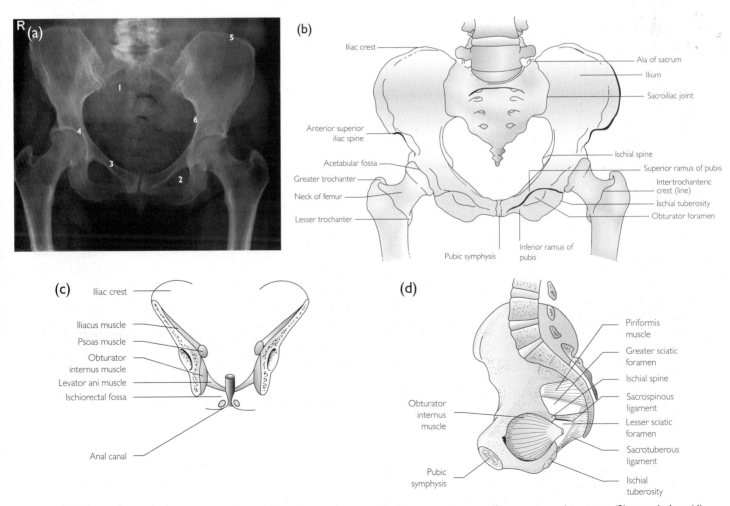

Fig. 9.1 (a) Pelvic radiograph: the sacrum and sacral foramina can be seen (1). Obturator foramen (2), superior pubic ramus (3), acetabulum (4), iliac crest (5) and iliopectineal line (6). (b) Diagram of pelvis in coronal plane. (c) Diagram of pelvic muscles in coronal plane. (d) Diagram of pelvis in sagittal plane.

Pelvic muscles

- The obturator internus muscle forms the pelvic side wall which is important for staging cancer (Fig. 9.2). The muscle passes through the lesser sciatic foramen and inserts into the greater trochanter of the femur.
- The pectineus is the most anterior muscle arising from the superior pubic ramus and attaches to the greater trochanter of the femur (Fig. 9.3a).
- The piriformis muscle is a long muscle arising from S2–4, passing through the greater sciatic foramen and inserting into the greater trochanter of the femur. It is involved in vascular disorders in the gluteal region.
- The sartorius muscle arises from the anterosuperior iliac spine and runs down across the thigh to insert into the medial tibial shaft. It stands out as the most anterior muscle at the top of the thigh (Fig. 9.3b).
- The iliopsoas muscle can be identified due to the fatty tendons centrally (Fig. 9.3b). It inserts into the lesser trochanter of the femur.
- The gluteal muscles form the buttock arising from the ilium and inserting into the greater trochanter of the femur or iliotibial tract.
- There are differences between the male and female pelvis (see Box 9.1).

Box 9.1 Differences between the male and female pelvis

Male pelvis	Female pelvis
Heart shape	Oval shape
Narrower pubic arch	Wider pubic arch
Shorter ala of the sacrum	Wider ala of the sacrum
Narrow pelvic brim	Wider pelvic brim

Pelvimetry

The true conjugate is the pelvic inlet. This is formed from the sacral promontory to the back of the symphysis pubis (Fig. 9.4). This is assessed for trial of labour.

Femur

- The femur is the strongest bone in the body. It has a hemispherical head that lies within the joint capsule.
- There is a small central depression within the femoral head called the fovea to which the ligamentum teres is attached. A small amount of the blood supply is derived via the fovea from vessels in the ligamentum teres. Most blood, however, comes from the capsule of the hip joint and through the shaft of the femur. A fracture of the neck of the femur may disrupt the blood supply via the neck and result in avascular necrosis of the femoral head. Fractures of the neck of femur may be difficult to evaluate. The trabecular pattern of the neck of the femur can aid diagnosis of a subtle fracture (Fig. 9.5).
- The mediolateral angle that the neck forms with the femoral shaft is 160° at birth decreasing to 125° on average in the adult.
- The neck of the femur is normally anteverted with respect to the shaft by 10° in the adult. This angle is greater in the non-weight-bearing neonate.
- The greater and lesser trochanters lie at the junction with the shaft and are separated by the intertrochanteric line. The hip joint capsule attaches to this line anteriorly.
- Inferiorly are the femoral condyles. On the lateral femoral condyle is a groove for the popliteus tendon insertion.

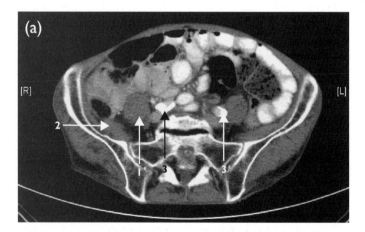

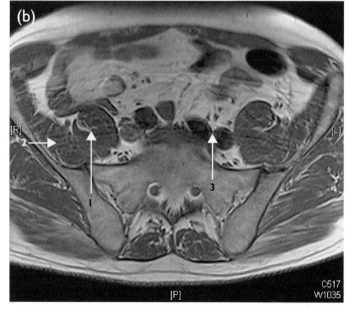

Fig. 9.2 (a) CT axial post-contrast and (b) MR axial T1-weighted of the pelvis. Iliopsoas is recognized by the fatty tendon (1). Iliacus (2) and left common iliac vessels (3).

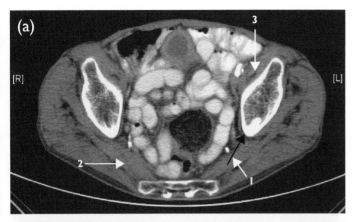

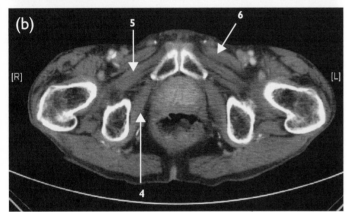

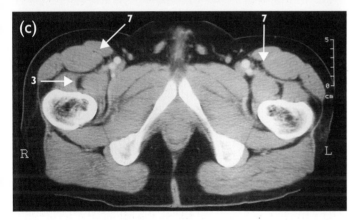

Fig. 9.3 CT of the pelvis: (a) level of greater sciatic foramen. The greater sciatic foramen (1), piriformis (2), iliopsoas with central fatty tendon (3). (b) Level of obturator foramen. Obturator internus (4), obturator externus (5), pectineus seen anteriorly (6), iliopsoas (3) and sartorius (7). (c) CT scan of the pelvis. Axial CT shows sartorius anteriorly in the thigh. The iliopsoas is seen inserting in the lesser trochanter, recognized by the fatty tendon (3).

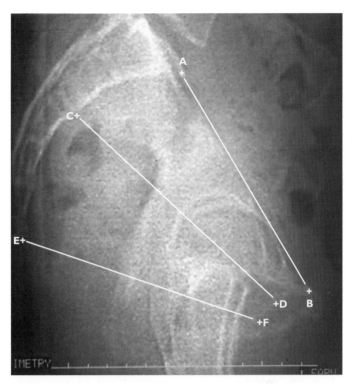

Fig. 9.4 CT pelvimetry: a scanogram is used. The pelvic inlet or AP diameter is the most important thing called the true conjugate, which runs from the sacral promontory to the back of symphysis pubis (A to B).

- The adductor tubercle arises from the medial aspect of the distal femur. The adductor magnus muscle inserts to the tubercle.
- In a child aged 4–7 years the lower femoral epiphysis is irregular.

At birth
- The long bones in the newborn consist radiologically of the diaphyses; with increasing age, the epiphyses appear which then fuse to the diaphyses at puberty. The metaphyses lie at the ends of the diaphyses with the epiphyseal growth plate between the epiphyses and the diaphyses. Various secondary ossification centres also form around bones.
- The femoral epiphysis proximally forms the head, which normally ossifies by age 1 year. Before ossification of the femoral head, hip ultrasound can be performed to assess the acetabulum and the labrum for congenital dislocation of the hip.

Ossification centres of the femur
- The femoral head should ossify between 6 months and 1 year (Fig. 9.6).
- The greater trochanter of the femur should ossify by age 5 years.
- The lesser trochanter should ossify by age 10.

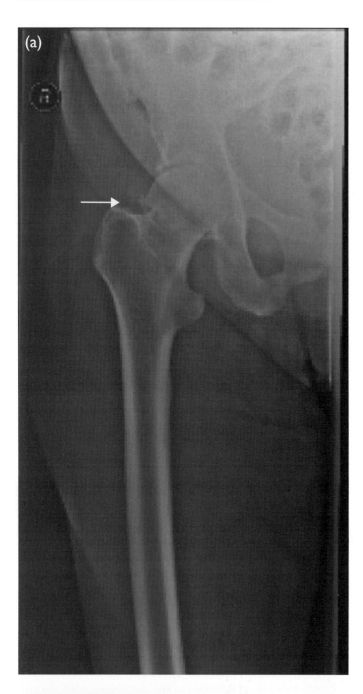

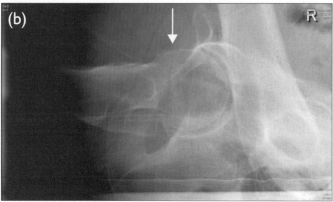

Fig. 9.5 (a) AP and (b) lateral views of the right femoral head and neck. There is a femoral head fracture (arrows) seen on both views.

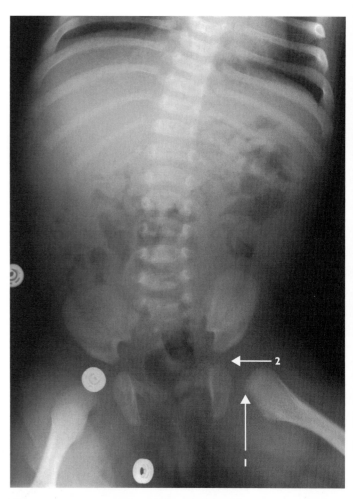

Fig. 9.6 AP pelvis radiograph in infant. Femoral head epiphysis: no femoral head is seen (1), indicating that the child is <1 year old. The triradiate cartilage is demonstrated (2).

Hip joint (Fig. 9.7)

- The hip joint is a synovial ball-and-socket joint.
- The femoral head sits in the acetabulum which is deepened by the labrum.
- The transverse ligament forms the acetabular foramen.
- The ligament of the head, the ligamentum teres, attaches to the pit on the femoral head and then extends inferiorly to attach to the transverse acetabular ligament (Fig. 9.8).
- The fibrous capsule of the hip joint becomes very thick in part forming the iliofemoral ligament.
- In older children Perthes' disease and slipped epiphysis may be encountered so the normal radiological appearance of the hip is important.

The thigh

The thigh is divided into three main muscle compartments (Figs 9.9 and 9.10):

- Anterior: quadriceps – vastus medialis, lateralis, intermedius, rectus femoris and sartorius, and pectineus proximally, and iliopsoas proximally.

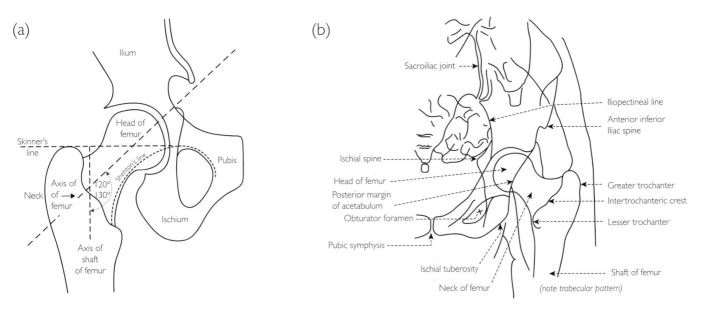

(a)

Ilium

Head of femur

Skinner's line

Neck

Axis of Neck of femur

120° 130°

Shenton's line

Pubis

Ischium

Axis of shaft of femur

(b)

Sacroiliac joint

Iliopectineal line

Anterior inferior Iliac spine

Ischial spine

Head of femur

Posterior margin of acetabulum

Obturator foramen

Greater trochanter

Intertrochanteric crest

Lesser trochanter

Pubic symphysis

Ischial tuberosity

Neck of femur

(note trabecular pattern)

Shaft of femur

Fig. 9.7 Pelvic diagrams showing (a) Shenton's line and (b) the iliopectineal line.

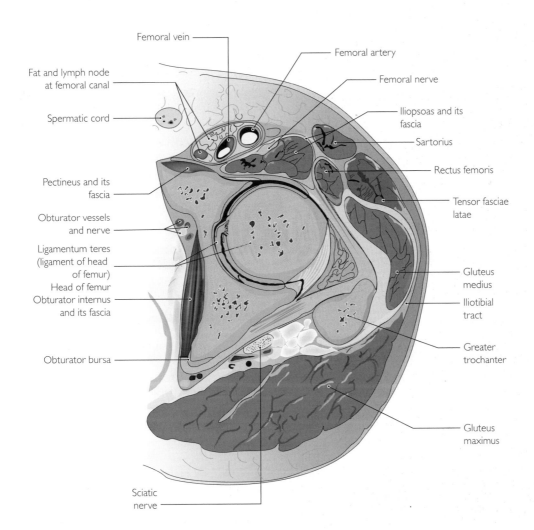

Femoral vein

Femoral artery

Fat and lymph node at femoral canal

Femoral nerve

Spermatic cord

Iliopsoas and its fascia

Sartorius

Pectineus and its fascia

Rectus femoris

Obturator vessels and nerve

Tensor fasciae latae

Ligamentum teres (ligament of head of femur)

Head of femur

Obturator internus and its fascia

Gluteus medius

Iliotibial tract

Greater trochanter

Obturator bursa

Gluteus maximus

Sciatic nerve

Fig. 9.8 Diagram of axial section of the thigh and hip.

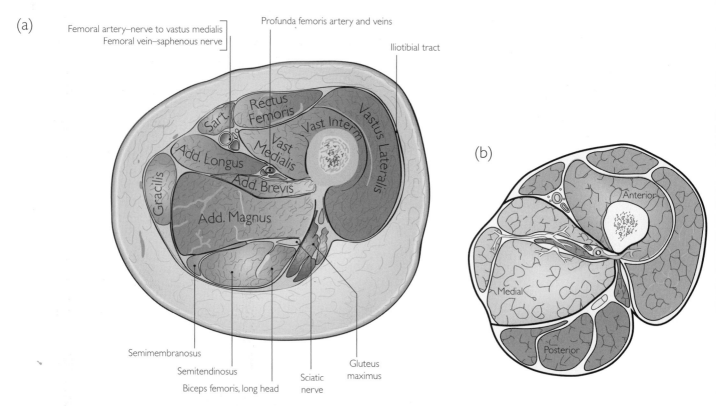

Fig. 9.9 Diagram of the thigh showing the muscles of the thigh.

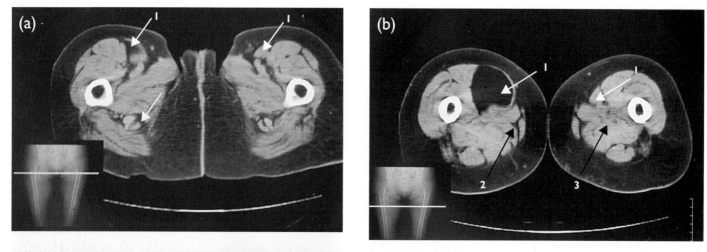

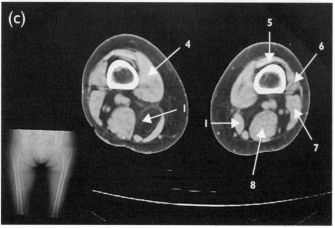

Fig. 9.10 Axial sections through the thigh. The sartorius muscle is identified on the right due to the presence of a lipoma and its course from lateral to medial across the anterior aspect of the thigh can be seen clearly (1). (7) Gracilis (2), adductor magnus (3), vastus medialis (4), rectus femoris muscles (5), vastus lateralis (6), biceps femoris (7) and semimembranosus (8).

- Medial or adductor compartment: the adductor magnus is a large muscle belonging to the adductor group and the hamstring group; adductor longus, adductor brevis, gracilis and obturator externus proximally.
- The posterior thigh, often called the hamstrings, is created by biceps femoris laterally, semitendinosis centrally and semimembranosus medially. Semitendinosus becomes tendinous for much of its length.

The tibia and fibula

- The tibia articulates with the femoral condyles and the fibula at its upper end, and with the talus and distal fibula distally.
- The tibia lies medially and forms the medial malleolus.
- The tibial tuberosity can be seen as a dark band across the middle third of the tibia 2 cm distal to the knee joint. It receives the attachment of the patellar tendon.
- The fibula takes no part in the knee articulation, but forms the lateral malleolus distally.

The patella (Fig. 9.11)

- The patellar ossification centre appears at age 3–5 years.
- The patella is a sesamoid bone lying in the quadriceps tendon.
- The patella has a roughened anterior surface from nutrient vessels.
- The lateral facet of the patella is larger and longer than the medial facet.
- The patella can be bipartite. The bipartite patella is seen superolaterally.
- Bipartite patella can be bilateral but unilateral is more common.
- Bipartite patella is more common in men than in women.
- Bipartite patella may be symptomatic.
- The large lateral femoral condyle and the lower fibres of vastus medialis, forming the medial retinaculum of the patella, help prevent lateral dislocation of the patella.

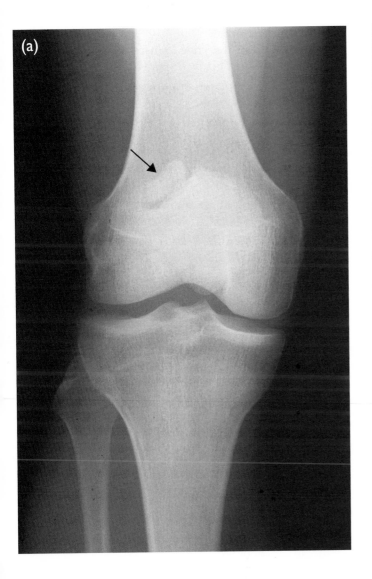
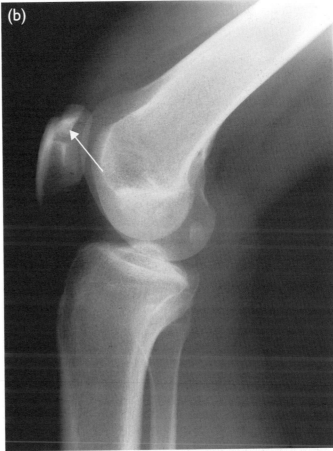

Fig. 9.11 (a) AP knee radiograph; (b) lateral knee radiograph showing a bipartite patella in the superolateral aspect (arrows).

The knee joint

- The condyles of the femur articulate with the tibial condyles and their menisci. Anteriorly is the articulation between the femur and the patella. The menisci are fibrocartilaginous C-shaped discs that are triangular in cross-section.
- The medial meniscus: this is larger and broader posteriorly than the lateral meniscus and is attached to the knee capsule. This means that it is more likely to be torn.
- The lateral meniscus is smaller and more circumscribed in shape and of uniform width (Fig. 9.12).
- The transverse ligament runs anteriorly connecting the two anterior menisci (Fig. 9.13).
- Three bursae are seen around the knee: the suprapatellar bursa, 9% of individuals have a popliteal bursa and 4% have a gastrocnemius bursa.
- The fabella is a small accessory bone in the lateral head of gastrocnemius. It is commonly seen on a lateral or anteroposterior (AP) view of the knee (Fig. 9.14).
- Hoffa's fat pad or the infrapatellar fat pad lies behind the patellar tendon and inferior to the patella. It is best seen on a sagittal view.
- The knee is supported by strong ligaments. The intravascular ligaments are the cruciates which cross each other within the joint cavity.

- The anterior cruciate ligament arises from the anterior intercondylar area and attaches to the medial aspect of the lateral femoral condyle. It prevents the femur from sliding posteriorly on the tibia and hyperextension of the knee and from medial rotation of the femur (Fig. 9.15).
- The posterior cruciate ligament arises from the posterior intercondylar area and attaches to the lateral aspect of the medial femoral condyle. It prevents the femur from sliding anteriorly on the tibia particularly when the knee is flexed.
- On the lateral side of the knee there are three main supporting structures: first the lateral collateral ligament or fibular collateral ligament is band like, arising from the lateral epicondyle of femur and attaching to the fibula. It does not attach to the lateral meniscus (Fig. 9.16); second the iliotibial tract; third the popliteus tendon lies behind the lateral meniscus running from the fibula to the femur (Fig. 9.17).
- On the medial side of the knee there is one main supporting ligament: the medial collateral ligament is a band running from medial epicondyle of femur to tibia. It is attached to the medial meniscus and best seen on a coronal view.
- The patellar ligament attaches from the lower border of the patella to the tubercle of the tibia. It is separated from the synovium of the knee joint by the infrapatellar fat pad and from the tibia by a small bursa.

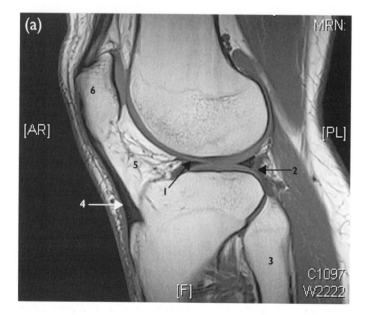
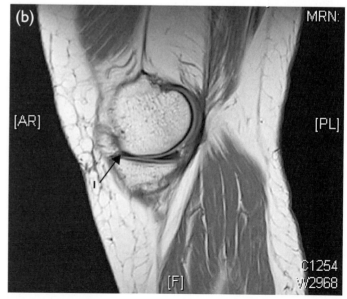

Fig. 9.12 Sagittal T1-weighted MRI: (a) sagittal section through the patella and lateral meniscus and (b) sagittal section through the medial meniscus. The menisci should appear as sharp black bow-ties, with pointed ends (1). The lateral meniscus is separated from the joint capsule by popliteus (2). In the lateral aspect the fibula is present (3). Patellar tendon (4), Hoffa's fat pad (5) and patella (6).

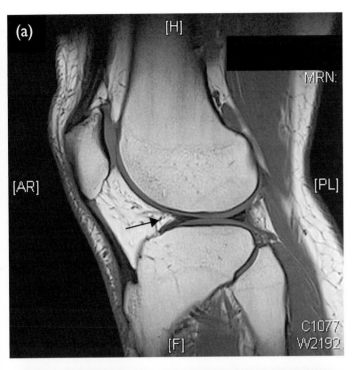

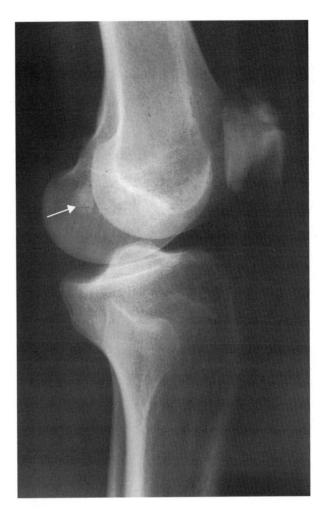

Fig. 9.14 Lateral knee radiograph: a fabella is a sesamoid bone in the lateral head of gastrocnemius (arrow).

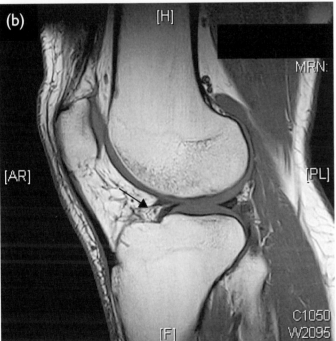

Fig. 9.13 MRI sagittal T1-weighted images: three sections all showing the transverse ligament connecting the two anterior horns of the medial and lateral meniscus (arrow).

The lower leg muscles

The lower leg is divided into three muscle groups by the interosseous membrane and intermuscular septa. Each has its own blood supply and nerve (Fig. 9.18): anterior, lateral and posterior. The posterior compartment is subdivided into three groups:

- Anterior tibiofibular compartment contains tibialis anterior, extensor digitorum longus and extensor hallucis longus, and anterior tibial vessels.
- The lateral compartment contains peroneus longus and brevis, and the peroneal nerve.
- The posterior compartment is subdivided into three with (1) deepest muscles: tibialis posterior; (2) intermediate muscles containing flexor digitorum longus, flexor hallucis longus, and posterior tibial vessels and nerve; and (3) most superficial muscles containing soleus, gastrocnemius and plantaris. The soleus inserts into gastrocnemius and inferiorly this thickens to become the Achilles tendon, which in turn inserts on to the posterior calcaneum.

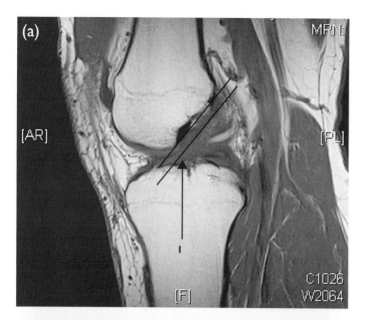

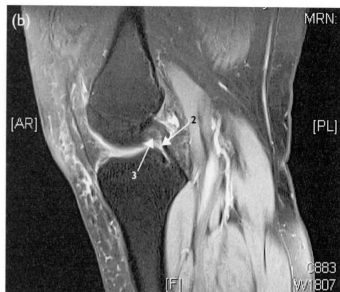

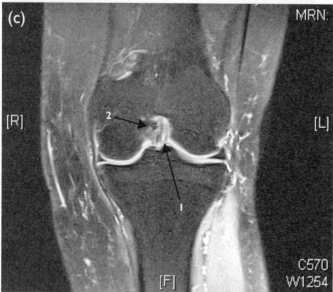

Fig. 9.15 (a) Sagittal T1 MRI: the anterior cruciate ligament is seen (1) as a fan of fibres, which should be parallel to the intercondylar roof (black lines). (b) Fat-suppressed proton density sagittal MRI. The posterior cruciate ligament (PCL) (2) is seen as a black band arising from the posterior intercondylar area. The ligament of Humphrey (3) can be seen anterior to the PCL. (c) Fat-suppressed coronal proton density. Only two structures should be present in the intercondylar region: the anterior cruciate ligament (ACL) (1) seen as a band running up laterally and the PCL (2) seen as a dark spherical structure medially. Further structures may represent bucket-handle fragments.

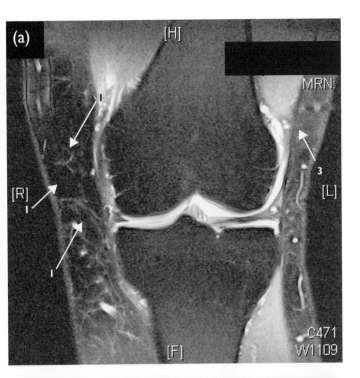

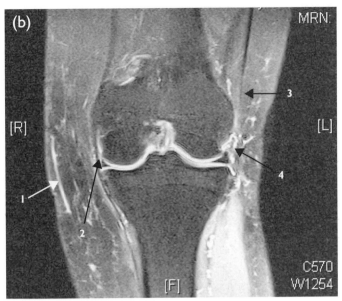

Fig. 9.16 (b) Middle

Fig. 9.16 (a) Anterior coronal fat-suppressed proton density images showing the collateral ligaments. The medial aspect of the knee is identified by the large amount of fat (1). The medial collateral ligament is seen as a band of fibres (2). Anteriorly on the lateral aspect the iliotibial tract is seen (3). More posteriorly towards the fibula (b) the lateral collateral ligaments (4) can be demonstrated and (c) popliteus (5).

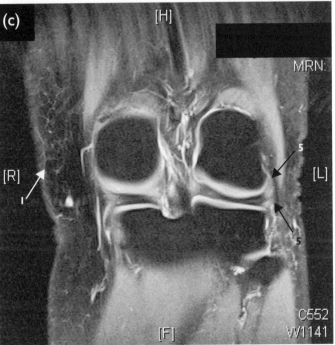

Fig. 9.16 (c) Posterior

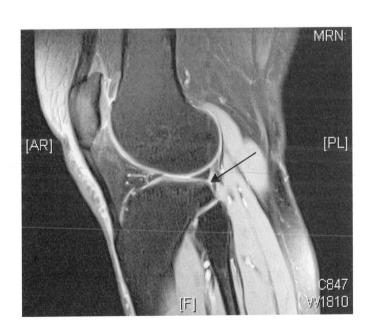

Fig. 9.17 Sagittal MRI proton density weighted: popliteus is seen arising from the fibula and can cause confusion with a tear in the lateral meniscus (arrow). This is a fat-suppressed proton density image.

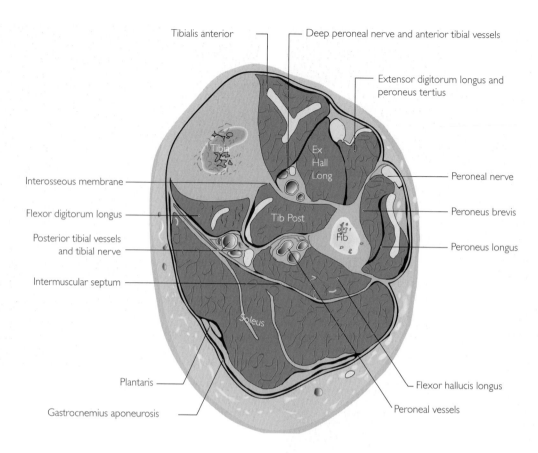

Tibialis anterior

Deep peroneal nerve and anterior tibial vessels

Extensor digitorum longus and peroneus tertius

Interosseous membrane

Peroneal nerve

Flexor digitorum longus

Peroneus brevis

Posterior tibial vessels and tibial nerve

Peroneus longus

Intermuscular septum

Plantaris

Flexor hallucis longus

Gastrocnemius aponeurosis

Peroneal vessels

Fig. 9.18 Diagram of the calf. It shows the interosseous membrane, defining the anterior and posterior compartments of the calf.

Ankle (Fig. 9.19)

- The distal tibiofibular joint is a syndesmosis or fibrous joint connected by the interosseous membrane.
- The ankle joint itself or tibiotalar joint is a synovial hinge articulation of the distal tibia, two malleoli and body of the talus.
- The ankle joint has a fibrous capsule that attaches to the articular margins of the tibia, fibula and talus. The capsule is thin anteriorly and posteriorly is reinforced by strong collateral ligaments.
- The deep fascia of the ankle is thickened to form a series of retinacula, which serve to keep the tendons in position and act as pulleys. The superior extensor retinaculum attaches to the distal tibia and fibula. The inferior extensor retinaculum is Y-shaped and attaches from the calcaneum to the medial malleolus and medial border of the foot. The flexor retinaculum extends from the medial malleolus to the medial calcaneum. Laterally are the superior and inferior peroneal retinacula.
- A series of ligaments supports the ankle joint.
- The medial ligament is called the deltoid ligament and is a strong band attached to the medial malleolus; it is triangular in shape with superficial and deep fibres. Superficial fibres pass to the navicular, calcaneum and

talus. The deep fibres have a strong anterior and posterior component called the anterior and posterior tibiotalar ligaments (Fig. 9.20).
- The lateral ligament is weaker and made up of three distinct bands: the anterior talofibular, calcaneofibular and posterior talofibular ligaments.
- The posterior ankle is strengthened by the posterior talofibular and tibiofibular ligaments.
- The subtalar joint is the posterior talocalcaneal joint. It is separated from the anterior calcaneal joint by the interosseous ligament.
- The tarsal tunnel or tarsal sinus lies between the anterior and posterior tarsal joints.
- The posterior tendons of the calf run medially behind the medial malleolus deep to the flexor retinaculum, in this order: posterior tibialis, flexor digitorum, then most posteriorly flexor hallucis longus: mnemonic 'Tom, Dick, Harry' (Fig. 9.21).
- Anterolaterally peroneus longus and brevis enter a common sheath above the ankle. They pass posterior to the lateral malleolus and deep to the retinacula. Peroneus brevis insets into the base of the fifth metatarsal and peroneus longus passes under the foot, inserting into the base of the first metatarsal.

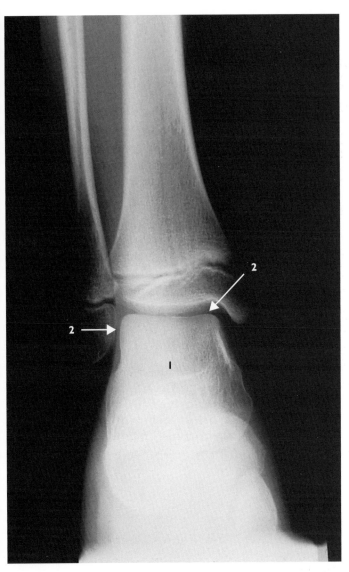

Fig. 9.19 Radiograph of the ankle mortice. Talus (1). The ankle mortise should have an even space of less than approximately 4 mm (2).

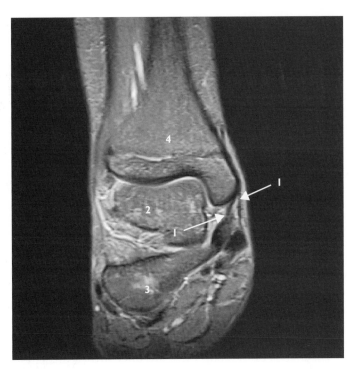

Fig. 9.20 MRI coronal STIR of the ankle shows the medial ligament of the ankle called the deltoid ligament (1). Talus (2), calcaneum (3) and distal tibia (4).

• Anteriorly on axial imaging in the ankle on the dorsum of the ankle the tendons from medial to lateral are 'Tom, Harry, Dick', i.e. anterior tibialis, extensor digitorum longus and extensor hallucis longus.

Foot

Foot development

At birth the talus calcaneum cuboid (TCC) ossify in this order:

• Last bone in the tarsus to appear is the navicular by age 4 years.

• In the metatarsals the first metatarsal has a proximal epiphysis whereas the second to fifth metatarsals have distal epiphyses.

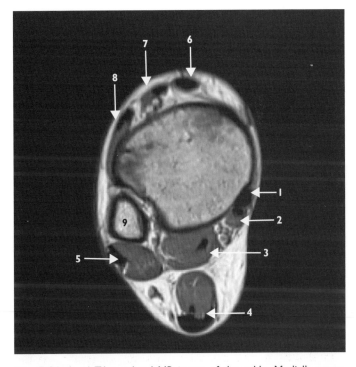

Fig. 9.21 Axial T1-weighted MR image of the ankle. Medially posterior to the medial malleolus are 'Tom, Dick and Harry'; Tom = tibialis posterior (1); Dick = extensor digitorum longus (2); Harry = extensor hallucis longus (3). Achilles tendon (4), peroneal tendons (5), tibialis anterior (6), flexor hallucis longus (7), flexor digitorum longus (8) and distal fibular (9).

Tarsal bones

- The talus articulates with the tibia, navicular and calcaneum.
- The calcaneum articulates with the talus and cuboid, and with the navicular at the talocalcaneonavicular joint (Fig. 9.22).
- The cuboid bone articulates with the fourth and fifth metatarsals (Fig. 9.23).
- It is important to assess for the articulations between the tarsal bones in the context of flat feet, which may occur due to a tarsal coalition. Tarsal coalitions are most common between the talus and calcaneum or calcaneum and navicular.
- Each cuneiform articulates with its own metatarsal. Loss of the alignment between the cuneiforms and the metatarsals occurs in Lisfranc's fractures (Fig. 9.24).
- The calcaneum is the largest tarsal bone. It can show sclerosis posteriorly as a normal variant in a child within the secondary ossification centre. It has a large medial process called the sustentacalum tali, which articulates with the talus.
- The arches of the foot: there are three arches present at birth that support the body's weight; the medial longitudinal, the most important, the lateral longitudinal and transverse.
- The plantar fascia is the fascia of the deep sole of the foot which can be evaluated on MRI for inflammation.

The vessels:

Arteries

- The aorta divides into the common iliac arteries, which in turn divide into the external and internal iliac arteries.
- The external iliac becomes the common femoral at the inguinal ligament.
- The common femoral divides into the superficial femoral artery which runs medially and gives off no branches in the thigh and profunda femoris.
- The profunda femoris passes laterally and deep within the thigh and gives off branches. It arises 4 cm inferior to the inguinal ligament.
- The superficial femoral artery has no branches in the thigh and becomes the popliteal artery at the adductor hiatus or, radiologically, at the medial bony border where the artery crosses the femur.
- At the inferior border of the popliteal fossa, the popliteal artery divides into anterior and common tibioperoneal arteries.
- The anterior tibial artery descends laterally and becomes dorsalis pedis in the foot, which runs over the dorsal aspect of the ankle into the foot.
- The common tibioperoneal trunk divides into posterior tibial artery and descends medially, and peroneal artery. The posterior tibial passes behind the medial malleolus.
- The peroneal artery continues into the foot behind the lateral malleolus.

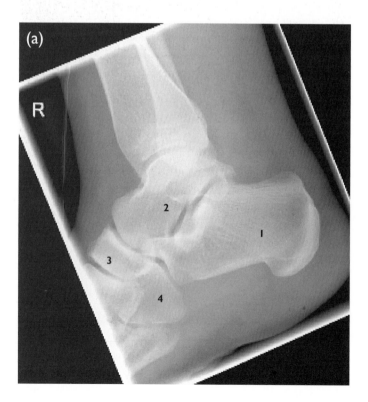

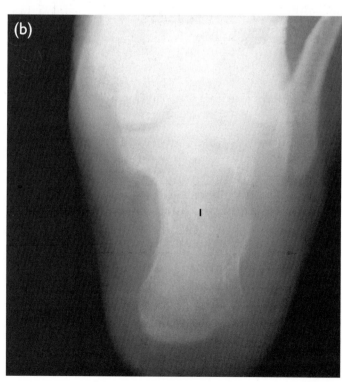

Fig. 9.22 Calcaneum: (a) lateral radiograph views and (b) axial radiograph. Calcaneum (1), talus (2), navicular (3), cuboid (4). The trabecula should be seen running in a parallel distribution through the calcaneum.

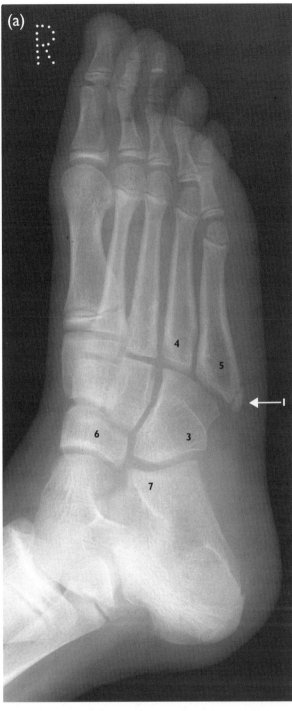
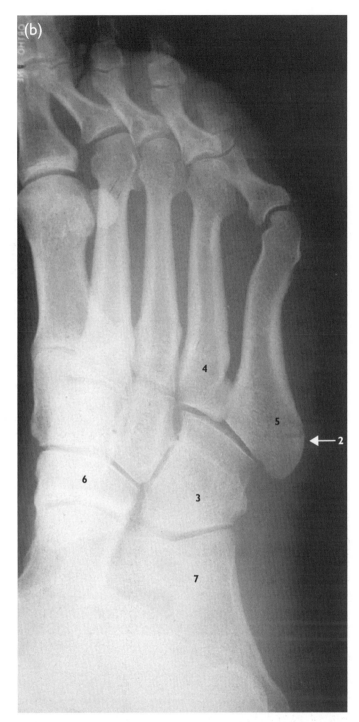

Fig. 9.23 (a) Oblique radiograph of the foot. At the base of the fifth metatarsal the secondary ossification centre can be seen running in a linear direction (1). (b) A fracture (2), which is running in a transverse plain, and shows no cortication. Note the cuboid bone (3) articulating with the fourth (4) and fifth (5) metatarsals. Navicular (6) and calcaneum (7).

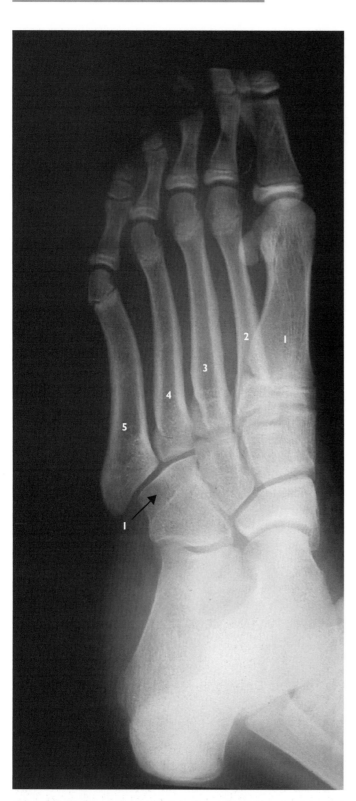

Fig. 9.24 Oblique radiograph of the foot shows the cuboid (arrow) articulating with the fourth (4) and fifth (5) metatarsals. The cuneiforms should articulate with a metatarsal bone each.

IMAGING

Plain film

Pelvis

Indications
Trauma, joint pain in an adult with joint disease or a child suspected of slipped epiphysis or Perthes' disease.

Technique
A pelvic radiograph shows both hip joints. Dedicated hip views in two planes – AP and lateral – are performed for trauma. A frog's leg view with the hips abducted is used for congenital dislocation of the hip and slipped epiphysis (Fig. 9.25).

Findings
- Shenton's line is a line along the inferior margin of the neck of the femur, which forms a continuous arch with the superior and medial margins of the oburator foramen of the pelvis. Disruption of the line can be seen in congenital dislocation of the hip and trauma (Fig. 9.26).
- The femoral line is the line drawn along the superior neck of the femur. This transects the femoral head in both the AP and lateral projections. One-third of the femoral head should lie lateral to the line. If less than this is present on the AP view, then a slipped epiphysis must be suspected.
- Perthes' disease usually occurs in 8-year-old children whereas slipped epiphysis tends to occur in older adolescent children.
- The iliopectineal line is important to assess when reviewing a pelvic film. This can be thickened in Paget's disease (Fig. 9.27).
- Os acetabuli is a small ossicle adjoining the superior lip of the acetabulum.

Knee

Technique
- AP view sometimes taken in the standing position.
- Lateral view or in trauma a horizontal beam lateral to show a lipohaemarthrosis.
- Skyline view of the patella and an intercondylar view to look for loose bodies.

Findings
- On an AP view the groove for popliteus can be seen laterally in the femur. The fabella can be seen laterally.
- A lipohaemarthrosis is a fat–fluid collection that occurs above the patella in the suprapatellar bursa after trauma to the knee and a tibial plateau fracture. The fat settles on top of the blood/haemorrhage because it is lighter (Figs 9.28 and 9.29).

(a)

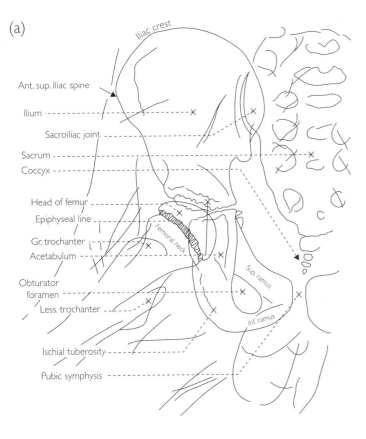

Fig. 9.25 (a) Diagram of frog's leg view and (b) frog leg's radiograph.

(b)

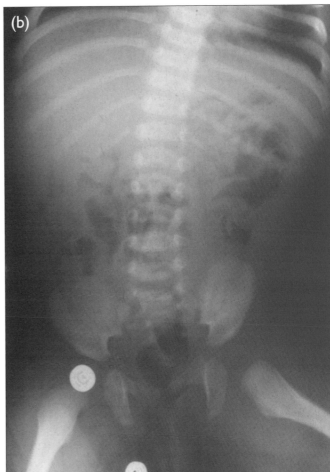

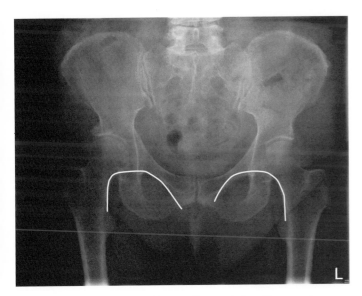

Fig. 9.26 Pelvic radiograph showing Shenton's line (drawn on).

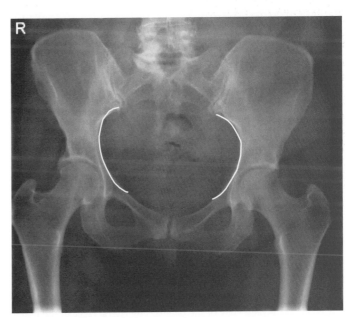

Fig. 9.27 Radiograph of pelvis showing iliopectineal line (drawn on).

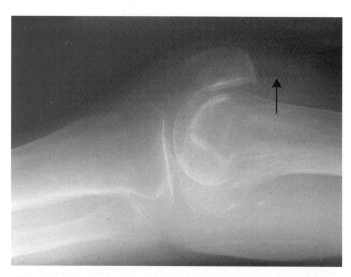

Fig. 9.28 Horizontal beam lateral knee showing a lipohaemarthrosis. Trauma to the knee may cause a fat blood collection in the suprapatellar bursa. This can be seen on the horizontal beam lateral view as a fat fluid level above the patella (arrow). A tibial plateau fracture is often associated with this.

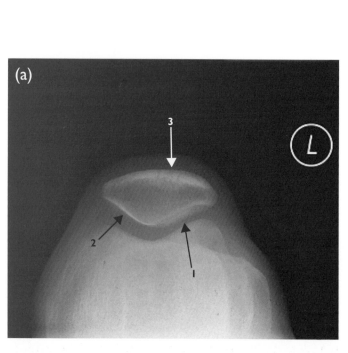

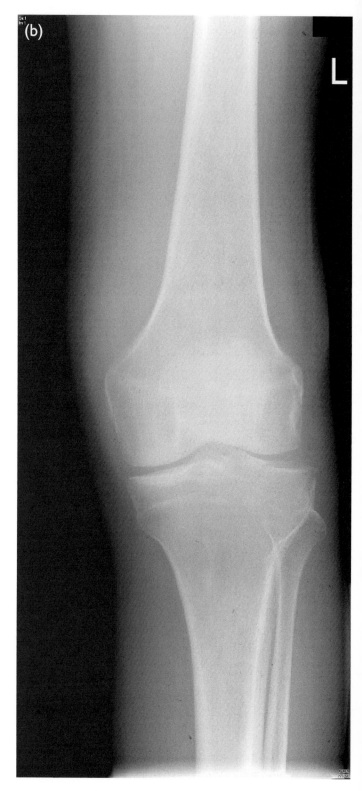

Fig. 9.29 (a) Skyline view of the patella. The lateral facet of the patella (1) is longer than the medial facet (2). There are often grooves (3) on the anterior surface of the patella from nutrient vessels. (b) AP view of the patella.

Ankle

Technique

- AP view.
- Lateral view.
- Externally rotated oblique view.
- Stress views in external and internal rotation can assess for ligamentous disruption.

Findings

- On plain film the medial and lateral malleolus and the dome of the talus can be seen for ankle mortise. The space around the dome of the talus should be around 4 mm in all directions on the mortise view.
- Well-corticated fragments can be seen around the malleoli, which are ossicles and cause confusion with fractures
- The subtalar joint is the posterior articulation between the talus and calcaneum.

Foot

Technique

Standard views of the foot are AP and oblique:

- A lateral may be performed to look at the arches of the foot.
- Dedicated calcaneal views are indicated in trauma to the heel from a height.

Findings

- The calcaneum can be fractured by a fall from a height. Boehler's angle can help detect a fracture. The angle is normally is 28–40°. If there is a calcaneal fracture then the angle decreases and becomes abnormal, i.e. an angle <28° is abnormal. This is due to flattening of the subtalar portion of the calcaneum. Boehler's angle is formed by the intersection of lines drawn on a lateral view from the anterosuperior and posterosuperior edges of the calcaneum to the highest point of the articular surface.
- The calcaneum has a secondary ossification centre that appears at the heel by age 10 and may appear dense, i.e. sclerotic.
- The base of the fifth metatarsal has a secondary ossification centre that is linear and vertical. Note that a fracture through the base of the metatarsal at this site is transverse; this helps differentiate the two (Fig. 9.30).
- Accessory ossicles around the foot: the most common ossicles are the os peroneum, os vesalianum, os tibiale externum and os trigonum. The ossicles are important to be aware of so as not to confuse them with fractures. In addition some of the ossicles, particularly the os trigonum, may be symptomatic (Fig. 9.30).
- The os trigonum is seen posterior to the talus.
- The os tibiale externum is seen adjacent to the navicular medially.
- The os peroneum is seen lateral and next to the cuboid, lying in the peroneal tendons. The os vesalianum is more

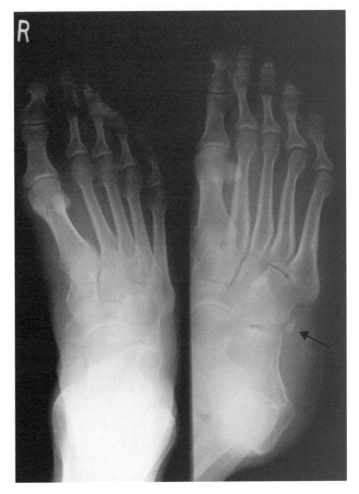

Fig. 9.30 Oblique radiograph foot showing the os peroneum lying within the peroneal tendons (arrow).

anterior in the V of the bones. The os vesalianum is seen at the base of the fifth metatarsal.

- Secondary ossification centres for the metatarsals such as the metacarpals occur at the base of the first metatarsal and heads of the second to fifth metatarsals

Arthrography

Indications

Arthrography of the knee has been superseded by MRI. MRI hip arthrography is used to assess the acetabular labrum for tears.

Technique

- Plain films must be performed before any arthrogram to detect any calcific or radio-opaque loose bodies in the joint (Fig. 9.31).
- A 22-gauge lumbar puncture needle is used. Very dilute gadolinium is used for the arthrogram and is usually injected under fluoroscopic control.

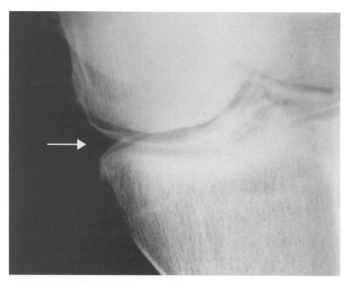

Fig. 9.31 Conventional knee arthrogram showing the meniscus (arrow).

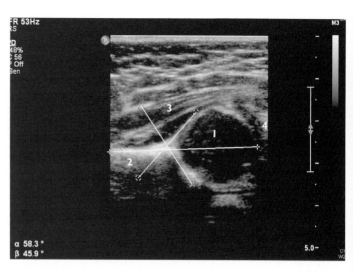

Fig. 9.32 Hip ultrasound: coronal view. The unossified femoral head is seen (1). Ilium (2), gluteal muscles (3) and diaphysis of the femur (4).

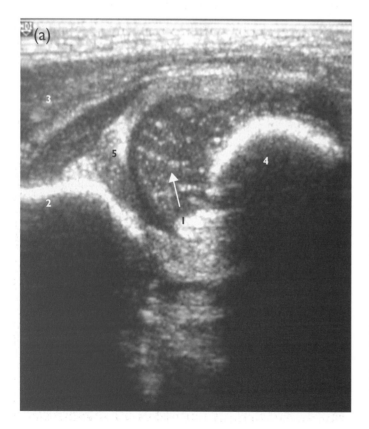

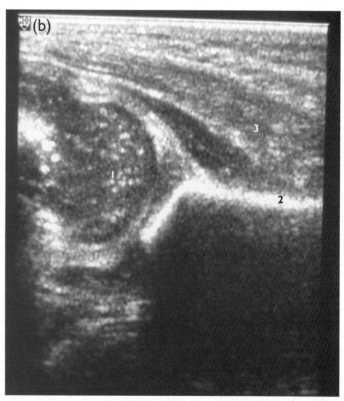

Fig. 9.33 Hip ultrasounds: (a) right and (b) left hips. Coronal views. The unossified femoral head is seen (1). Ilium (2), gluteal muscles (3), diaphysis of the femur (4) and labrum (5).

Ultrasound

Indications
- Paediatric hip ultrasound, soft-tissue trauma, Achilles tendon injury.
- The hip is the most frequently scanned joint in the child. It is the investigation of choice for developmental hip dysplasia. It is also useful in an older child with hip pain or a limp, or when an irritable hip is suspected.

Technique
Use a linear-array probe with as high a frequency as possible while allowing sufficient depth. Remember that there is an inverse relationship between frequency of the probe and depth (Figs 9.32 and 9.33).

Findings
In an irritable hip the patient should be scanned supine to look for an effusion anterior to the femoral neck.

CT

Indications
- Pelvic trauma and to assess for acetabular fracture and fragments that may make relocating a hip joint difficult. CT has superseded Judet's views, which were dedicated plain films taken of the acetabulum (Fig. 9.34).
- In the knee CT shows the position and number of fragments in fractures of the tibial plateau. Depression of fragments greater than 8–10 mm is commonly surgically lifted.
- CT is indicated to study complex calcaneal fractures and their relationship to the subtalar joint.

Technique
Fine cuts with a bony algorithm are used and multiplanar reformatting is used to visualize the bone or joint in all planes.

MRI of the hip and pelvis

Indications
Hip pain, suspected fracture of the femur, avascular necrosis, labral abnormality (Fig. 9.35).

Technique
Axial, coronal and sagittal images using a balance of T1-weighted, T2-weighted and STIR images.

Findings
- Variations in the marrow pattern in the proximal femur are confusing and mimic marrow pathology.
- Well-defined areas of low signal called herniation pits can be seen as a normal variant in the femoral necks in 5% of adults. These are about 1 cm in size and occur in the femoral neck.

MR of the knee

MR is the investigation of choice to examine the ligaments and soft tissues of the knee joint. Series are routinely taken in the coronal and sagittal plane and are supplemented by axial images to view the patellofemoral joint.

The following are the most important anatomical structures to identify. Form a system and use the same order each time when reporting. On the sagittal plane identify:

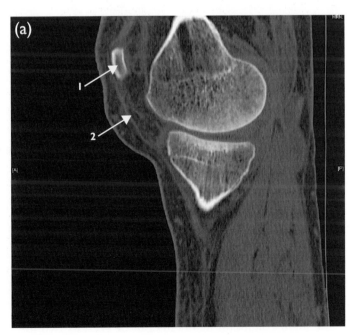 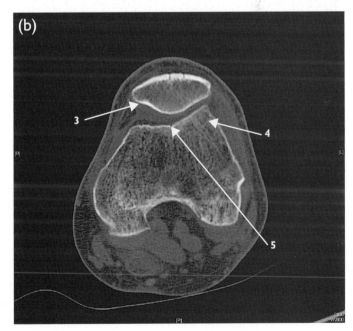

Fig. 9.34 Tibial plateau: (a) sagittal and (b) axial CT using high-resolution bony algorithm. Used to demonstrate tibial plateau fractures. Patella (1), Hoffa's fat pad (3), medial facet (3), lateral facet patella (4) and truchlea (5).

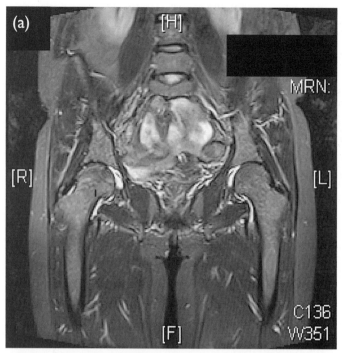

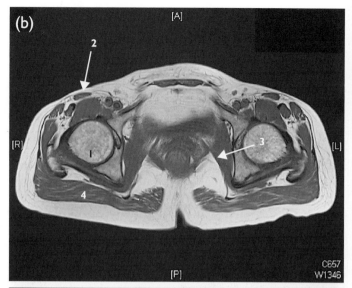

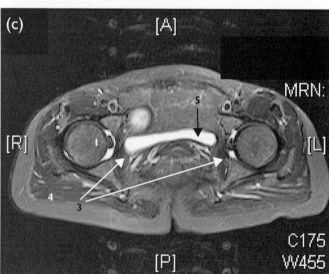

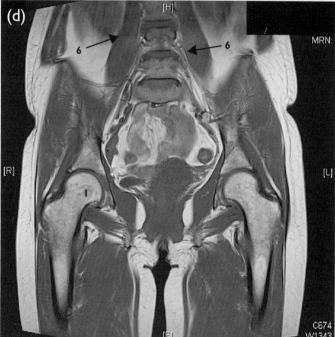

Fig. 9.35 MRI of the hips: (a) coronal STIR; (b) axial T1; (c) axial STIR; (d) coronal T1. Femoral head (1), sartorius (2), obturator internus (3), gluteal muscles (4), fluid in the bladder (5) and psoas muscle (6).

- ACL: the anterior cruciate ligament is a band of fibres and it may not be well seen if the knee is in the wrong angle. It can be seen on sagittal and coronal planes; on the sagittal images it is seen in the midline. Only one fibre needs to be seen to see if it is present. The ACL should run parallel to the intercondylar roof. Loss of this normal alignment indicates a tear or disruption (Fig. 9.36a).
- The ACL is of higher signal intensity on MRI than the posterior cruciate ligament (PCL) on MR (Fig. 9.36b).
- Once the ACL has been seen on the sagittal plane, look at the coronal plane and the ACL can be seen running from anteriorly to the lateral condyle.

- There are no attachments to the tibial spines.
- It is intracapsular extrasynovial.
- PCL: this is low signal on all sequences. It runs up from posteriorly, and is again seen on the sagittal images and shaped like a shepherd's hook. As a soft sign there may be an ACL tear if the PCL has a sigmoid shape. Look at the coronal images and the PCL is seen as a round low-signal ligament adjacent to the ACL.
- On the sagittal images anterior and posterior to the PCL, the meniscofemoral ligaments can be seen as two low-signal round lesions, which are called the ligaments of Humphrey and Wisberg. These lie on either side of the

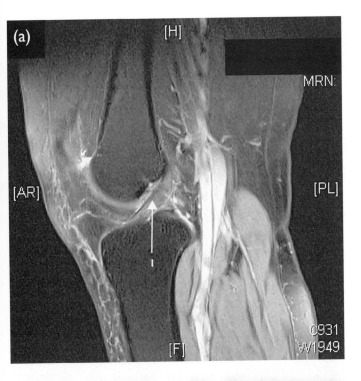

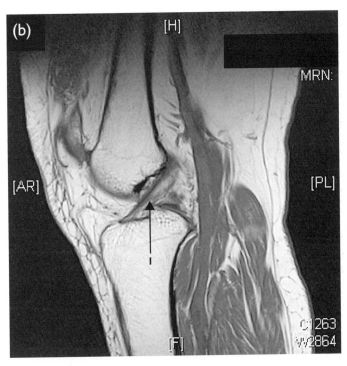

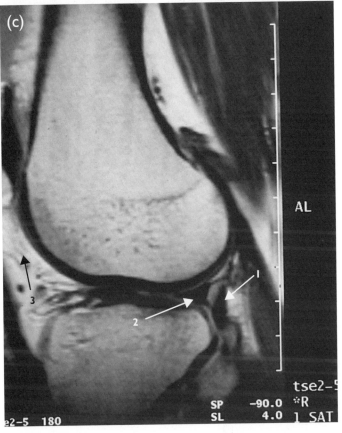

Fig. 9.36 Sagittal MRI of the anterior cruciate ligament. (a) Proton density fat-suppressed and (b) T1-weighted. A band of fibres is seen running parallel to the intercondylar roof of the femur (1). Only a single band needs to be detected. The anterior cruciate ligament is of intermediate-signal intensity. (c) MRI sagittal T1-weighted image of the popliteus tendon. Running to insert into the femur just behind the lateral meniscus (1). Lateral meniscus (2) and Hoffa's fat pad (3).

PCL and can cause confusion with pathology such as tears, bucket-handle fragments and torn menisci if their normal presence is unknown (Fig. 9.37).

- The ligaments of Humphrey and Wisberg are seen on either side of the posterior cruciate ligament. The ligament of Humphrey lies anterior to the ligament and the ligament of Wisberg posterior to the ligament on the sagittal view. This is remembered by remembering that H comes before W in the alphabet. The meniscofemoral ligaments attach to the knowing and the menisci.
- The menisci are low signal on MRI and should have a bow-tie/triangular appearance. The horns should have a sharp pointed appearance and not be truncated on all images sagittal.
- The lateral meniscus has a bow-tie shape. The medial meniscus is fatter and at least two bow-ties should be seen on the sagittal images. It is important to view the menisci of both planes on every image.
- Note that lateral geniculate vessels can give the appearance of a tear near the menisci because the vessels cause a small high-signal focal lesion adjacent to the menisci.
- The transverse meniscal ligament can mimic an anterior tear of the lateral meniscus just as it inserts into the meniscus.

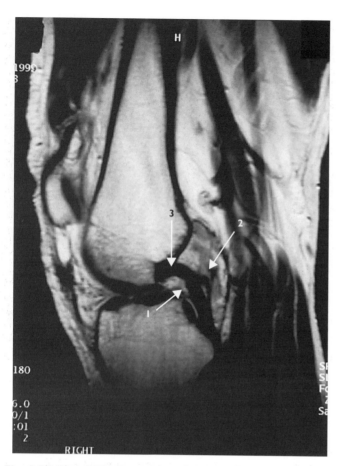

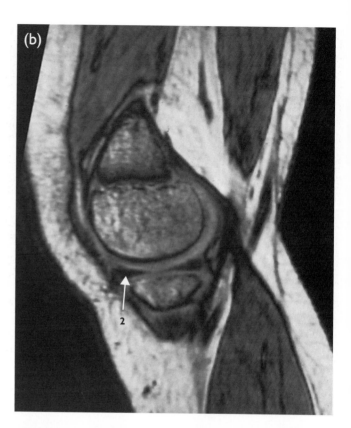

Fig. 9.37 Sagittal MRI T1-weighted: ligaments of Humphrey (1) and Wisberg (2) are seen on either side of the posterior cruciate ligaments (3) and may lead to confusion with bucket-handle tears at the meniscus.

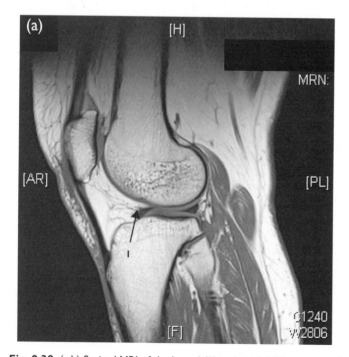

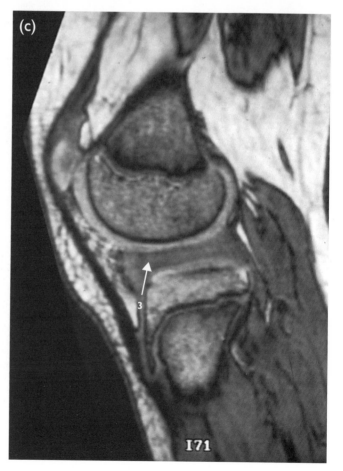

Fig. 9.38 (a,b) Sagittal MRI of the lateral (1) and medial (2) meniscus. (c) Discoid lateral meniscus (3). Bow-ties are normally seen in the mid-aspect of the menisci. A discoid meniscus shows no bow-ties with a very thick medial aspect – this is prone to tearing.

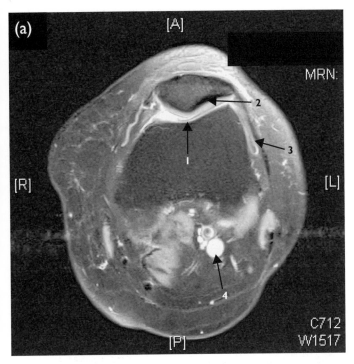 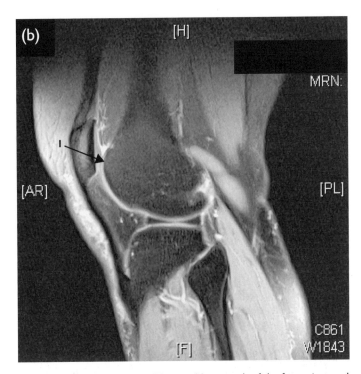

Fig. 9.39 (a) Axial and (b) sagittal fat-suppressed proton density images showing the patellofemoral joint. The trochlear notch of the femur is noted (1). Longer lateral facet of the patella (2). The patellar retinacular (3) and popliteal vessels (4).

- The popliteus tendon runs adjacent to the lateral meniscus on the sagittal images and can mimic a tear.
- The magic angle phenomenon can cause a high signal lesion mimicking a tear seen at 55°.
- Discoid meniscus: this is more common laterally and is a congenital variant of a thick meniscus prone to tears (Fig. 9.38).
- The patellar tendon is seen anteriorly on the sagittal images and variations in position can lead to buckling (Fig. 9.39).
- Hoffa's fat pad: should be clean and fat containing on the sagittal plane.

- The bones: marrow changes in the distal femur may be a normal variant, which is very common. The STIR images are useful for bone marrow oedema.
- On the coronal plane look at the ACL, PCL and menisci as above and review.
- Medial collateral ligament: this is a band of fibres seen running medially from the femur to the tibia. High signal within it can indicate pathology but some things may mimic a tear. Fat between the medial collateral ligament or the collateral ligament and the capsule can be confused with tears (Fig. 9.40).

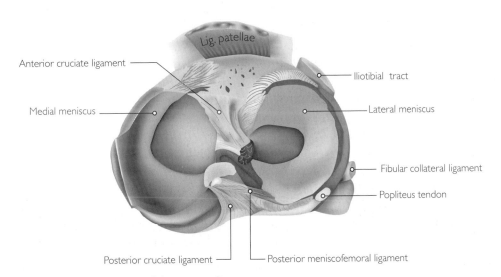

Fig. 9.40 Diagram of the tibial plateau and origin of the cruciate ligaments.

- Lateral collateral ligament: on the coronal plane three structures can be seen from anterior to posterior: the ilio-tibial tract is a band of fibres running from lateral femur to lateral tibia, the lateral collateral ligament is a short ligament seen more posteriorly deep within the knee joint, and lastly the popliteus tendon can be seen both sagittally and coronally. All three structures constitute the lateral supporting ligaments.
- The intercondylar notch should contain only two structures the ACL and the PCL. On the coronal plane loose bodies and bucket-handle fragments can be seen in the notch.
- The axial plane is for looking at the patellofemoral joint.
- The lateral facet of the patella is longer than the medial facet. The patella sits in the trochlear notch of the femur.
- The patella retinacula are small reflections of the capsule that are strengthened by expansions of vastus lateralis and medialis.
- Dislocation of the patella is more common laterally, resulting in trauma to the lateral facet of the patella and the medial femoral condyle. The integrity of the retinacula may be disrupted.

MRI of the ankle

Indications

Ankle pain, ligamentous damage, Achilles tendon trauma, subtalar joint pain.

Technique

Three planes are used: coronal, sagittal and axial using a mixture of T1-weighted, T2-weighted and STIR (short T1 inversion and recovery) images (Figs 9.41 and 9.42).

Findings

- On coronal imaging the normal ligaments that can be identified are, medially, the tibiotalar, tibionavicular, tibiocalcaneal and, laterally, the anterior and posterior talofibula and calcaneal fibular ligaments.
- On sagittal images the tibialis posterior tendon can be clearly seen medially under the malleolus and peroneal tendons longus and brevis laterally (Fig. 9.43c,d).
- On the axial image anterior and posterior structures can be seen.

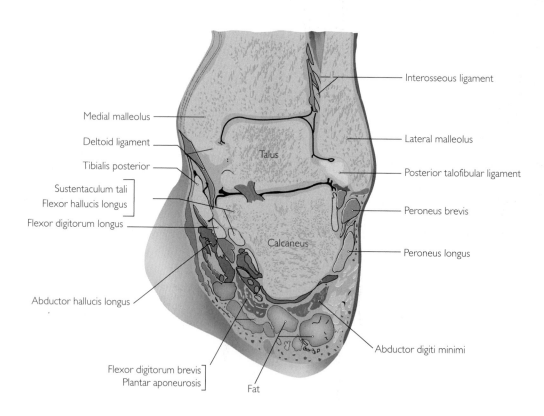

Fig. 9.41 Diagram of ankle, coronal plane, showing origin of the ligaments.

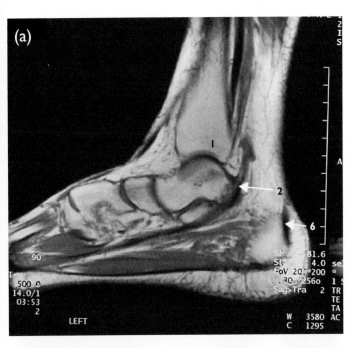

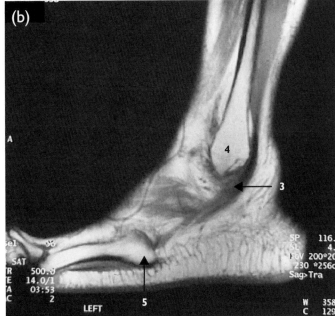

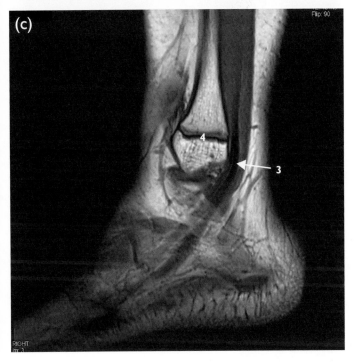

Fig. 9.42 Lateral ankle MRI: (a) relates to the medial malleolus (1) which is related to the posterior tibial tendon (2); (b) relates to the lateral malleolus showing the peroneal tendons (3) running round the fibular (4) towards the head of the fifth metatarsal (5). (c,d) Zoomed sagittal MR T1-weighted images of the lateral ankle. The peroneal tendons (3) are seen running behind the fibular (4). Achilles (6).

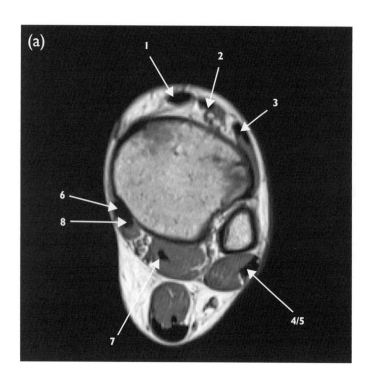

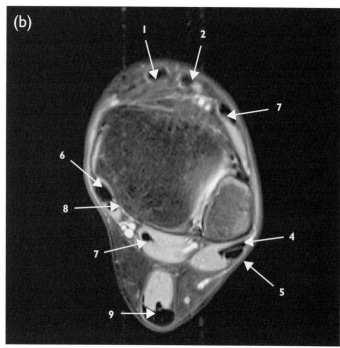

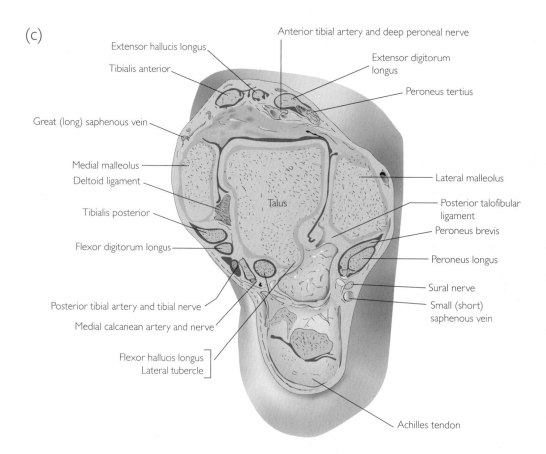

Fig. 9.43 (a) Axial MRI of the ankle; (b) axial T1-weighted proton density fat-suppressed image. Anterior tibialis (1), flexor hallucis longus (2), flexor digitorum longus (3), peroneus longus (4), peroneus brevis (5), posterior tibialis (6), extensor hallucis longus (7), extensor digitorum longus (8) and Achilles tendon (9). (c) Diagram of the axial ankle.

Posterior structures

- Medially behind the medial malleolus the tendons are in order, from medial to lateral, Tom, Dick, Harry, i.e. tibialis posterior, flexor digitorum longus and flexor hallucis longus (Fig. 9.43). These lie deep to the flexor retinaculum. The posterior tibial artery lies between flexor digitorum longus and flexor hallucis longus.
- Achilles tendon and the pre-Achilles fat pad are located posterior to the ankle. Achilles tendon is identified in cross-section as a low-signal thick structure with a convex posterior and flattened anterior surface (Figs 9.44 and 9.45).
- The peroneal longus and brevis tendons pass posterior to the lateral malleolus deep to the superior peroneal retinaculum.

Anterior structures

- Tibialis anterior tendon, extensor hallucis longus tendon, anterior tibial artery, extensor digitorum longus tendon pass deep to extensor retinaculum in a medial to lateral direction, Tendons are Tom, Harry, Dick.
- The tarsal canal and tarsal sinus are found between the posterior and lateral subtalar joint and the anterior subtalar joint. They run from anterolateral to posteromedial. The tarsal canal extends posterior to sustentacalum tali. Several important ligaments including the cervical and interosseous ligaments lie in the canal and sinus. In patients with sinus tarsi syndrome with lateral ankle pain, diffuse low signal may be seen in the sinus representing fibrosis.

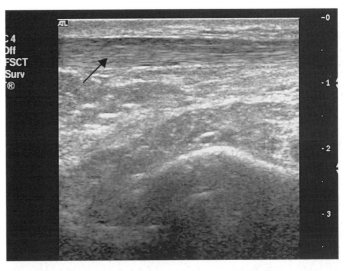

Fig. 9.45 Longitudinal ultrasound of the heel. The Achilles tendon is well visualized with ultrasound (arrow).

Systemic approach to the ankle

- Look at the bones for oedema and alignment.
- Identify the tendons – medial, lateral and anterior (Fig. 9.46).
- Look at the ligaments – anterior and posterior.
- Look at the sinus tarsi.
- Look at the Achilles tendon.
- Look at the plantar fascia.

MRI of the foot

The plantar fascia lies on the sole or plantar aspect of the foot. It may become inflamed, leading to plantar fasciitis.

Femoral angiography

Indications

Most peripheral angiography is performed using CT or MR for diagnosis of stenosis. Direct femoral angiography is used for intervention to perform angioplasty or stent insertion (Fig. 9.47).

Technique

- Angiography: a femoral artery puncture is performed at the groin. An anterograde study can be performed to visualize both legs, and a retrograde for intervention. The diagnostic angiograms have been superseded by CTA and MRA.
- Ultrasound can be performed at the groin to look for pseudoaneurysms using a high-frequency linear-array probe.
- CT angiography (CTA).
- MR angiography (MRA).

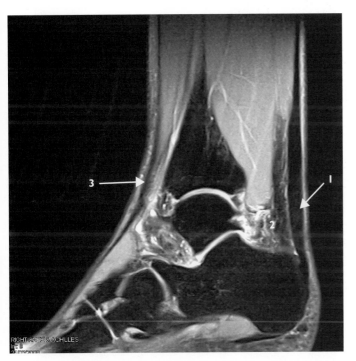

Fig. 9.44 Sagittal MRI fat-saturated image: the Achilles tendon is seen with Karger's fat pad (2) anterior to the Achilles tendon (1). Tibialis anterior running anterior over the dorsum of the foot (3).

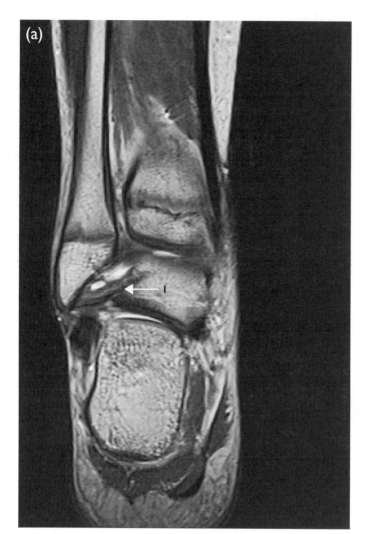

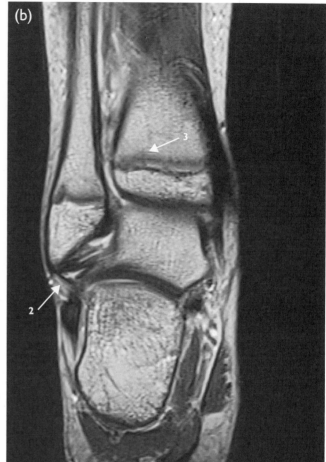

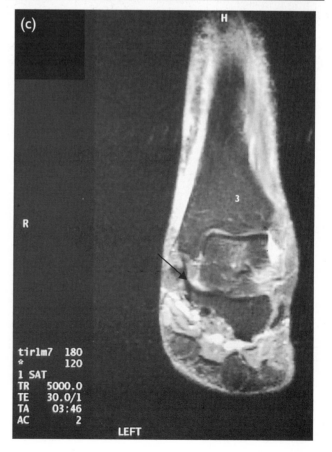

Fig. 9.46 (a,b) MRI of the ankle: coronal T1-weighted images showing the talofibular ligaments (1) and the fibulocalcaneal (2) lying laterally. Tibialis (3). (c) Part of the deltoid medial ligament. The tibiocalcaneal ligament is well seen (4).

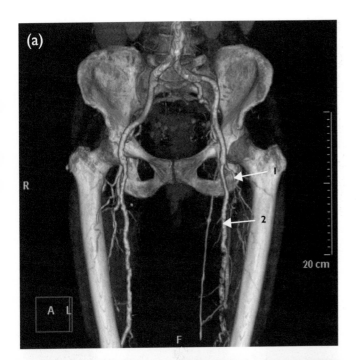

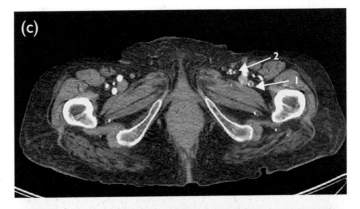

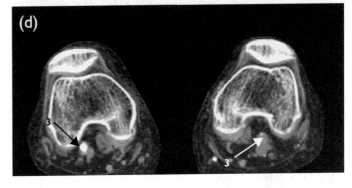

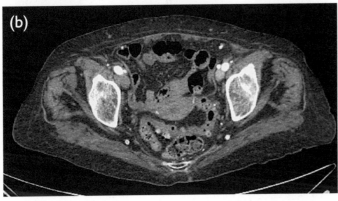

Fig. 9.47 CT femoral angiogram: (a) volume-rendered, reconstructed, coronal CT peripheral angiogram. (b) CT angiogram femoral images. (c,d) Conventional and digital images of the femoral angiogram. Profunda femoris (1), superficial femoral (2) and popliteal (3).

Findings
- The femoral vein lies medial to the femoral artery in the groin.
- The femoral artery lies medial to the lymph node.
- Within the groin the relationship from medial to lateral is VAN – vein, artery, nerve.
- The femoral sheath contains vein, artery and lymph nodes. The nerve lies outside the sheath.
- The great saphenous vein pierces the fascia laterally to enter the femoral vein in the femoral sheath.
- The external iliac vessel becomes the common femoral vessel at the inguinal ligament.
- The communal femoral artery becomes the superficial femoral artery and profunda femoris artery.
- The profunda femoris artery has branches and lies lateral and deep to the superficial femoral artery (see Fig. 9.47).

- The superficial femoral artery becomes the popliteal artery at the adductor canal or the medial border of the femur (Fig. 9.48).
- In the popliteal fossa the popliteal artery divides into the common tibioperoneal artery and the anterior tibial artery which runs laterally.
- The tibioperoneal trunk divides into the posterior tibial artery and the peroneal artery (Fig. 9.49).
- Within the calf the posterior tibial artery is the most medial.
- The peroneal artery is the middle artery.
- The anterior tibial artery is the most lateral and becomes the dorsalis pedis.

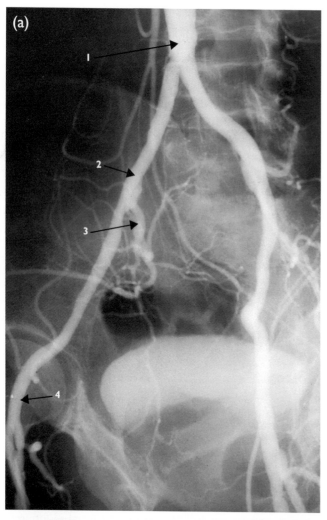

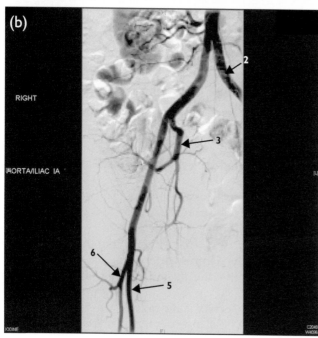

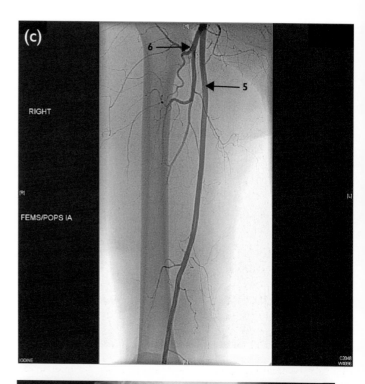

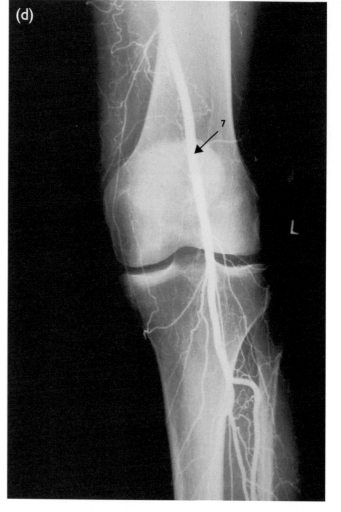

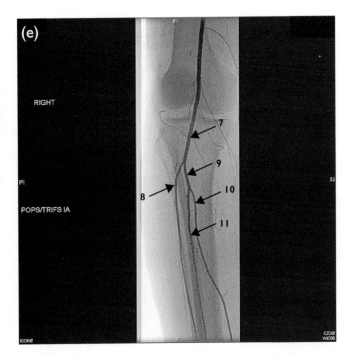

Fig. 9.48 Femoral angiogram. Aorta (1), common iliac (2), internal iliac (3), common femoral (4), superficial femoral (5), profunda femoris (6), popliteal (7), anterior tibialis (8), common tibial peroneal trunk (9), post tibial artery (10) and peroneal artery (11).

Venography

- Superficial veins in the lower limb drain into the deep veins, both containing valves.
- The short saphenous vein runs laterally, draining into the popliteal vein behind the knee and the long or great saphenous vein runs medially draining into the femoral vein in the inguinal triangle.
- In the calf there are three pairs of deep calf veins which join to form the popliteal vein in the popliteal fossa.

Technique

- Venography: contrast is injected into a vein or the dorsum of the foot after applying tourniquets above the ankle and putting the foot in warm water to vasodilate the veins.
- Doppler ultrasound.

CASES

Case 9.1

A patient has had a skiing knee injury. Initially plain films are taken with a horizontal beam lateral looking for a lipohaemarthrosis.

- Plain films: these show a fluid level above the knee in the suprapatellar bursa. This is a fat–fluid level with the fat rising above the fluid. When seen, suspect a fracture of the tibial plateau. The plain film shows a tibial plateau fracture, but CT is performed for better delineation of the fragments and amount of depression of the plateau.
- CT confirms the tibial plateau fracture. Its extent, number of fragments and amount of depression are well demonstrated.

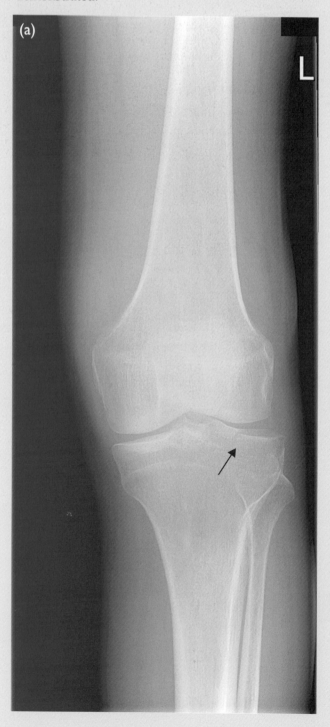

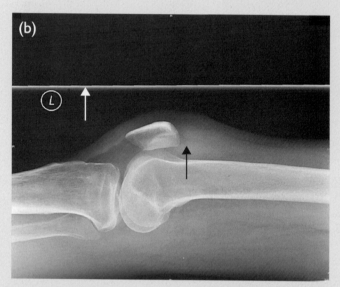

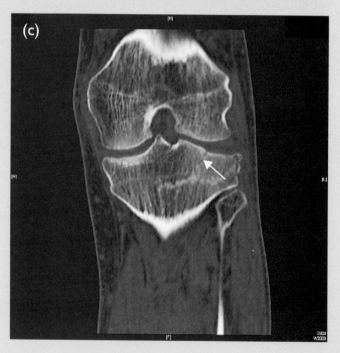

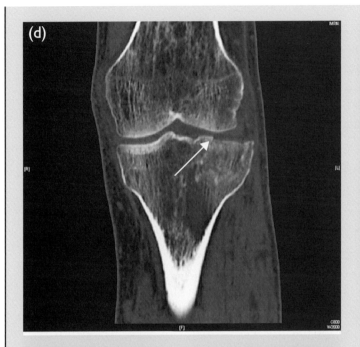

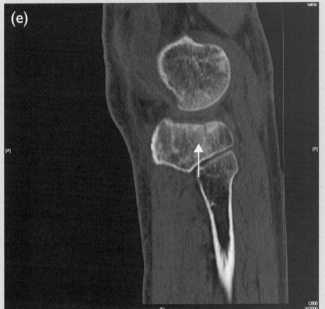

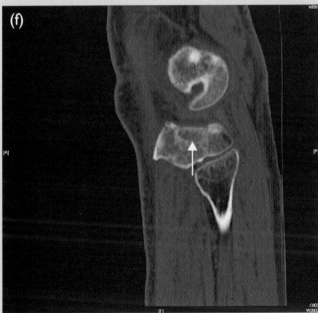

Fig. 9.49 Fracture of the tibial plateau: plain films (b). Horizontal beam shows a small lipohaemarthrosis (arrow) above the supra-patellar bursa. (a) A lucency is seen running through the lateral tibial plateau on the AP view (arrow). (c,d) Coronal MPR (magnetic proton resonance) CT and (e,f) sagittal MPR CT. The CT of the tibial plateau confirms a fracture of the lateral tibial plateau with some depression seen (arrow).

Case 9.2

A teenage boy presents with knee pain. A knee radiograph is performed initially, which is the modality of choice for bony abnormalities. The AP view shows a bony prominence projecting from the femur pointing away from the joint.

This cannot be seen on the lateral radiograph. Two views of bony lesions and injuries are indicated for accurate delineation of the lesion and any displacement of joints or fracture ends. An MRI was performed to show any associated soft-tissue abnormality, and the extent of the lesion and any underlying signal abnormality in the marrow. MRI will show bone oedema.

With bones, usually two or three orthogonal planes are performed with STIR images and T1-weighted images pre- and post-contrast.

The MRI is a coronal STIR image. This suppresses the fat but shows the fluid or oedema as high signal. Vessels also appear as high signal. The MRI shows the abnormality but no abnormal signal in the lump or oedema. There is no associated soft-tissue abnormality.

Diagnosis

The diagnosis is a benign lump called an osteochondroma. This is different to a bony spur. Osteochondromas grow away from a joint and have a small malignant potential. Bony spurs point towards the joint.

The importance of this case is the correct use of plain films, the use of two views and the correct indication for MRI to delineate extent of a lesion.

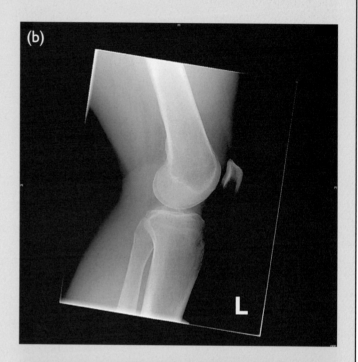

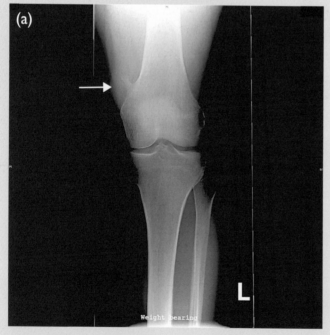

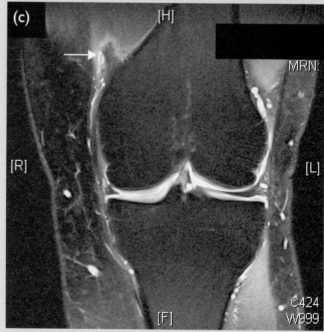

Fig. 9.50 (a,b) Plain films shows a bony exostosis projecting away from the joint, suggestive of an osteochondroma. (c) MRI showing this with a normal knee joint and no high signal within it to suggest any tumour.

Case 9.3

A 10-year-old is referred with limping. At this age a differential diagnosis includes Perthes' disease, congenital dislocation of the hip, and in a slightly older child slipped epiphysis. A plain radiograph of the pelvis is performed initially. Use Shenton's line to check for alignment of femoral head. The normal femoral head ossifies by age 1, the greater trochanter by age 5 and lesser trochanter by age 10.

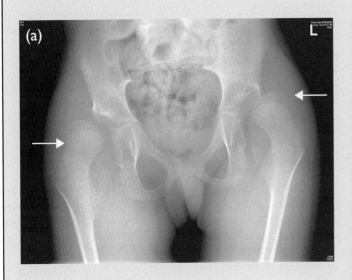 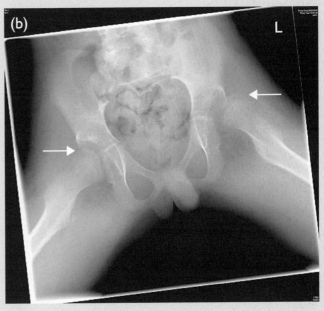

Fig. 9.51 (a) AP and (b) frog's leg lateral views showing bilateral acetabular dysplasia and dislocation of the left hip on the frog's leg lateral view.

Findings

The plain pelvic AP view shows dysplastic femoral heads and acetabula. The left femoral head is dislocated and the right is to a lesser extent. The acetabula are shallow and dysplastic.

This is better seen on the frog's leg lateral view. A normal pelvis is shown for comparison. Shenton's line shows the dislocation.

Diagnosis

Bilateral acetabular dysplasia and dislocation of the left and right hip.

10 On-call top tips

NEUROIMAGING

CT

Indications

In June 2003 the National Institute (for Health) and Clinical Excellence (NICE) issued guidance on the management of head injuries in the UK. The key features of this guidance were that the indications for computed tomography (CT) should include minor head injury.

The NICE guidelines are followed by A&E and make it difficult to refuse most neurological requests on call.

NICE guidelines

Skull radiograph indications
(1) Suspicion of intentional injury to a child less than 5 years of age and (2) penetrating trauma.

CT of the brain – NICE indications
According to NICE guidelines, a CT brain should be performed immediately when requested if:
- Glasgow Coma Scale (GCS) score <13 at any point since injury.
- GCS <15 2 hours after the injury.
- Suspected open or depressed skull fracture.
- Any sign of basal skull fracture: panda eyes, blood from tympanic membrane, cerebrospinal fluid (CSF) leak from the nose – otorrhoea.
- Post-traumatic seizure.
- Focal neurological deficit.
- More than one episode of vomiting since head injury.
- Amnesia for more than 30 min before impact.

CT should also be immediately requested when there is some loss of consciousness or post-traumatic amnesia in the following:
- Age >65 years.
- Following a dangerous mechanism of injury (e.g. ejected from motor vehicle, fell more than five stairs or hit by a motor vehicle).
- Coagulopathy.

Urgency of CT
- Immediately if GCS score <9 at any point since injury
- Within 1 hour of request and 8 hours in the remainder.
- If there is only amnesia and a dangerous mechanism of injury the scan can be performed between 2 and 8 hours.

NICE guidelines for when to refer to neurosurgeons
All new surgically significant lesions should be discussed with a neurosurgeon but not:
- a solitary contusion <5 mm
- thin localized subarachnoid blood if a primary subarachnoid haemorrhoid (SAH) is not suspected
- isolated pneumocephaly
- closed depressed skull fracture not through the inner table
- smear subdural haematoma <4 mm thick.

Technique
- Intravenous contrast: use in cases of immunosuppression, focal fitting or suspected cerebral metastases, although MRI is superior in the detection of metastases. Contrast is required for CT arteriography studies but requires neuroradiology review.
- Routinely review the images with bony windows to become familiar with normal skull markings. This aids detection of skull fractures.

Findings
The findings will vary according to the history and the image interpretation should be tailor-made to the request.

The Glasgow Coma Scale

The GSC is a neurological scale that aims to objectively record the conscious state of a person based on three responses, which can be verbal, motor and eye opening. It is score out of 15 with 3 being the worst score and 15 the best, when a person is fully awake. It is modified for infants when the Paediatric Glasgow Coma Scale is used:
- Best eye response: 4 grades.
- Best motor response: 5 grades.
- Best verbal response: 6 grades.

The NICE guidelines suggest that a CT of the brain should be performed if the GCS score is 13 at any point since injury or 13 or 14 2 hours after injury. This implies that there may only be confusion or disorientation at 2 hours that reduces the GCS to 14, indicating that a CT of the brain has to be performed within an hour of request to comply with NICE. The NICE guidelines have been written and the emergency staff are following them only so that it is better to be cooperative rather than obstructive when on call.

Trauma

Quick tips for interpreting the CT of the brain
- In the context of trauma, look for a scalp haematoma. The position of the scalp haematoma will guide you often to

the site of a skull fracture and any subtle contusions or extra-axial haemorrhage. A contre-coup injury is usually directly opposite the impact site (Fig. 10.1).

- Deep to the scalp haematoma look for haemorrhage, both parenchymal and extra-axial (Fig. 10.1).

- Always apply the bony windows, using a sharp filter to sharpen the images to assess for skull fractures. A fracture appears as an asymmetrical black line not seen on the opposite side of the skull with no marginal cortication, i.e. sclerosis of the edges. Follow a fracture by

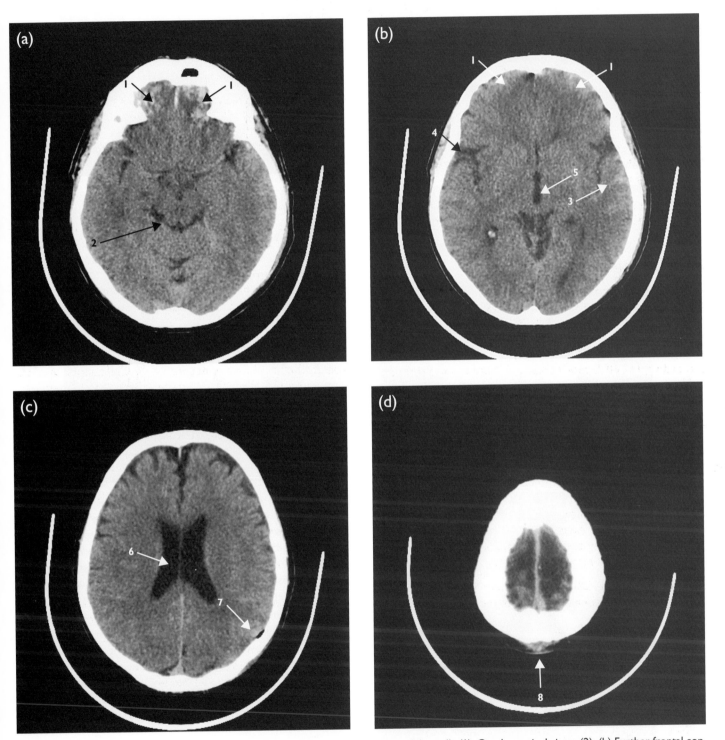

Fig. 10.1 (a) Axial CT at the level of the circle of Willis showing frontal contusions bilaterally (1). Quadrageminal cisem (2). (b) Further frontal contusion seen (1). Axial CT at the level of the third ventricle shows a small amount of subarachnoid haemorrhage laterally on the left side (3). Sylvian fissure (4) and third ventricle (5). (c) Level of the body of the lateral ventricles (6) shows some air within the cranial vault (7). This is indicative of a skull fracture. Bony windows need to be applied with a high-resolution bony algorithm or sharp filter to assess for skull fractures. (d) There is a scalp haematoma posteriorly (8). Axial CT at the level of the vertex.

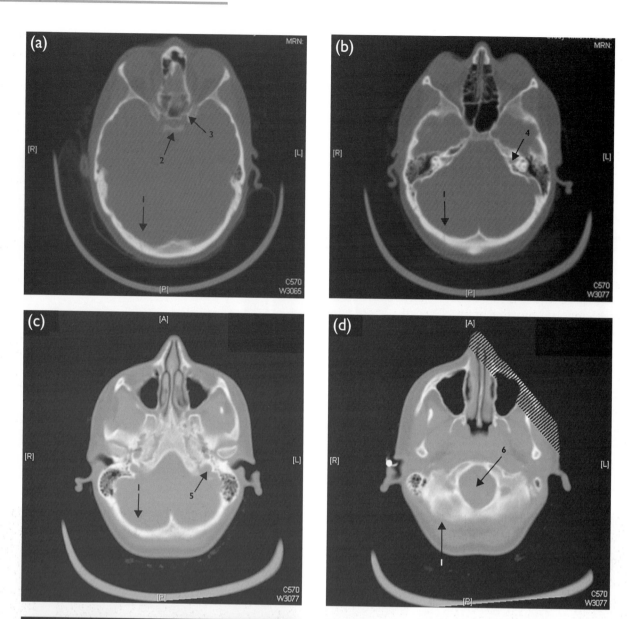

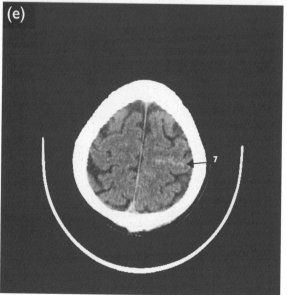

Fig. 10.2 Level of the anterior clinoid processes. (a–d) Axial CT bony windows: a skull fracture (1) in the right occipital region, which could be followed right down to the skull base. Fracture should be followed to see if they extend into foramina in the skull base. Dorsum sellae (2), anterior clinoid process (3), IAM (4), jugular trauma (5) and foramen magnum (6). (e) Axial CT unenhanced: this shows foci in the left cerebral hemisphere, with high density compatible with haemorrhage within the sulci (7).

scrolling through the images to assess the superior and inferior limit, in case the fracture extends into the petrous bone, sinuses or skull base (Fig.10.1b). This may lead to damage to nerves VII or VII or the ossicular chain.

- The bony windows also reveal the sites of old trauma and the site of any burr holes or neurosurgery previously performed.
- Look for haemorrhage extra-axially, i.e. outside the brain. It is important to look for a contre-coup injury. This is an injury incurred to the opposite side of the brain as a result of a deceleration injury (Fig. 10.1).
- Due to the narrow window range and the centre value, acute haemorrhage appears as high density on CT pf the brain. This remains high density for 2 weeks; it becomes isodense for the next 2 weeks and then hypodense at 4 weeks.
- Assess the sulci. This may be the only sign of some oedematous change within the brain. The sulci should be symmetrical around the brain including the vertex. Is there loss of sulci? Scroll through every image carefully looking for asymmetry and loss of the sulci associated with swelling (Fig. 10.12).
- Look for midline shift and measure the degree of shift at the level of the foramen of Monro in millimetres.
- Decide if the abnormality is intra-axial, i.e. within the brain, or extra-axial. If unsure it is important to put this in the provisional report and get a senior opinion.

- Look for contusions, in particular in the inferior frontal lobes and the anterior aspects of the temporal lobes (Fig. 10.3).
- Look for haemorrhage within the ventricles themselves, which is seen as a fluid–fluid level in the posterior horn of the lateral ventricle. Look for dilatation of the ventricles due to secondary hydrocephalus from the intraventricular haemorrhage (see Fig. 10.6).
- Look for fluid levels in the middle ear, mastoid air cells and paranasal sinuses, which may indicate blood after a fracture. Is there opacification of the external auditory canal suggesting blood?
- Look for tiny pockets of extradural air, which is associated with a fracture into the sinuses or skull. Apply a lung window to make this easier (Fig. 10.4).
- Look at the facial bones for associated trauma.

Acute stroke

NICE guidelines published in July 2009 stipulate that brain imaging should be performed immediately on all people suspected of a cerebrovascular accident (CVA). They qualify that 'immediately' should be the next available slot or within an hour in those:

- indicated for thrombolysis or early anticoagulation treatment
- with a known bleeding tendency

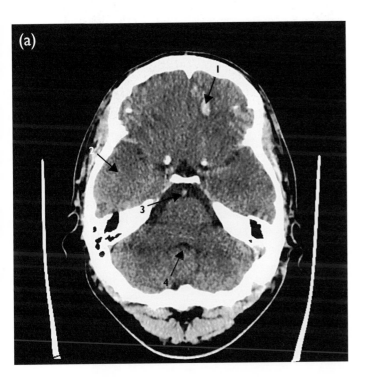
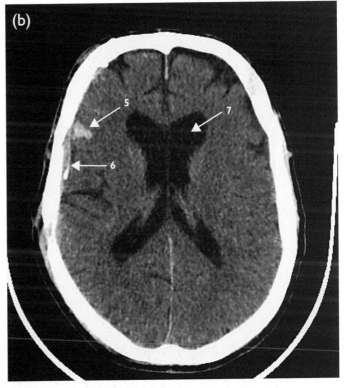

Fig. 10.3 (a) Axial unenhanced CT at the level of the suprasellar cistern showing frontal contusions (1). Temporal lobe (2), basilar artery (3) and fourth ventricle (4). (b) Axial CT unenhanced, at the level of the body of the lateral ventricles, showing a right-sided contusion (5) and a small amount of acute-on-chronic extra-axial haemorrhage (6). Left ventricle (7).

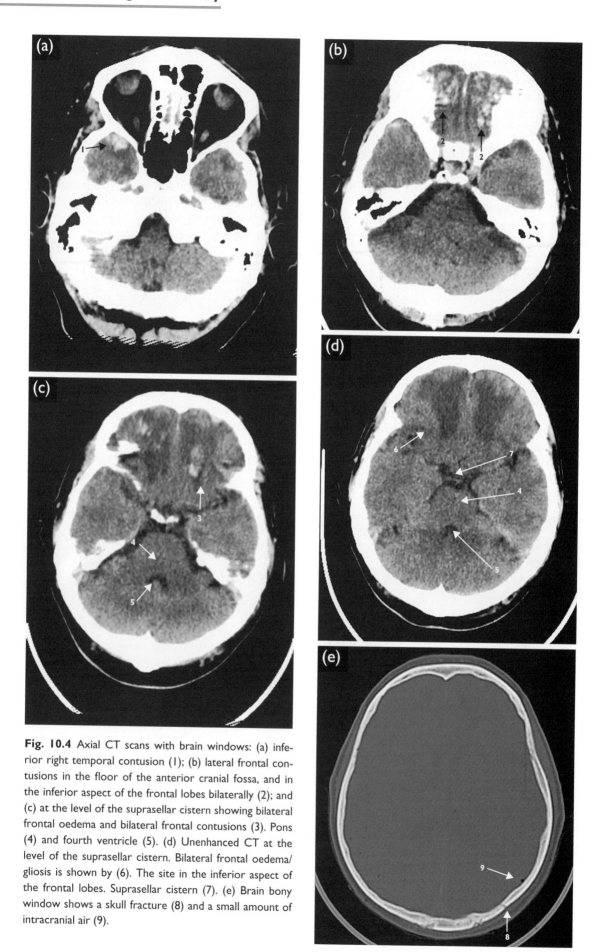

Fig. 10.4 Axial CT scans with brain windows: (a) inferior right temporal contusion (1); (b) lateral frontal contusions in the floor of the anterior cranial fossa, and in the inferior aspect of the frontal lobes bilaterally (2); and (c) at the level of the suprasellar cistern showing bilateral frontal oedema and bilateral frontal contusions (3). Pons (4) and fourth ventricle (5). (d) Unenhanced CT at the level of the suprasellar cistern. Bilateral frontal oedema/gliosis is shown by (6). The site in the inferior aspect of the frontal lobes. Suprasellar cistern (7). (e) Brain bony window shows a skull fracture (8) and a small amount of intracranial air (9).

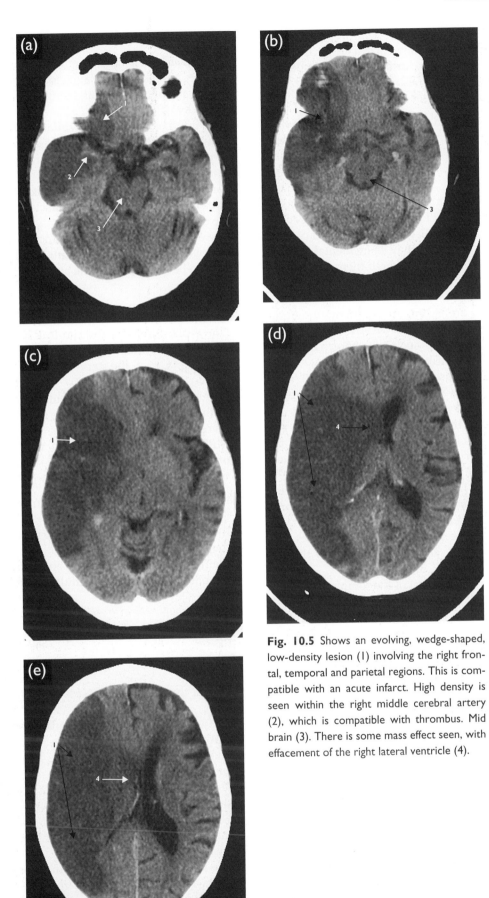

Fig. 10.5 Shows an evolving, wedge-shaped, low-density lesion (1) involving the right frontal, temporal and parietal regions. This is compatible with an acute infarct. High density is seen within the right middle cerebral artery (2), which is compatible with thrombus. Mid brain (3). There is some mass effect seen, with effacement of the right lateral ventricle (4).

- on anticoagulants
- a depressed level of consciousness, i.e. a GCS <13
- with unexplained progressive or fluctuating symptoms
- with papilloedema, neck stiffness or fever
- with severe headache at onset of stroke symptoms.

The guidelines state that diffusion-weighted MRI is the modality of choice for transient ischaemic attacks (TIAs) and give a full description of when and in which patients.

Findings in stroke
- The clinical details are important and should be correlated with the radiological findings; a patient presenting with left-sided weakness will have a right-sided cerebral event in most cases. Changes may be incidental if on the incorrect anatomical side. However, if there is a discrepancy check that the physicians have given the correct findings.
- Unenhanced scans are taken. If a patient undergoes thrombolysis, a follow-up scan is performed to look for improvement, complications such as haemorrhage or the development of an established infarct.
- In a suspected stroke, use the stroke window 40/40 to look for subtle asymmetry with low density or subtle loss of sulci. The loss of a few sulci may be the only clue.
- In a thrombotic CVA there may be an associated hyperdense vessel. Look closely at the circle of Willis and middle cerebral artery (MCA) for the hyperdense linear sign of thrombus in a vessel (Fig. 10.5).
- In an SAH the only finding may be loss of sulci. Every sulcus must be reviewed and compared with the opposite side to see asymmetry.
- In SAH blood may be seen layering in the ventricles with a fluid–fluid level due to blood layering below the less dense cerebrospinal fluid (CSF) (Fig. 10.6).
- The inferior images at the level of the foramen magnum may show coning. The cerebellar tonsils should not be projecting through the foramen magnum on CT (Fig. 10.7).
- Further supporting signs of raised intracranial pressure is loss of the basal cisterns, i.e. the prepontine cistern is effaced.

Global ischaemia

- On CT normally there should be grey/white differentiation, with the grey matter being denser than the white. This normal reversal of grey/white matter differentiation is due to white matter being fattier as a result of the presence of sphingomyelin.
- In severe global oedema/ischaemia there is complete loss of the grey/white matter which appears featureless supratentorially with no visible sulci. The cerebellum in the posterior fossa may then appear bright like a 'white triangle' (Fig. 10.8).

Facial bones trauma – orbital blow-out fracture
- CT is indicated in assessment of orbital blow-out fracture.
- Images are taken in the axial plane with coronal and sagittal reformatted images using multiplanar reformated images (MPR).
- The inferior and medial orbital wall and any displaced bony fragments can be easily visualized with CT.
- The medial wall or lamina papyracea is commonly fractured due to its thin nature.
- Any intraconal haemorrhage that is haemorrhage in the area enclosed by the rectus muscles behind the globe can be detected.
- Associated facial injuries are documented.
- Displacement of the globe with enophthalmos or proptosis can be measured on the axial images (Fig. 10.9).

Cervical spine – NICE guidelines
- Three plain films of the cervical spine are indicated in trauma. If an area is not well seen using conventional imaging, CT of the cervical spine is the modality of choice.
- In multi-trauma the whole spine can be quickly assessed with CT if the patient is having other body areas imaged using CT.
- MRI is indicated if there are neurological symptoms attributable to the cervical spine or if there is suspicion of ligamentous or disc injuries.

Cervical spine imaging is also recommended when:
- GCS <13
- there is clinical suspicion of injury, despite normal X-ray
- the patient is intubated
- plain films are inadequate or abnormal
- the patient is scanned for multiregion trauma.

Technique
Images are taken in the axial plane and reconstructed using MPR.

Findings
- Use all three planes to assess the spine for a fracture on CT.
- The joints of Lushka are posterolateral lips to the bodies that can be seen on axial images.
- The distance between the facets should be symmetrical an axial CT.
- The basivertebral veins causing a Y shape in the bodies should be differentiated from fractures (Fig. 10.10).
- The prevertebral soft tissues are usually widened in trauma and aid in locating the level of trauma when widened.
- The anterior and posterior spinal lines can be seen well on the reconstructed sagittal images, as can the spinolaminar and pillar line and atlantoaxial distance.

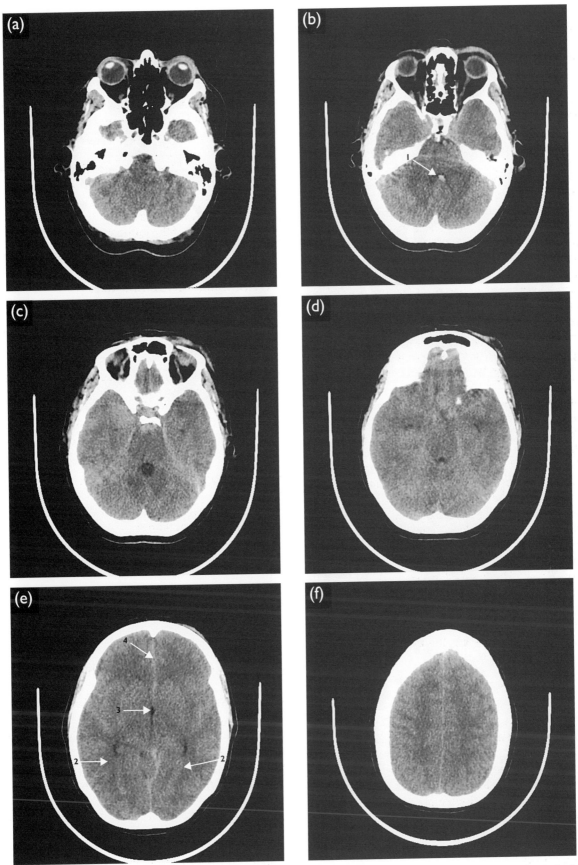

Fig. 10.6 (a–f) Complete lack of sulci and ventricles for patient's age. Subarachnoid haemorrhage can cause generalized loss of sulci if extensive. The white arrow marks haemorrhage within the fourth ventricle (1). Layering of blood within the occipital horn of the lateral ventricles (2). Third ventricle (3) and blood in talx (4).

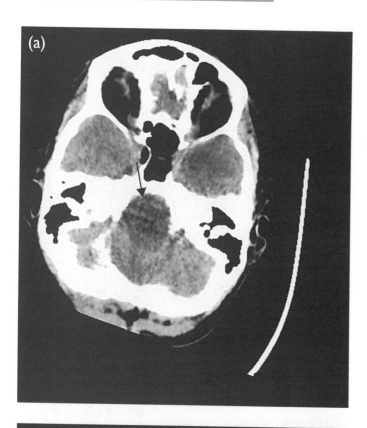

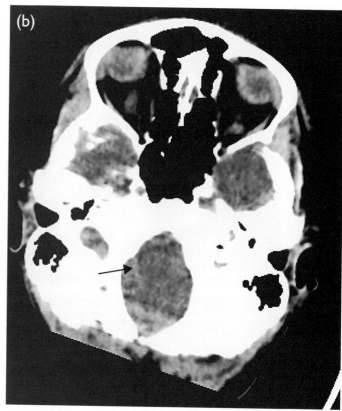

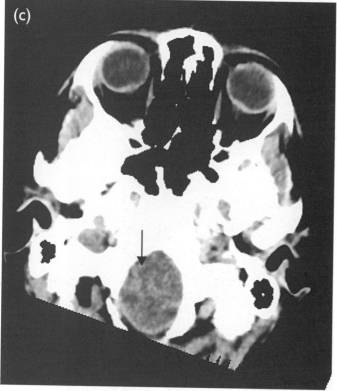

Fig. 10.7 Axial CT through the skull base, showing three images of complete loss of cerebrospinal fluid (CSF) space at the level of the foramen magnum, consistent with raised intracranial pressure; the patient is at risk of coning (arrow). The cerebellar tonsils may be seen protruding into the foramen magnum.

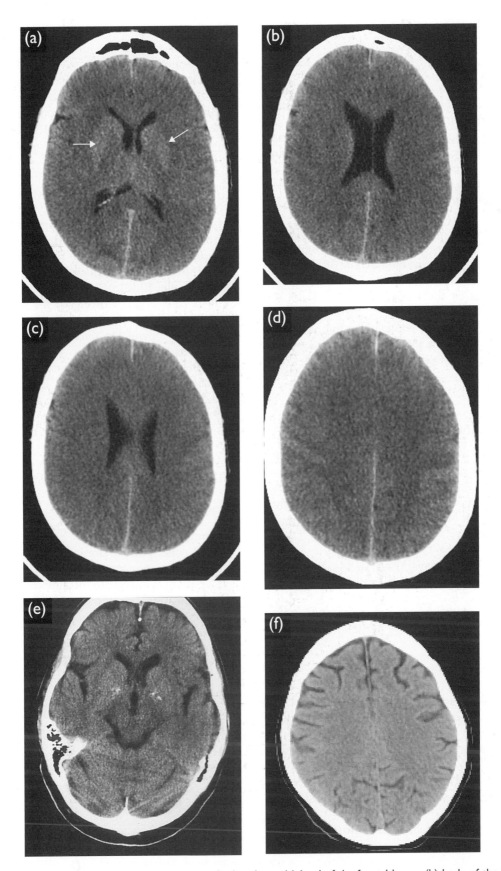

Fig. 10.8 Images taken at various levels showing extensive cerebral oedema: (a) level of the frontal horns; (b) body of the lateral ventricles; (c) more superior section at the level of the body of the lateral ventricles; and (d) centrum semiovale. Axial CT unenhanced images show a loss of grey/white matter differentiation and sulci, consistent with generalized oedema. Note that the basal ganglia are very prominent on (a) (arrow). This is due to the featureless remaining brain losing grey/white matter differentiation. Compare (e) and (f) which show normal sulci and grey/white matter from a different patient.

CHEST

CT pulmonary angiogram

- Indication: breathlessness, chest pain, raised D-dimers.
- Technique: bolus tracking is used to find the best timing for optimal opacification of the pulmonary arteries.
- Findings: to look for a pulmonary embolus (PE), initially start by zooming in on one lung in the axial plane and carefully scrolling through each level. Then zoom in on the other lung. Follow the vessels from the hila. Beware of confusing the pulmonary veins, which drain into the left atrium.
- Review the lung windows for interstitial lung disease, pneumothorax, airspace or ground-glass shadowing.
- Review the mediastinum for mediastinal lymphadenopathy.
- Review the images in the coronal plane and thicken the slices using maximum intensity projection (MIP) to about 7–8 mm and again zoom in on one lung at a time. As one improves this may seem unnecessary, but it focuses the eye when on call and is a good safety check (Fig. 10.11).

CT for chest and body trauma

CT rapidly evaluates the multi-trauma victim and is the modality of choice. Blunt trauma is the most common injury and is usually due to a road traffic accident (RTA). Chest trauma, alone or in combination with other injuries, accounts for almost half of all traumatic deaths.

Technique

Intravenous contrast is always used unless there is a contrast allergy or contrast is contraindicated for other reasons.

Use a system for reviewing the scans.

Chest

- Look at the mediastinum for haematoma on soft-tissue windows.
- Check that the main vessels are intact and the trachea.
- Look at the lungs for contusions and the pleural spaces for fluid/haemothorax.
- Review lung windows for pneumothorax and pneumomediastinum.
- Look at the bony windows for rib fractures, especially where multiple fractures to the same ribs constitute a flail segment.
- Look at the scapulae and vertebrae for fractures. Although these may seem irrelevant in the context of multiorgan trauma, when the patient has recovered from the acute event, the radiologist will be criticized for not mentioning trauma to the remaining skeleton.
- Look for unsuspected incidental pathology such as a lung tumour or aortic aneurysm.

Abdomen

- In trauma always use intravenous contrast unless contraindicated in allergy.
- Trauma to the abdominal organs is more common if there are fractures of the lower three ribs.
- The spleen is the most commonly injured intra-abdominal organ. CT is the modality of choice for assessing splenic trauma.

Findings

- The presence of free fluid, i.e. ascites, haemoperitoneum or urine in the peritoneal cavity. The peritoneal cavity consists of the subphrenic spaces, paracolic gutters and pelvis. Free intra-abdominal fluid in the context of trauma indicates that there has been significant trauma and the source of haemorrhage or a urine leak must be located (Fig. 10.12).
- Check each organ thoroughly for laceration, fracture to an organ or damage to the vascular pedicle.
- Check the bowel for thickening which may be due to haemorrhage.
- Use a lung window to look for free peritoneal air.
- If just the abdomen has been imaged, review the lung bases for pleural collections, contusions and pneumothorax.
- Review the vertebra and pelvis for bony injury.

URINARY TRACT

CT KUB

Indications

1. Renal colic: patient presents with acute loin pain and haematuria on urinalysis.
2. If a patient is allergic to intravenous contrast and cannot undergo an intravenous urogram (IVU).

Technique

No intravenous contrast required. Unenhanced images detect calcification.

Findings

Fig. 10.13 shows a dilated left renal pelvis and ureter. A stone is seen at the distal end on the left ureter.

When reviewing the images

In the case in Fig. 10.13, the lung bases are clear. The unenhanced liver, spleen, pancreas and adrenal glands appear normal.

There is no free fluid in the abdomen or pelvis. CT findings in acute obstruction from a ureteric calculus include:

- Perirenal stranding, although this can be seen bilaterally as a normal finding with increasing age.
- A dilated ureter or renal pelvis.
- A dense stone in the ureter.

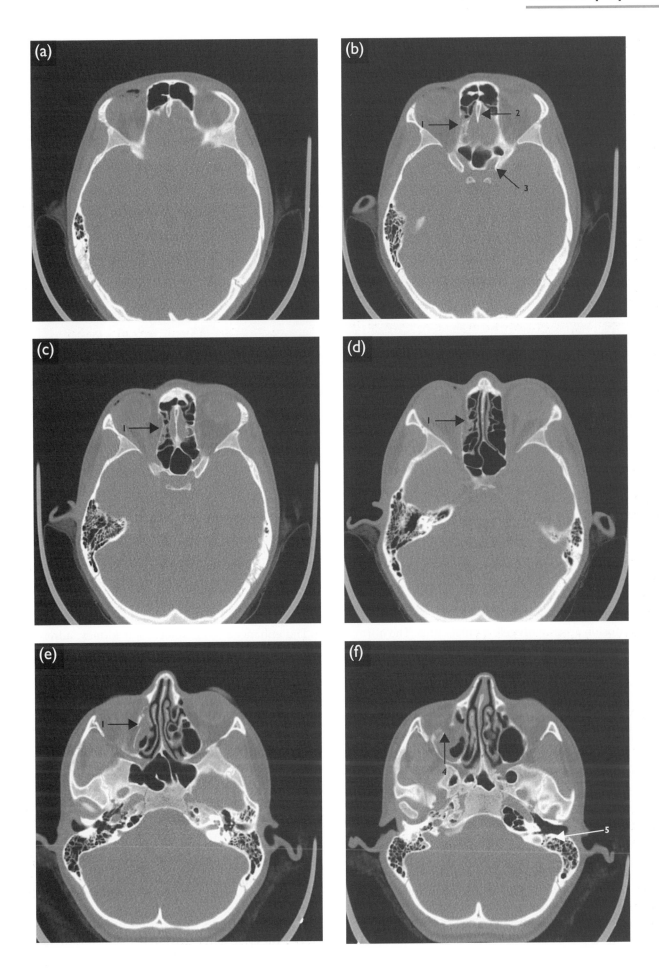

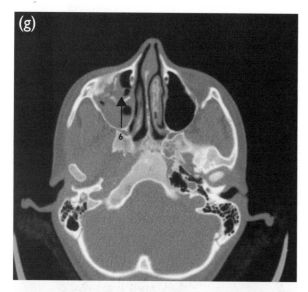

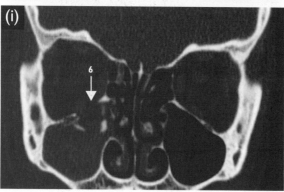

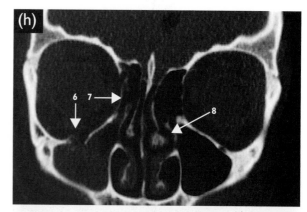

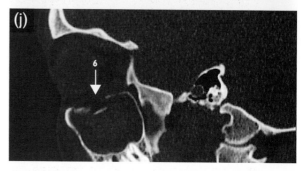

Fig. 10.9 (a–e) Axial CT images through the orbit with bony windows showing a blow-out fracture of the lamina papyracea (1). Crista galli (2) and anterior clinoid process (3). (f,g) A fracture through the inferior orbital margin and fragments of bone within the right maxillary antrum (4). Eam (5) and inferior blow-out fracture of the orbit (6). (h–j) Coronal reconstructed images on bony window and ostimeatal complex marks the fracture of the right lamina papyracea (7).

- The normal ureter can be hard to follow into the pelvis and confusion arises with pelvic phleboliths. The normal ureter has quite a medial course in the pelvis. Following the course of the ureter on the coronal and sagittal images helps differentiate phleboliths from calculi.
- The ovaries, gallbladder, bowel and appendix can be assessed for unsuspected pathology or a different diagnosis to ureteric colic.

CT of pyelonephritis

A patient presents with acute loin pain and sepsis. There are pus cells in the urine on urinalysis. There may also be some haematuria.

Technique
Give intravenous contrast in suspected pyelonephritis. Occasionally the history may be confused with renal colic and a pre-contrast CT KUB may also be performed, but, when the findings of perirenal fluid and stranding are seen and pyelonephritis is suspected, a post-contrast phase can be performed.

Findings (Fig. 10.14)
- The enhanced liver, spleen, left kidney, adrenal glands and bowel appear normal.
- The right kidney is abnormal with a striated nephrogram appearance. This is a finding associated with acute pyelonephritis.
- There is a small amount of free fluid in the right perirenal space and the right paracolic gutter.
- The fat is hazy and slightly stranded around the right kidney.
- This is the appearance of acute right pyelonephritis.

ABDOMEN

CT: abdominal collection

Indications
Suspected collection, obstruction to the bowel, ischaemic bowel, colitis, acute pancreatitis and its follow-up.

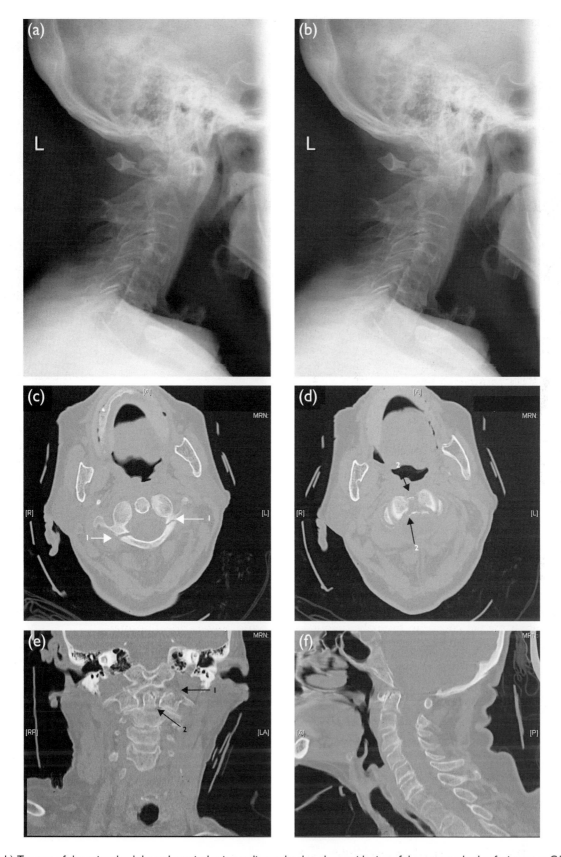

Fig. 10.10 (a,b) Trauma of the spine: both lateral cervical spine radiographs that show widening of the prevertebral soft tissues at C1–2 and loss of alignment. (c,d) Axial CT through C1–2 showing a fracture of the atlas (1) and the axis (2). (e) MPR (multiplanar reformatted) coronal and (f) MPR sagittal images showing the fractures of C1 (1) and C2 (2).

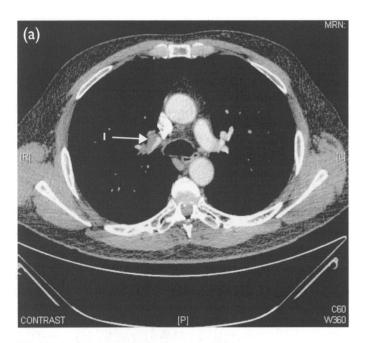

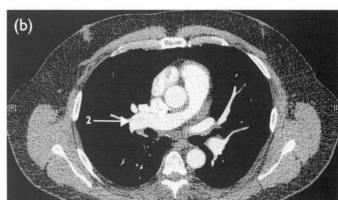

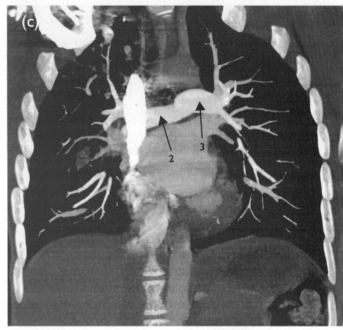

Fig. 10.11 (a) CT pulmonary angiography (CTPA) axial post-contrast image showing a thrombus in the right main pulmonary artery (1). Compare with (c) CTPA axial post-contrast image, which shows a normal right pulmonary artery (2). (b) Coronal maximum integrated projection (MIP) image of a patient with no pulmonary embolism showing the detail obtained with an MIP image. Left pulmonary artery (3).

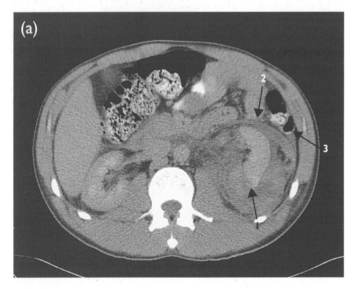

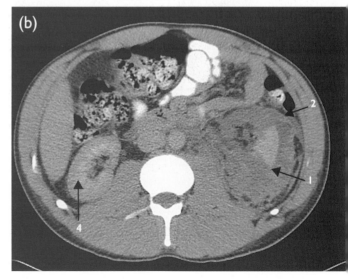

Fig. 10.12 (a) An extensive heterogeneous perirenal haematoma is seen on the left. Block arrow shows the fracture of the left kidney (1), which is displaced anteriorly. (2) demarcates Gerota's fascia, which is confining the haematoma. (3) shows some free fluid. The right kidney (4) shows the normal perirenal appearance. (b) (1) shows the fracture of the left kidney. (2) again marks Gerota's fascia.

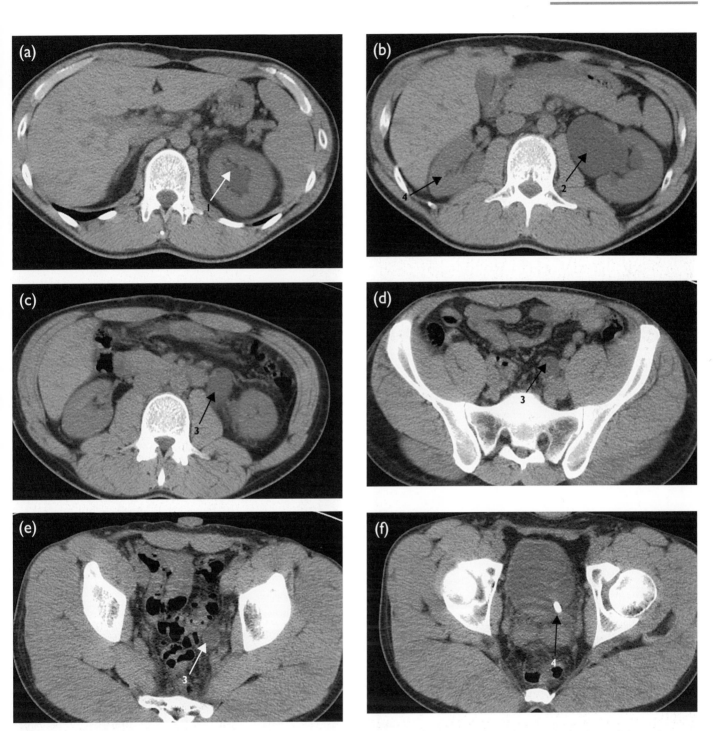

Fig. 10.13 Unenhanced CT KUB images: (a) (1) marks the dilated upper pole calyx. (b–f) The (2) marks the dilated renal pelvis and shows the cause of the dilated ureter (3) down into the pelvis, where on (f) there is a stone at the left vesicoureteric junction (4).

Technique

Intravenous contrast is given unless looking for calcification when a pre-contrast study is also taken.

If a patient is vomiting or has bowel obstruction then oral contrast is omitted. Dilated bowel has its own contrast because it distends with water.

Findings

Develop a routine for reporting the examination:
- Start reviewing the lung bases. A pneumothorax or lung metastases can be missed without using lung windows.
- Review the whole liver, then the biliary tract and gall-bladder.

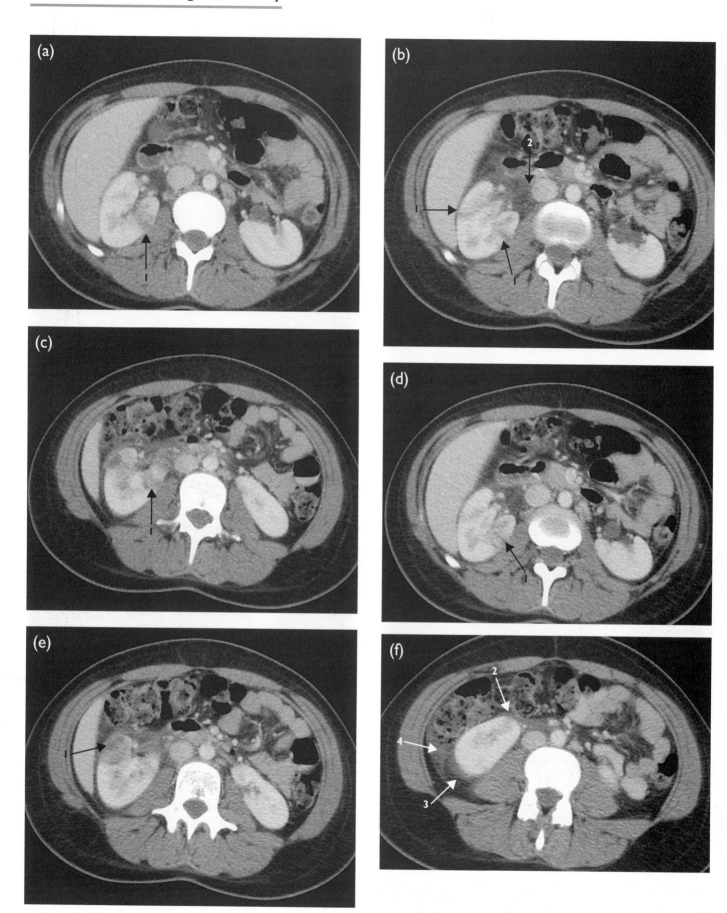

Fig. 10.14 Enhanced axial CTs through the renal tract: (1) marks striations visible within the right kidney, (2) marks some perirenal stranding, (3) shows perirenal fluid, (f) (4) shows free intra-abdominal fluid.

- Then review the spleen for size and enhancement.
- Review the kidneys, adrenals and para-aortic region for enlarged nodes.
- Review the bowel for dilatation and wall thickening. Again it is best to develop a system. One system is to start following the rectum and to scroll up and down, following the rectum to the sigmoid, then to the descending, transverse and ascending colon. Starting with the axial plane and using the coronal plane, which looks similar to barium enema images, is helpful. Any bowel thickening or pericolonic stranding is more apparent if the whole bowel is checked in a systematic order. The small bowel also needs systematic following, starting at the stomach and following down to the duodenum and then the jejunum.
- Review the abdomen and pelvis for free fluid under the diaphragms, in the paracolic gutters and the pelvis (Fig. 10.15).
- Assess the spine on bony windows.
- Review the corners of the film for thrombus in the femoral veins, for peritoneal deposits. These are seen in the areas were there is usually fat such as the greater omentum anteriorly and the gastrosplenic ligament.
- Review the abdominal wall for hernias and any herniated bowel.
- Try to correlate the clinical history with any findings. A patient with right iliac fossa pain is more likely to have radiological signs in the right iliac fossa than the left upper quadrant, so closely scrutinize the appendix and caecum and right adnexal structures if such a history.

Left iliac fossa pain

Investigation: CT

Indications
Diverticulitis is a very common reason for referral for CT on call. CT can show the complications of acute diverticulitis such as abscess or perforation.

Technique
- Intravenous contrast should be administered.
- Careful scrutiny of the pericolonic fat for stranding in the pelvis should be made and search of any small pockets of free fluid.
- Lung windows when applied to the abdominal images, aid detection of any free air and perforation.

Findings (Fig. 10.16)
A patient presented with acute left iliac fossa (LIF) pain. A CT of the abdomen/pelvis was performed.

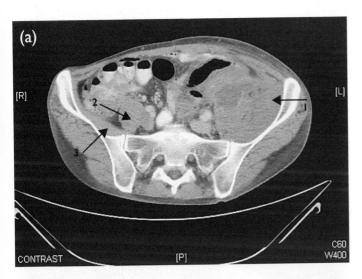

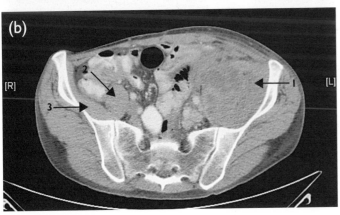

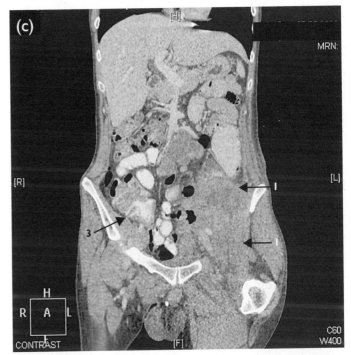

Fig. 10.15 There is a collection in the left iliopsoas muscle (1). (a,b) Axial enhanced CT; (c) a coronal reconstructed CT. (b) The normal right psoas (2) and iliacus muscles (3).

- Look for bowel wall thickening: the CT scan shows thickened sigmoid colon.
- Look for stranding: there is stranding in the fat around the sigmoid colon.
- Look for any free fluid or collections: these may look like

loops of bowel so, by carefully scrolling up and down following the loops, any collections and abscesses become more apparent. In this case there is a left-sided pelvic abscess. There may be more than one abscess so look for multiple walled-off abscesses.

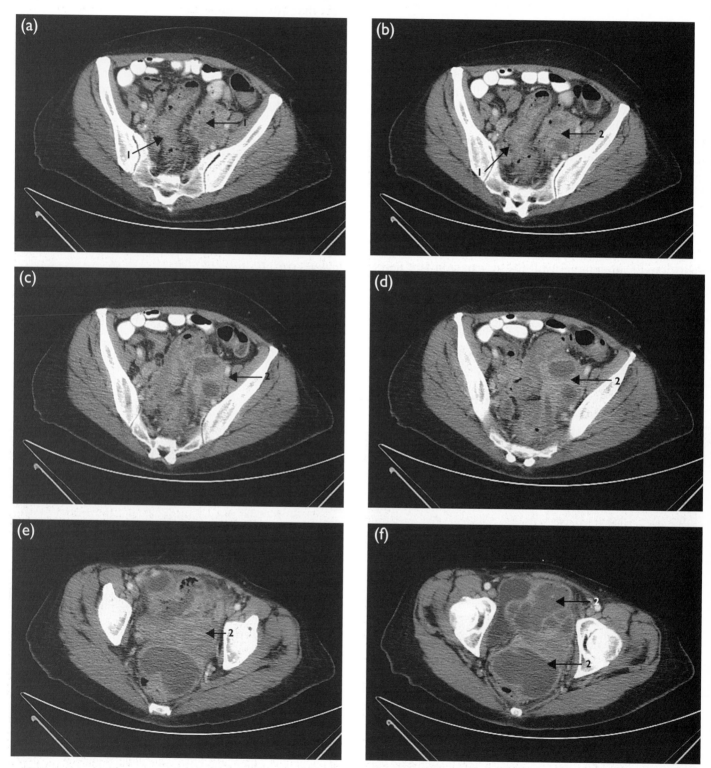

Fig. 10.16 Enhanced axial CT images through the pelvis: (1) shows the thickened sigmoid colon on (a) and (b), with diverticular disease and some stranding around the fat, (2) shows an abscess in the left adnexal region. Tracing the lumen of the bowel, extra-axial air and collections can be identified.

CT for trauma

In trauma conventional plain films are often initially performed, but CT precisely assesses the fracture extent, bony fragment location and identification of any intra-articular fragments.

- CT for thoracolumbar spine trauma: CT is useful for characterizing posterior element fractures and spinal canal impingement. It aids in the assessment of stability.
- CT for acetabular fractures: use the axial plane and multiplanar reformatting to show the fracture and its relation-

ship to the joint and displacement of any bony fragments (Fig. 10.17).
- CT in tibial plateau fractures: displacement of fragments by more than 3–5 mm warrants open reduction. Again axial imaging with MPR shows three orthogonal planes.
- CT in complex ankle trauma: again the relationship of fractures to the ankle mortise and subtalar joint and other foot joints is aided with multiplanar CT.
- CT in shoulder, elbow and wrist trauma aids bony fragment definition.

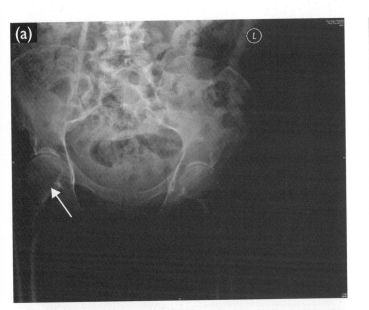
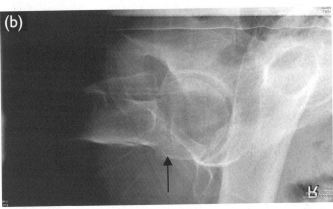
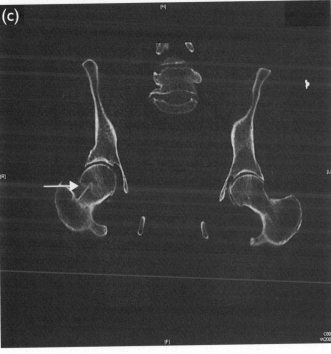
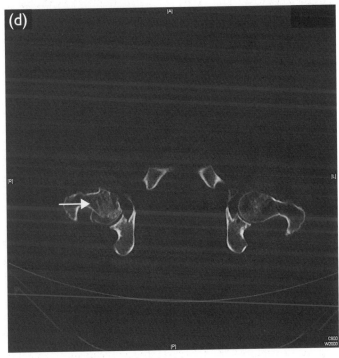

Fig. 10.17 (a) Coronal pelvic radiograph; (b) lateral right hip radiograph; (c) coronal CT; and (d) axial CT. (a–c) There appears to be an impacted fracture, marked by the arrow of the right femoral neck. (c,d) Confirmation of a fracture.

CASES

Case 1

- A 79-year-old presents with confusion and a history of a fall. Confusion decreases the GCS score in the verbal category from 5 down to 4.
- NICE guidelines indicate that a CT of the brain is required initially.

What is the diagnosis?

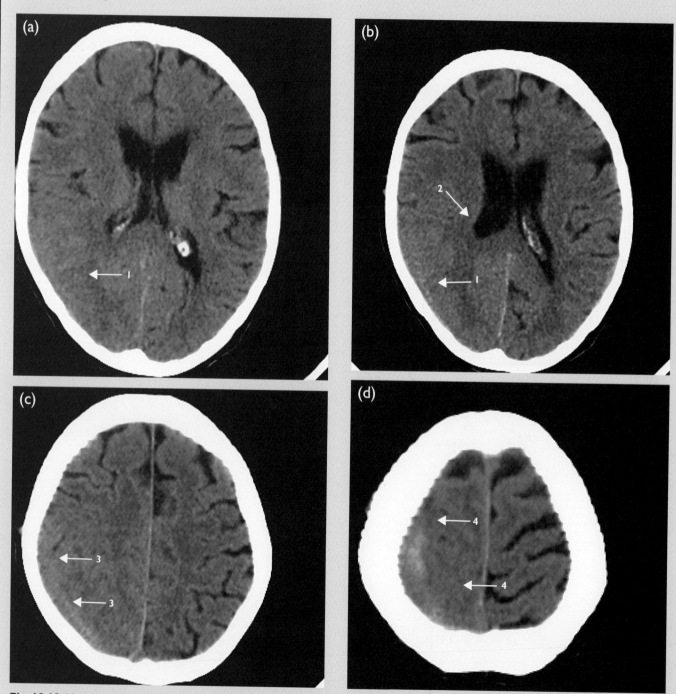

Fig. 10.18 Unenhanced axial CTs: (a) shows the first sign (1), which is a loss of sulci when comparing with the other side in the right parieto-occipital region. (b) (1) again shows asymmetry with loss of sulci. (2) shows compression or effacement of the occipital horn of the right lateral ventricle. (c) (3) show an extra-axial collection, causing loss of sulci and a small collection outside the brain. (d) A relatively acute subdural (4), showing the importance of assessing the vertex. Look at the loss of sulci.

Systematic analysis
- Is there a scalp haematoma?
- Is there a fracture deep to haematoma?

Use post-processing to sharpen the images
- Are there any contusions deep to scalp haematoma or fracture or in a contrecoup distribution?
- Is there an extraxial collection?
- Are there any loss of sulci?

Findings
- There is no scalp haematoma and there is no skull fracture on bony windows.
- The abnormality can be seen only on the top axial images towards the vertex, hence the importance of reviewing the vertex images very carefully. In this case, there is loss of sulci and asymmetry of the sulci in the right parieto-temporal region, and the subdural haemorrhage can be seen on the uppermost two images.
- Answer: acute right subdural haemorrhage.

Case 2

A 65-year-old man presents with acute right-sided weakness. An infarct is suspected and CT is performed.

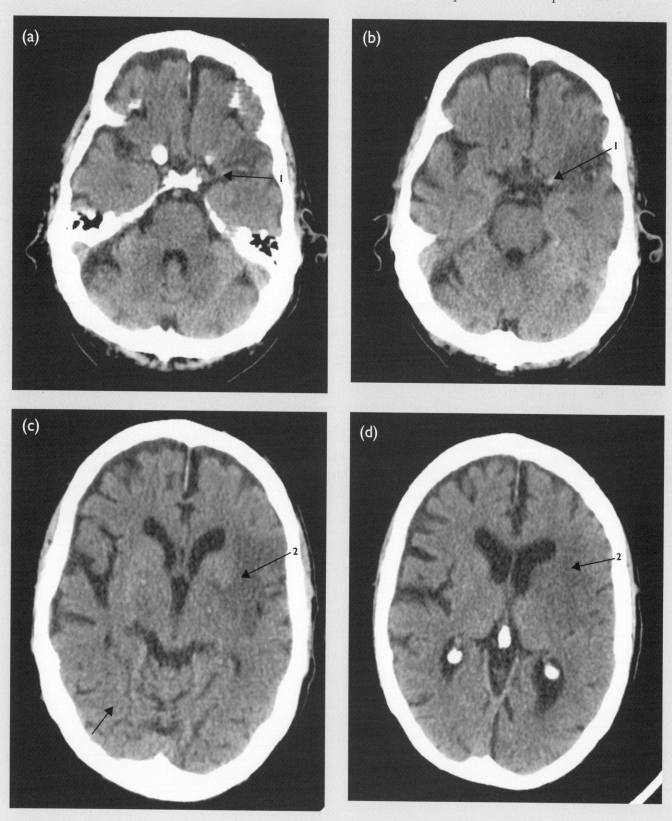

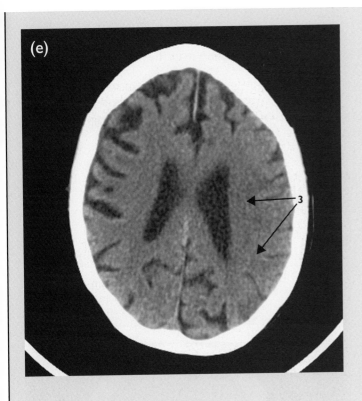

Fig. 10.19 Axial CT images of the brain showing a hyperdense (1) left middle cerebral artery (a, b), a wedge-shaped low density lesion (2) extending to the cortex with loss of sulci (c, d), and further loss of density and loss of sulci in the left cerebral hemisphere (3) (e).

Systematic analysis
- In the context of a possible CVA look for a hyperdense vessel around the circle of Willis or in the sylvian fissure.
- Look for loss of sulci and a low density wedge-shaped area.
- Use stroke windows.

Findings
There is a hyperdense left MCA. There is a loss of sulci and a wedge-shaped low density region in the right front temporal region.

Answer
Acute right MCA infarct.

Case 3

An 84-year-old woman from a nursing home presents with recent onset of confusion over the past month. CT of the brain is indicated.

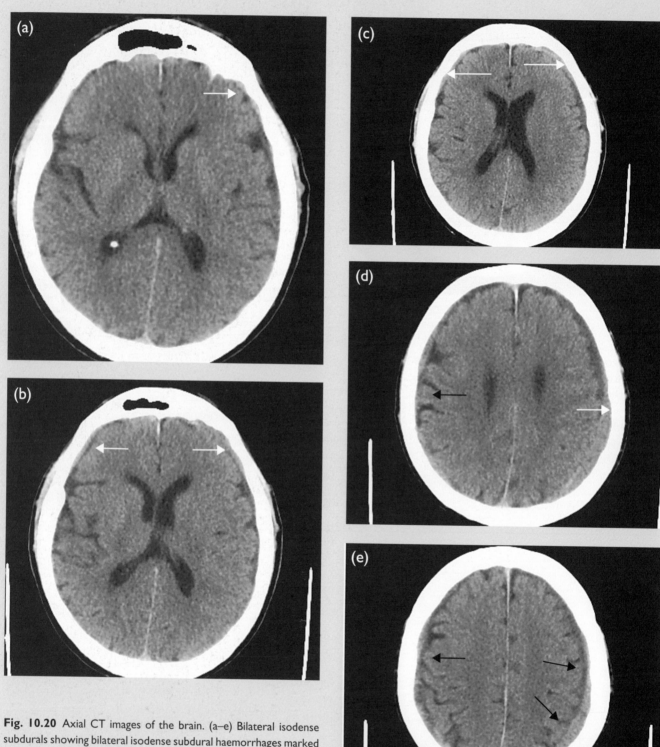

Fig. 10.20 Axial CT images of the brain. (a–e) Bilateral isodense subdurals showing bilateral isodense subdural haemorrhages marked by the arrows. The sulci do not extend to the skull surface, which should be a review area to look for subtle or isodense subdural collections. The collections are between 2 and 4 weeks old.

Findings
- The sulci do not go to the edge but stop some distance before the skull, suggestive of an extra-axial collection.
- There are bilateral, isodense, subdural collections. Blood is isodense between about 2 and 4 weeks on CT brain windows.
- The basal cisterns should be reviewed for any mass effect and the temporal horns for dilatation.
- Bilateral subdurals can be missed due to their symmetry. The sulci are the clue, not extending to the skull surface.
- Note: smear subdurals <4 mm thick do not need discussing with a neurosurgeon.

Answer
Bilateral subdural haemorrhages.

Case 4

A 35-year-old presents with a first grand mal fit. The patient had been complaining of headaches for some months before the fit. The management of a first fit under the age of 50 years depends on the unit. Some would book an MRI of the brain as an outpatient because it is superior in the detection of abnormalities associated with fitting. In our institution, as in others, a CT of the brain is performed to exclude any gross abnormality.

- In this example pre- and post-contrast CT images of the brain were performed due to the abnormality seen on the unenhanced images.

What is the diagnosis?

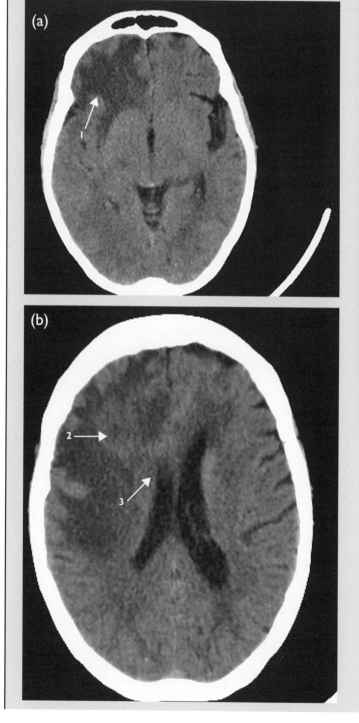

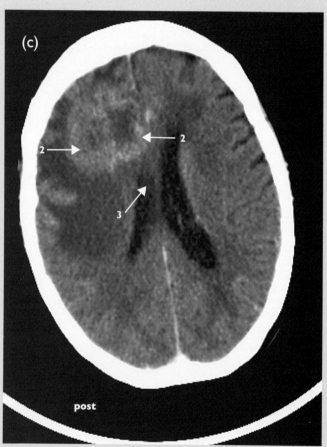

Fig. 10.21 CT of a glioblastoma: (a,b) pre-contrast and (c) post-contrast CT scans of the brain showing extensive low density consistent with oedema in the right frontal region. There is effacement of the right sylvian fissure, more noticeable when comparing with the other side (1). The post-contrast images show a ring-enhancing (2) ill-defined lesion centrally, extending into the corpus callosum. There is effacement of the right lateral ventricle (3). The findings have a differential, including a glioblastoma or primary brain tumour and a secondary deposit or brain abscess.

Findings
- On the unenhanced images there is a ring-like lesion that enhances after contrast in the right frontal region, which extends into the corpus callosum – quite typical of butterfly gliomas.
- It has marked surrounding oedema.
- The right lateral ventricle is squashed or 'effaced' by the mass and there is midline shift to the contralateral side.
- A ring-like enhancing lesion could be a primary brain tumour, as in this case, or a secondary deposit or an abscess, and the history is pertinent to aid the diagnosis.
- In a febrile immunosuppressed patient, infection such an abscess would have to be in the differential.
- Glioblastoma

Answer
Glioblastoma.

Case 5

- A 78-year-old patient presents with bilateral weakness of arms and legs of acute onset. A CT of the brain is performed.
- Symmetrical abnormalities are often hard to detect initially.
- In suspected CVAs look for wedge-shaped low-density lesions extending to the cortex. In this case there are bilateral, low-density, extensive, wedge-shaped lesions extending to the cortex (Fig. 10.22e – block arrows). This is the territory for infarcts in the right MCA territory (Fig. 10.22f).
- Routinely look at the circle of Willis and main cerebral vessels because a hyperdense vessel due to thrombus may be visible as in this case on the left (Fig. 10.22a–d). This can be helpful if other changes are not apparent.
- Apply stroke windows of 40/40 if no obvious abnormality is seen because this exaggerates any loss of grey/white matter differentiation.
- The vascular territories are shown and correlation with clinical signs is important. Anterior cerebral event should have changes abutting the midline anteriorly and posterior cerebral events should have changes abutting the midline posteriorly (Fig. 10.22f).

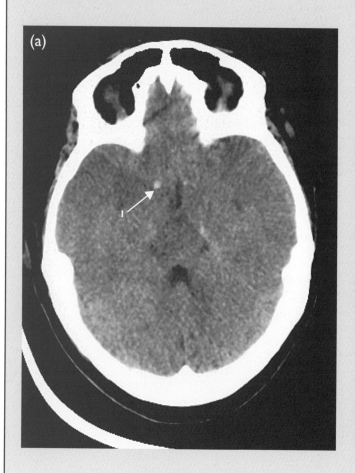

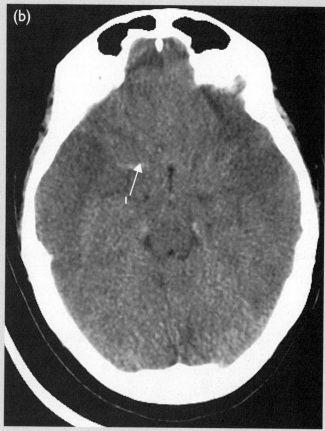

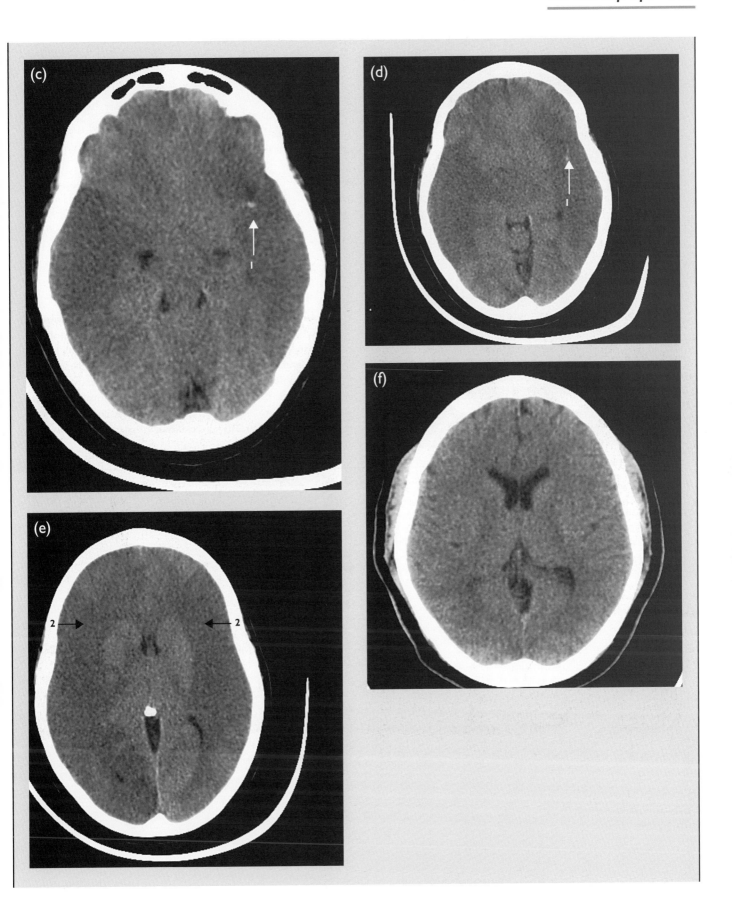

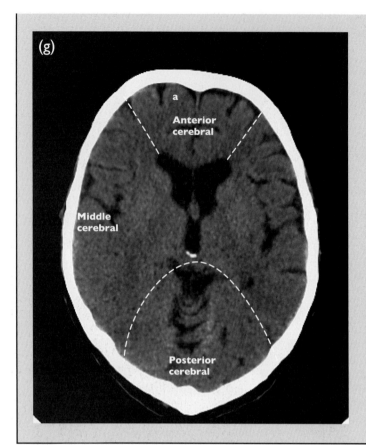

(g)

Anterior
cerebral

Middle
cerebral

Posterior
cerebral

Answer
Acute bilateral CVA.

Fig. 10.22 Cerebrovascular accident (CVA): (a–e) two bilateral axial CT brain images showing bilateral, low-density, wedge-shaped lesions in both cerebral hemispheres. There is high density in both middle cerebral arteries (MCAs) (1). (2) shows wedge-shaped, large low-density lesions, which are consistent with extensive bilateral MCA infarcts. Compare with (f) which shows normal brain. Symmetrical abnormalities can be difficult to detect due to their symmetrical nature. (g) The approximate vascular territories of the three cerebral arteries.

Case 6

- A 64-year-old man on warfarin presents with a decreased GCS after an RTA. A CT of the brain is indicated.
- The CT shows small, rounded, high-density lesions in the temporal and frontal regions. These are typical contusions and this is a typical location for them.
- There is also a rounded, well-demarcated, low-density lesion in the left basal ganglia/lentiform nucleus. This is an established lacunar infarct. It is possible to be distracted by the incidental infarct and not search thoroughly for the small contusions in their typical location.
- Bony windows should automatically be reviewed for a fracture.

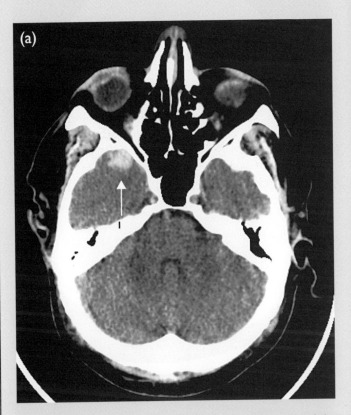

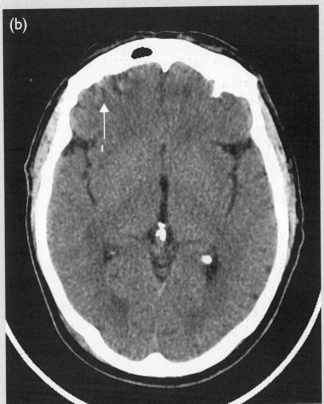

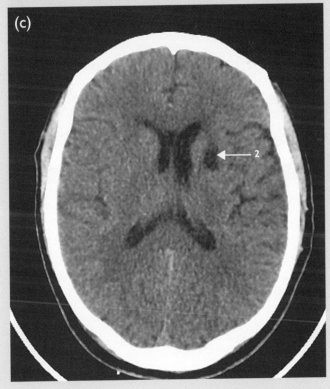

Fig. 10.23 Contusions on warfarin: (a,b) axial CT images of the brain show small round foci of high density consistent with contusions (1) in the right frontal and temporal lobes anteriorly a typical site for trauma. (c) An incidental lacunar infarct (2) in the left lentiform nucleus. Perivascular spaces can also mimic infarcts.

Answer

Small contusions and incidental, left, long-standing lacunar infarct.

A solitary contusion <5 mm in size does not need referral to the neurosurgeons but in this case there are several contusions, so a referral is indicated.

Case 7

- A 27-year-old woman presents with a severe headache after a bout of severe diarrhoea and vomiting.
- A CT of the brain was performed to look for a subarachnoid haemorrhage.
- Some high density is seen in a linear distribution in the superior sagittal sinus region.
- This should be a review area to look for thrombus on a CT of a patient with headache, particularly if dehydrated.
- An MRI of the brain was performed showing the filling defect (block arrow on Fig. 10.24) in the superior sagittal sinus, extending into the right transverse sinus. This is seen by comparing the two sides. The normal left transverse sinus has a black signal void (no. 1 on Fig. 10.24) whereas the abnormal right transverse sinus has intermediate-signal intensity within (no. 2 on Fig. 10.24). Axial flair MRI shows changes in the parieto-occipital region which is bilateral ((1) on Fig. 10.24) and commonly seen in venous infarction and may be haemorrhagic.

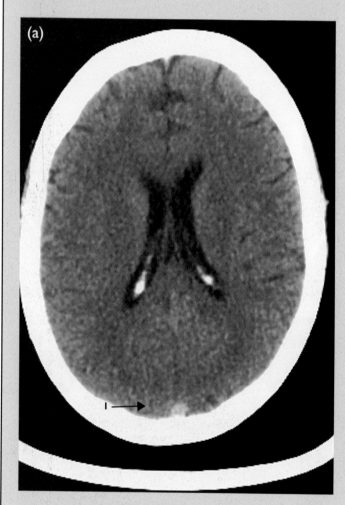

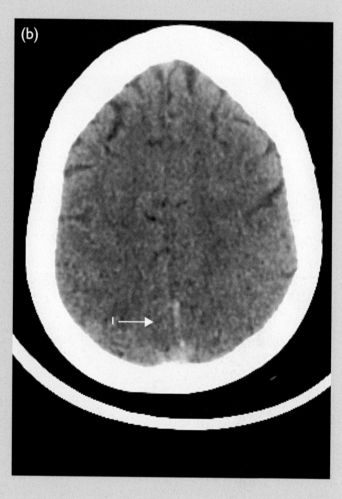

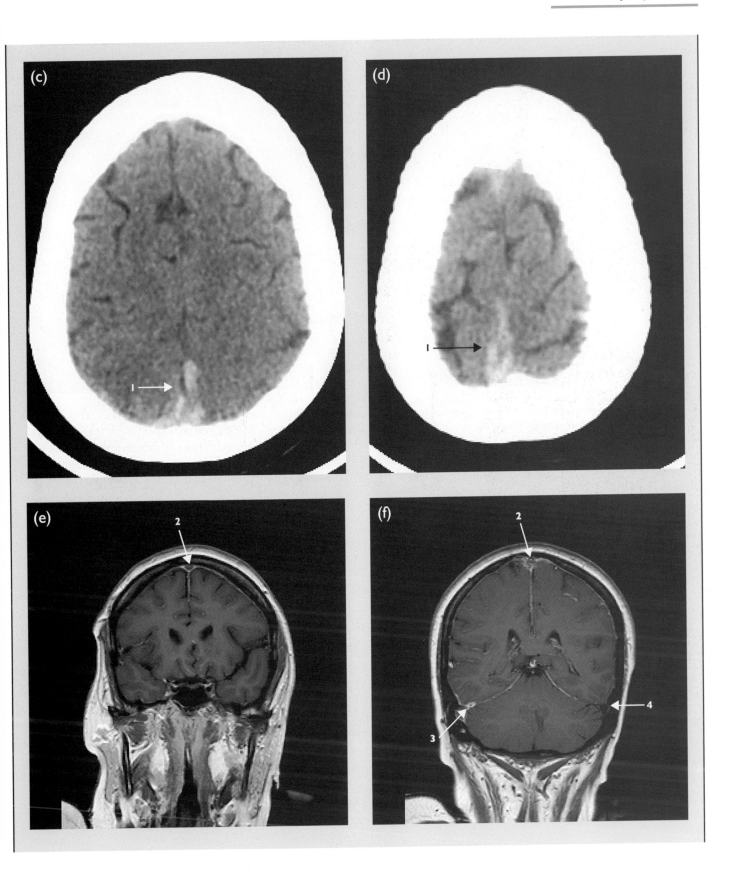

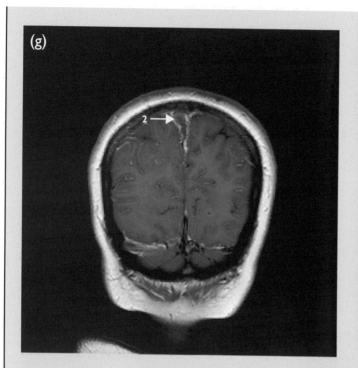
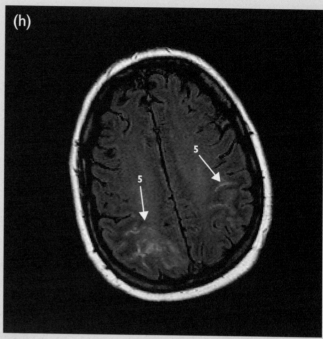

Fig. 10.24 Superior sagittal thrombosis: (a–d) axial unenhanced CT images of the brain show linear high density in the region of the superior sagittal sinus (1), another area to review always on CT for thrombus. In retrospect there may be subtle effacement of the sulci posteriorly. (e–g) Coronal post-contrast MR images of the brain and (h) an axial FLAIR image of the brain. MR confirms an extensive filling defect in the superior sagittal sinus, which should be of bright signal post-contrast. There are filling defects in the superior sagittal sinus (2). There is also thrombus in the right sigmoid/transverse sinus (3), but the left sigmoid sinus shows a normal signal void (4). (h) The axial FLAIR image shows oedema bilaterally and posteriorly (5) which may be more extensive due to venous infarction.

Answer
Superior sagittal sinus thrombosis.

Case 8

A 76-year-old patient known to have a left psoas collection presents on call with sudden new abdominal pain, abdominal distension and diarrhoea.

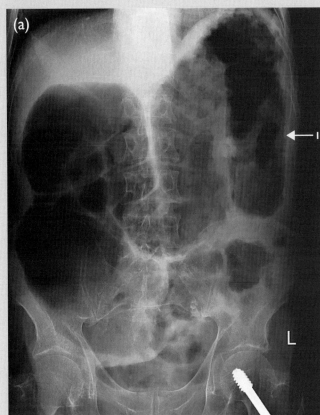

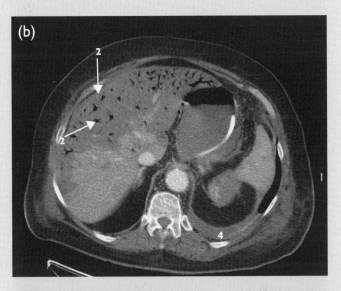

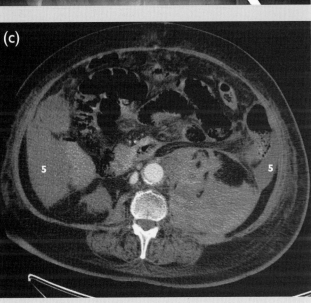

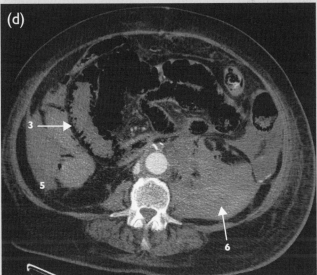

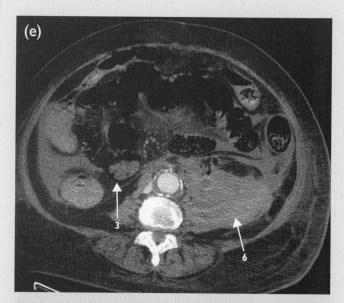

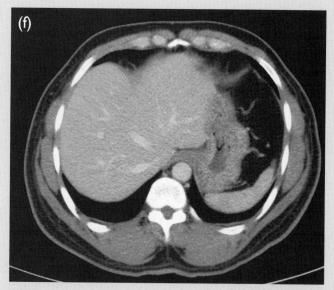

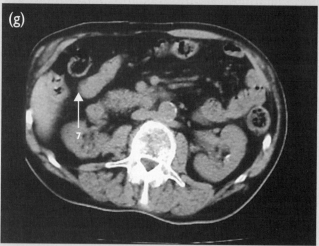

Fig. 10.25 Ischaemic bowel: (a) an abdominal radiograph showing dilated thick-walled large bowel with thumbprinting (1). Thumbprinting is the name given to the thick lumpy appearance of the oedematous bowel wall. (b–e) Images from an axial post-contrast CT of the abdomen: (b) portal venous gas in the liver (2); compare with the normal liver (f). (c–e) Thickened large bowel with intramural gas (3). There is a left pleural effusion (4), free intraperitoneal fluid (5) and a left psoas/retroperitoneal collection (6). (g) Normal large bowel (7) which reveals how abnormal the large bowel is in (c–e).

An abdominal radiograph is performed. This shows dilated colon, seen around the periphery of the abdominal radiograph, which is thick walled with thumbprinting suggestive of colitis.

A CT of the abdomen is performed. This will give more information about the extent of bowel dilatation and thickening and may show a cause such as a mesenteric thrombus.

Findings
Review the images in the standard order:

- The lung bases show a small left pleural effusion ((1) on Fig. 10.25) and should be reviewed on lung window settings.
- The liver is abnormal with linear air-density branching structures noted which extend to the periphery. This is portal venous gas that is seen in very sick adults, often with ischaemic colitis, and is associated with a poor prognosis. The liver also has a peripherally well-demarcated low density. The spleen and adrenal glands are unremarkable. Review the kidneys, aorta and retroperitoneum. Note the left known psoas collection and compare with old images if available.
- Review the bowel. There is air in the bowel wall seen concentrically around the bowel consistent with ischaemic colitis. The mesenteric vessels should be reviewed for filling defects.
- Look for free intra-abdominal fluid (no. 2 on Fig. 10.25).
- The portal gas and intramural colonic gas are consistent with ischaemic colitis.

Answer
Ischaemic bowel.

Case 9

A 36-year-old presents with acute right iliac fossa pain. CT of the abdomen is the modality of choice unless the radiologist is competent in ultrasound of the appendix.

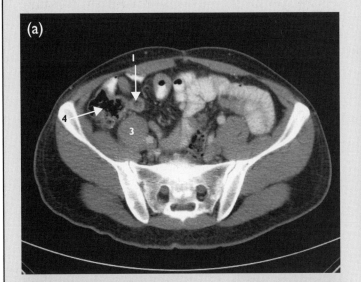

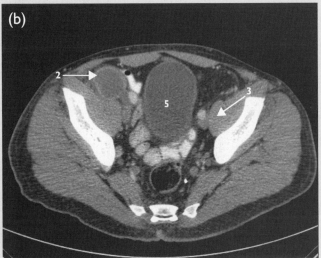

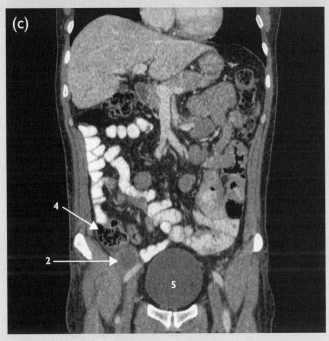

Fig. 10.26 CT of appendicitis, small bowel thickening: (a–b) axial post-contrast CT scans of the abdomen and (c) a coronal MPR (multiplanar reformatted) image. The images show a slightly thickened terminal ileum (1) and an appendix abscess (2). Iliopsoas (3), caecum (4) and bladder (5). To find the appendix, find the caecum and look at the pole in any direction. Any associated subtle stranding or fluid may aid detection of pathology.

Review the CT of the abdomen systematically looking at the organs in order for incidental findings. CT also shows other causes of right iliac fossa pain, e.g. in women it shows ovarian and tubal anomalies.

The CT shows thickened small bowel and a small abscess of the appendix. This could be mistaken for bowel, but, by following the caecum inferiorly and looking for the appendix, the abscess becomes apparent.

Answer
CT of appendicitis, thickening and right iliac fossa abscess.

Case 10

A 69-year-old man presents with a distended abdomen and absolute constipation. An abdominal radiograph showed dilated bowel. CT is the modality of choice on call for assessing the cause and level of obstruction. Oral contrast need not be given due to the negative contrast of water in dilated bowel. Use a system to interpret the scans, reviewing the lung bases, liver, spleen, pancreas, kidneys and adrenals in order. Then review the bowel. First, follow the small bowel to see if it is dilated and whether a transition point can be found. If the large bowel is also involved follow this down from the ascending colon, to the transverse, the splenic flexure and then into the sigmoid.

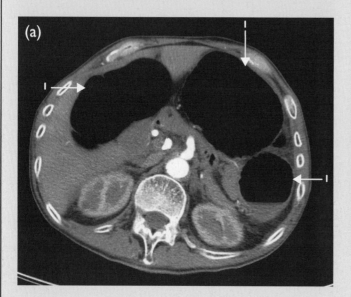
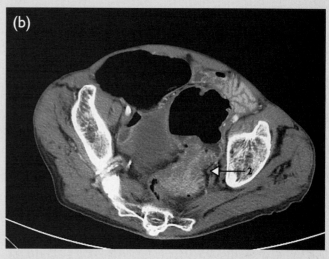

Fig. 10.27 Bowel obstruction carcinoma sigmoid colon. (a) Axial CT abdomen shows dilated large bowel (1) and (b) axial CT abdomen shows a stricture in the sigmoid colon with an associated mass (2). This is consistent with a carcinoma of the sigmoid colon.

This case shows dilated bowel on Fig. 10.27a. The large and small bowel is dilated right to the sigmoid colon. The sigmoid colon has a thick-walled irregular stricture which was a carcinoma. If a tumour is suspected, look for any metastatic disease in the liver or peritoneum and check the lung bases and bones for metastases.

Answer
Bowel obstruction due to carcinoma of the sigmoid colon.

Case 11

A patient presents with acute left iliac fossa pain. CT is the modality of choice for acute diverticulitis. Review the CT abdomen systematically looking at the lung bases and organs first. Then focus on the clinical problem and carefully review the sigmoid colon and large bowel. Look for any free fluid, even small pockets, and follow the rectum carefully image by image in order to detect small abscesses as here. Look for any stranding in fat surrounding the colon. Review the images on a lung window to check for any free air. There is an abscess in the left iliac fossa. Once an abscess has been found look carefully for a second one.

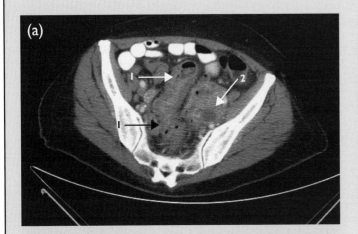

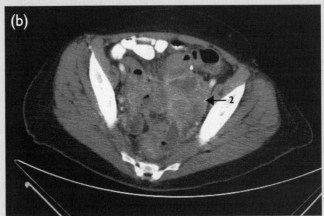

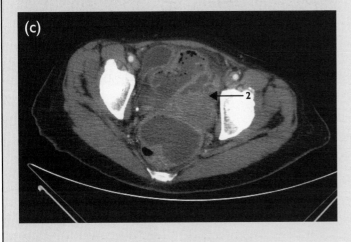

Fig. 10.28 CT – axial abdominal images of a patient with left iliac fossa pain and a temperature. CT shows a diverticular abscess: (a) a thickened sigmoid colon with diverticular disease (1) and a pericolic abscess (2); (b,c) the abscess shown more extensively (2).

Answer
Acute diverticular abscess.

Case 12

A patient presents with haematuria. A CT KUB is performed to look for renal colic. This is performed without intravenous contrast to look for calcification initially.

Some calcification and a mass are seen in the inferior pole of the left kidney. Intravenous contrast is given which shows a mass at the lower pole of the kidney. It is a common scenario, in many cases, to incidentally find a mass that is unsuspected. It is then important to try to get a little more information as in this case by giving intravenous contrast. However, some cases can wait for more complex imaging at a later date. Incidental findings should be reported to the clinicians in charge of the patient because these unexpected findings may be overlooked without alerting the clinicians. In this case a triple phase scan is performed to assess the renal parenchyma. The aorta is very dense or white in the early aortic phase and the aorta is the same as the other vessels on the late phase.

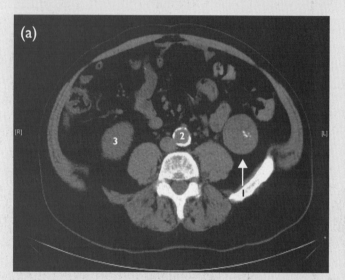

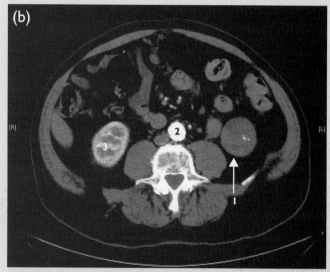

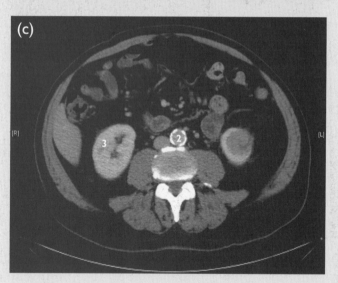

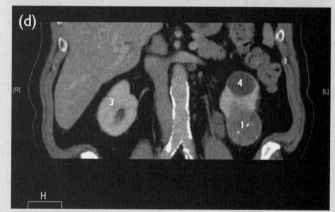

Fig. 10.29 Mass in the left kidney: (a) pre-contrast, (b) arterial and (c) delayed phase axial post-contrast CT of the kidney, and (d) coronal multiplanar reformatted (MPR) of the abdomen showing a mass at the lower pole of the left kidney (1). The aorta reveals the phase of contrast. In (a) the aorta is unenhanced, in (b) it is very dense and in (c) it is less dense. Aorta (2), normal right kidney (3) and simple cut (4).

Diagnosis
Mass at lower pole of left kidney – possible renal cell carcinoma. Urgent referral to urology is recommended.

Answer
Mass at lower pole of left kidney.

Case 13

A patient presents with symptoms of canal stenosis. An MRI was performed. Apply the A, B, C, D and E system of review.

- Alignment: the fourth lumbar vertebra has slipped forward on the fifth lumbar vertebra. The canal appears stenosed at L1–2 and L4–5.
- Bones: look at the T1-weighted images for marrow signal. The marrow should be brighter than the discs on T1-weighted images. The marrow appears normal in this case.
- Cord: the terminal cord is of normal calibre and signal intensity and terminates at the correct level.
- Discs: the discs have generally degenerated with dehydration change and loss of height. Discs can be assessed on axial images.
- Everything else: look at the uterus, bladder, adnexa, and aorta for an aneurysm, the bones and the lung bases.

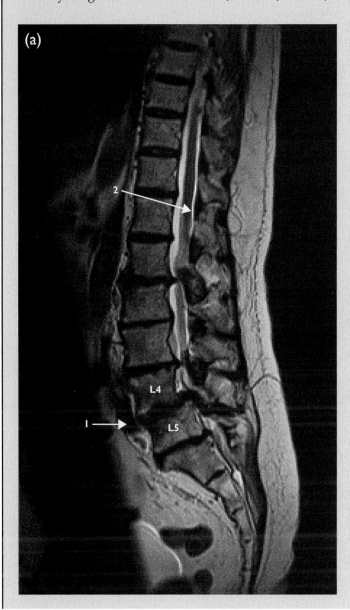

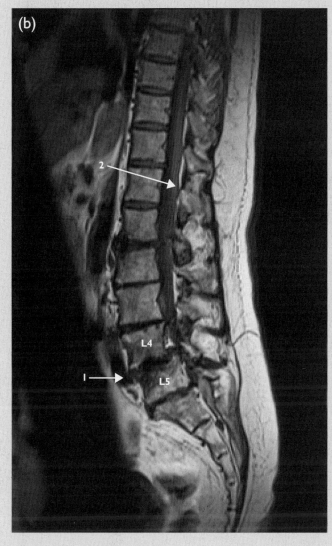

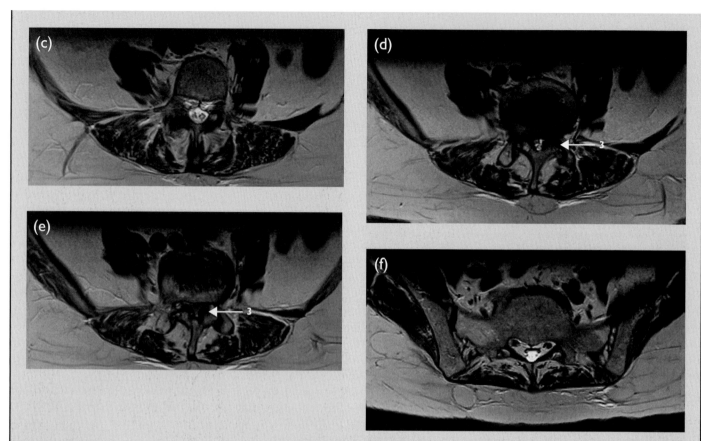

Fig. 10.30 Spondylolisthesis. MR lumbosacral spine images: (a) sagittal T2-weighted and (b) sagittal T1-weighted images showing a spondylolisthesis or slip of L4 on L5 (1). Conus (2). (c–f) Axial T2-weighted images showing marked narrowing of the spinal canal dimensions in (d) and (e) (3).

A spondylolisthesis causes a pseudo-disc bulge due to the vertebral slip. The canal can be encroached on due to a combination of ligamentous thickening of the ligamentum flavum, caused by disc bilges, spondylolisthesis, disc protrusions, osteophytes and facet joint hypertrophy

Answer
Spondylolisthesis of L4 on L5. Severe spinal stenoses caused at this level.

Case 14

- A young man has a pushbike injury with a cycle helmet on. He is knocked off his bike by a lorry. Initially he loses consciousness for 3 min but fully recovers by the time he reaches A&E. However, the NICE guidelines stipulate that a CT of the brain is indicated due to the loss of consciousness in someone with a dangerous mechanism of injury.
- On the axial slices again towards the vertex a few sulci contain SAH (arrow on Fig. 10.31).
- Bony windows need reviewing for a fracture.

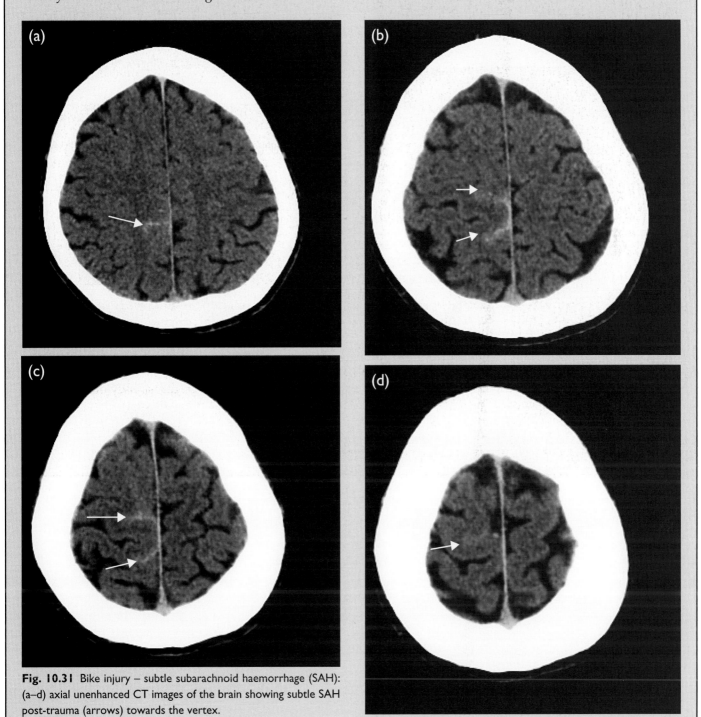

Fig. 10.31 Bike injury – subtle subarachnoid haemorrhage (SAH): (a–d) axial unenhanced CT images of the brain showing subtle SAH post-trauma (arrows) towards the vertex.

Answer

Subtle SAH.

Index